Pediatric Rheumatology

Editors

SUZANNE C. LI
GLORIA C. HIGGINS

PEDIATRIC CLINICS
OF NORTH AMERICA

www.pediatric.theclinics.com

Consulting Editor
BONITA F. STANTON

August 2018 • Volume 65 • Number 4

ELSEVIER

1600 John F. Kennedy Boulevard • Suite 1800 • Philadelphia, Pennsylvania, 19103-2899

http://www.theclinics.com

THE PEDIATRIC CLINICS OF NORTH AMERICA Volume 65, Number 4
August 2018 ISSN 0031-3955, ISBN-13: 978-0-323-64169-2

Editor: Kerry Holland
Developmental Editor: Casey Potter

Photocopying

Single photocopies of single articles may be made for personal use as allowed by national copyright laws. Permission of the Publisher and payment of a fee is required for all other photocopying, including multiple or systematic copying, copying for advertising or promotional purposes, resale, and all forms of document delivery. Special rates are available for educational institutions that wish to make photocopies for non-profit educational classroom use. For information on how to seek permission visit www.elsevier.com/permissions or call: (+44) 1865 843830 (UK)/(+1) 215 239 3804 (USA).

Derivative Works

Subscribers may reproduce tables of contents or prepare lists of articles including abstracts for internal circulation within their institutions. Permission of the Publisher is required for resale or distribution outside the institution. Permission of the Publisher is required for all other derivative works, including compilations and translations (please consult www.elsevier.com/permissions).

Electronic Storage or Usage

Permission of the Publisher is required to store or use electronically any material contained in this periodical, including any article or part of an article (please consult www.elsevier.com/permissions). Except as outlined above, no part of this publication may be reproduced, stored in a retrieval system or transmitted in any form or by any means, electronic, mechanical, photocopying, recording or otherwise, without prior written permission of the Publisher.

Notice

No responsibility is assumed by the Publisher for any injury and/or damage to persons or property as a matter of products liability, negligence or otherwise, or from any use or operation of any methods, products, instructions or ideas contained in the material herein. Because of rapid advances in the medical sciences, in particular, independent verification of diagnoses and drug dosages should be made.

Although all advertising material is expected to conform to ethical (medical) standards, inclusion in this publication does not constitute a guarantee or endorsement of the quality or value of such product or of the claims made of it by its manufacturer.

The Pediatric Clinics of North America (ISSN 0031-3955) is published bimonthly by Elsevier Inc., 360 Park Avenue South, New York, NY 10010-1710. Months of issue are February, April, June, August, October, and December. Periodicals postage paid at New York, NY and additional mailing offices. Subscription prices are $216.00 per year (US individuals), $613.00 per year (US institutions), $292.00 per year (Canadian individuals), $816.00 per year (Canadian institutions), $338.00 per year (international individuals), $816.00 per year (international institutions), $100.00 per year (US students and residents), and $165.00 per year (international and Canadian residents and students). To receive students/resident rare, orders must be accompanied by name of affiliated institution, date of term, and the signature of program/residency coordinator on institution letterhead. Orders will be billed at individual rate until proof of status is received. Foreign air speed delivery is included in all Clinics subscription prices. All prices are subject to change without notice. **POSTMASTER:** Send address changes to The Pediatric Clinics of North America, Elsevier Health Sciences Division, Subscription Customer Service, 3251 Riverport Lane, Maryland Heights, MO 63043. **Customer Service: 1-800-654-2452 (US and Canada). From outside of the US and Canada: 1-314-447-8871. Fax: 1-314-447-8029. For print support, E-mail: JournalsCustomerService-usa@elsevier.com. For online support, E-mail: JournalsOnlineSupport-usa@elsevier.com**.

Reprints. For copies of 100 or more, of articles in this publication, please contact the Commercial Reprints Department, Elsevier Inc., 360 Park Avenue South, New York, NY 10010-1710. Tel.: 212-633-3874; Fax: 212-633-3820; E-mail: reprints@elsevier.com.

The Pediatric Clinics of North America is also published in Spanish by McGraw-Hill Inter-americana Editores S.A., Mexico City, Mexico; in Portuguese by Riechmann and Affonso Editores, Rua Comandante Coelho 1085, CEP 21250, Rio de Janeiro, Brazil; and in Greek by Althayia SA, Athens, Greece.

The Pediatric Clinics of North America is covered in MEDLINE/PubMed (Index Medicus), Excerpta Medica, Current Contents, Current Contents/Clinical Medicine, Science Citation Index, ASCA, ISI/BIOMED, and BIOSIS.

Contributors

CONSULTING EDITOR

BONITA F. STANTON, MD
Founding Dean, Professor of Pediatrics, Hackensack Meridian School of Medicine at Seton Hall University, South Orange, New Jersey, USA

EDITORS

SUZANNE C. LI, MD, PhD
Professor, Pediatrics, Hackensack Meridian School of Medicine at Seton Hall University, Joseph M. Sanzari Children's Hospital, Hackensack, New Jersey, USA

GLORIA C. HIGGINS, MD, PhD
Professor Emeritus of Pediatrics, Division of Pediatric Rheumatology, The Ohio State University, Nationwide Children's Hospital, Columbus, Ohio, USA

AUTHORS

STACY P. ARDOIN, MD, MS
Associate Professor, Pediatric Rheumatology, Nationwide Children's Hospital, Columbus, Ohio, USA

TIMOTHY BEUKELMAN, MD, MSCE
Associate Professor, Department of Pediatrics, Division of Rheumatology, The University of Alabama at Birmingham, Birmingham, Alabama, USA

SHARON BOUT-TABAKU, MD, MSCE
Division Chief of Rheumatology, Department of Pediatric Medicine, Sidra Medicine, Qatar Foundation, Doha, Qatar

ROBERT A. COLBERT, MD, PhD
Pediatric Translational Research Branch, National Institute of Arthritis, Musculoskeletal and Skin Diseases, National Institutes of Health, USA

COURTNEY B. CRAYNE, MD
Fellow, Department of Pediatrics, Division of Rheumatology, The University of Alabama at Birmingham, Birmingham, Alabama, USA

POLLY J. FERGUSON, MD
Professor, Department of Pediatrics, University of Iowa Carver College of Medicine, Iowa City, Iowa, USA

KATHLEEN A. HAINES, MD
Section Chief, Pediatric Immunology, Section of Pediatric Rheumatology and Immunology, Professor, Department of Pediatrics, Hackensack Meridian School of Medicine at Seton Hall University, Hackensack University Medical Center, Hackensack, New Jersey, USA

GLORIA C. HIGGINS, MD, PhD
Professor Emeritus of Pediatrics, Division of Pediatric Rheumatology, The Ohio State University, Nationwide Children's Hospital, Columbus, Ohio, USA

ADAM M. HUBER, MSc, MD
Pediatric Rheumatologist, Division of Pediatric Rheumatology, IWK Health Centre, Professor of Pediatrics, Dalhousie University, Halifax, Nova Scotia, Canada

JENNIFER J.Y. LEE, MD
Rheumatology Clinical Fellow, Division of Rheumatology, The Hospital for Sick Children, University of Toronto, Toronto, Ontario, Canada

SUZANNE C. LI, MD, PhD
Professor, Pediatrics, Hackensack Meridian School of Medicine at Seton Hall University, Joseph M. Sanzari Children's Hospital, Hackensack, New Jersey, USA

KATHLEEN M. O'NEIL, MD
Professor of Clinical Pediatrics, Chief, Division of Rheumatology, Department of Pediatrics, Indiana University School of Medicine, Riley Hospital for Children at Indiana University Health, Indianapolis, Indiana, USA

RAYFEL SCHNEIDER, MBBCh
Professor and Associate Chair (Education), Department of Paediatrics, Staff, Division of Rheumatology, The Hospital for Sick Children, University of Toronto, Toronto, Ontario, Canada

JENNIFER N. STINSON, RN, PhD
Senior Scientist, Research Institute, Child Health Evaluative Sciences, The Hospital for Sick Children, Professor, Lawrence S. Bloomberg Faculty of Nursing, University of Toronto, Toronto, Ontario, Canada

KATHLEEN E. SULLIVAN, MD, PhD
Professor, Department of Pediatrics, Division of Allergy Immunology, The Children's Hospital of Philadelphia, Perelman School of Medicine, University of Pennsylvania, Philadelphia, Pennsylvania, USA

STACEY E. TARVIN, MD, MS
Assistant Professor of Clinical Pediatrics, Division of Rheumatology, Department of Pediatrics, Indiana University School of Medicine, Riley Hospital for Children at Indiana University Health, Indianapolis, Indiana, USA

JENNIFER E. WEISS, MD
Associate Professor of Pediatrics, Hackensack Meridian School of Medicine at Seton Hall University, Joseph M. Sanzari Children's Hospital, Hackensack University Medical Center, Hackensack, New Jersey, USA

PAMELA F. WEISS, MD, MSCE
Department of Pediatrics and Epidemiology, Perelman School of Medicine, University of Pennsylvania, Division of Rheumatology, Children's Hospital of Philadelphia, Philadelphia, Pennsylvania, USA

YONGDONG ZHAO, MD, PhD
Assistant Professor, Pediatric Rheumatology, Seattle Children's Hospital, University of Washington, Seattle, Washington, USA

Contents

> This article focuses on creating an orderly approach to history taking, examination, and ordering appropriate investigations when caring for a child with joint complaints. It classifies complaints as those with and without pain, swelling, or fever and of short or long duration. It recommends an approach to the physical examination and both suggests and discourages various laboratory and imaging studies.

> The pathogenesis of pediatric rheumatologic conditions varies with the specific disorder; however, certain commonalities are seen: altered migration of cells into tissues, production of inflammatory mediators, and enhanced activation of cells. Autoantibodies signal loss of tolerance, and B and T cells may be seen on pathologic evaluation. Neutrophils are commonly observed in tissues for many diseases and are recruited through the activation of endothelial cells. These cellular infiltrates define the inflammatory response character and, in some cases, provide a therapeutic framework. Increased knowledge of the interactions of these cells and their products allow targeted treatments for rheumatic diseases.

> Juvenile idiopathic arthritis (JIA) comprises a group of heterogeneous diseases further divided into various categories based on shared clinical presentation, laboratory markers, and disease prognosis. Extraarticular complications include uveitis and growth abnormalities. Disease course and prognosis vary with respect to each JIA category and subsequently guide respective treatment. Over the past few decades, considerable treatment advances have significantly reduced the morbidity associated with childhood arthritis. Nevertheless, the treatments are not curative; many children continue to have active disease into adulthood. Emphasis is placed on the initiation of early aggressive therapy in hopes of delaying disease progression and inducing remission.

Juvenile spondyloarthritis (SpA) is a distinct form of juvenile arthritis characterized by male predominance and adolescent onset. Clinical manifestations include lower extremity and sacroiliac joint arthritis, enthesitis, and subclinical gastrointestinal inflammation. Juvenile SpA is an immune-mediated inflammatory disease long recognized as associated with HLA-B27, which may be related to the microbial environment as suggested by its coexistence with reactive arthritis and psoriasis. Treatment of peripheral arthritis includes nonsteroidal antiinflammatory drugs, joint injections, and disease-modifying agents, whereas treatment of axial disease may necessitate a tumor necrosis factor inhibitor biologic agent. Fewer than half of children achieve remission off medication 5 years after diagnosis.

Systemic juvenile idiopathic arthritis (sJIA) is a distinctive subtype of juvenile idiopathic arthritis, characterized by fever and arthritis, often accompanied by rash, sometimes by generalized lymphadenopathy, hepatosplenomegaly, and serositis. The diagnosis requires adequate exclusion of infectious, oncologic, autoimmune, and autoinflammatory diseases. Macrophage activation syndrome, a serious and potentially fatal complication of sJIA, requires prompt evaluation and treatment. Newer biologic agents, particularly interleukin-1 and interleukin-6 inhibitors, are highly effective and have transformed the treatment approach by reducing the use of systemic glucocorticoids. Primary care providers have a crucial role in monitoring children with sJIA for disease-related complications and medication-related adverse events.

Juvenile systemic lupus erythematosus (jSLE), mixed connective tissue disease (jMCTD), and Sjögren syndrome (jSS) are systemic autoimmune and inflammatory disorders with distinct patterns of organ involvement. All are characterized by autoantibody formation, with antinuclear (ANA) and anti-double-stranded DNA common in jSLE, ANA with high-titer ribonucleoprotein antibody in jMCTD, and Sjögren syndrome A and Sjögren syndrome B antibodies + ANA in jSS. Recognition, monitoring, and management for primary care providers are discussed, focusing on the role of primary physicians in recognizing and helping maintain optimal health in children with these potentially life-threatening diseases.

The juvenile idiopathic inflammatory myopathies (JIIMs) are a group of rare, chronic, autoimmune illnesses that affect muscle and, to a lesser extent, skin. The presence of new-onset weakness and, in juvenile dermatomyositis, typical rashes should lead to consideration of these diagnoses. Careful evaluation to exclude alternative diagnoses is needed. Investigations include a variety of blood tests, imaging, and possibly muscle biopsy. Validated clinical assessments are available for monitoring. Standard treatment includes corticosteroids and methotrexate and often extends beyond 1 year. Outcomes are generally good, but disease persistence remains problematic. Early involvement of providers with expertise in JIIM is essential.

Scleroderma is a rare disease that has two main forms: localized scleroderma (LS) and systemic sclerosis (SSc). Both are chronic diseases, can present in different patterns (subtypes), and are associated with extracutaneous involvement in pediatric patients. Morbidity and mortality is much worse for juvenile SSc, with patients at risk for life-threatening lung, heart, and other visceral organ fibrosis and vasculopathy. Mortality is extremely rare in juvenile LS, but morbidity is common, with patients at risk for severe disfigurement and functional impairment. Scleroderma treatment is directed toward controlling inflammation and managing specific problems. Early diagnosis can greatly improve outcome.

Chronic nonbacterial osteomyelitis (CNO) is an innate immune system disorder that predominantly affects children. It can present as part of a syndrome or in isolation. It presents as bone pain with or without fever or objective swelling at the site. It is difficult to diagnose. Laboratory studies can be normal, whereas a biopsy reveals sterile osteomyelitis. Osteolytic or sclerotic bone changes may be seen on radiographs. However, MRI is more sensitive for detecting CNO and is considered the gold standard for monitoring the disease. Treatment depends on disease severity and includes nonsteroidal antiinflammatory drugs, bisphosphonates, and cytokine inhibitors.

Chronic musculoskeletal pain (CMP) is one of the main reasons for referral to a pediatric rheumatologist and is the third most common cause of chronic pain in children and adolescents. Causes of CMP include amplified musculoskeletal pain, benign limb pain of childhood, hypermobility, overuse syndromes, and back pain. CMP can negatively affect physical, social, academic, and psychological function, so it is essential that clinicians know how to diagnose and treat these conditions. This article provides an overview of the epidemiology and impact of CMP, the steps in a comprehensive pain assessment, and the management of the most common CMPs.

> Medications to treat children with rheumatic disease include disease-modifying antirheumatic drugs, glucocorticosteroids, and biologic response modifiers that target mediators and cells involved in autoimmunity and inflammation. Although usually well tolerated, such medications have many possible side effects, of which primary care and emergency providers should be aware. Both disease and immunosuppression contribute to susceptibility to unusual and opportunistic infections, in addition to usual childhood infections for which these children should receive all applicable nonlive vaccines. Close coordination between the rheumatologist and other medical care providers is essential, because medication side effects, infections, and disease flares are difficult to distinguish and may occur together.

> As a result of new medications and therapeutic approaches, most children with rheumatic diseases are no longer at risk for growth failure that results from chronic inflammation and prolonged corticosteroid treatment. However, obesity, poor nutrition, and insufficient exercise are still problems that increase risks for poor bone, cardiovascular, and general health. Diet should be monitored and modified as appropriate; supplemental calcium and vitamin D should be provided. Obesity and poor physical fitness can be ameliorated by an exercise program that should become part of a healthier lifestyle.

> Although it has been widely acknowledged for more than two decades that transition from pediatric to adult care is a vulnerable time for adolescents and young adults with rheumatic diseases, current primary and subspecialty care transition and transfer processes remain inadequate. Barriers to improving transition include complex health care systems, neurodevelopmental challenges of adolescents and young adults, and insufficient transition-related education and resources for health care providers. Standardized, evidence-based transition interventions are sorely needed to establish best practices. Quality improvement approaches such as the Six Core Elements of Health Care Transition offer opportunities to improve transition care for teens and young adults.

PROGRAM OBJECTIVE
The goal of the *Pediatric Clinics of North America* is to keep practicing physicians and residents up to date with current clinical practice in pediatrics by providing timely articles reviewing the state-of-the-art in patient care.

TARGET AUDIENCE
All practicing pediatricians, physicians and healthcare professionals who provide patient care to pediatric patients.

LEARNING OBJECTIVES
Upon completion of this activity, participants will be able to:
1. Review juvenile spondyloarthritis
2. Discuss systemic lupus erythematosus, sjögren syndrome, and MCTD in children and adolescents
3. Recognize treatment complications for pediatric rheumatic diseases

ACCREDITATION
The Elsevier Office of Continuing Medical Education (EOCME) is accredited by the Accreditation Council for Continuing Medical Education (ACCME) to provide continuing medical education for physicians.

The EOCME designates this enduring material for a maximum of 15 *AMA PRA Category 1 Credit*(s)™. Physicians should claim only the credit commensurate with the extent of their participation in the activity.

All other healthcare professionals requesting continuing education credit for this enduring material will be issued a certificate of participation.

DISCLOSURE OF CONFLICTS OF INTEREST
The EOCME assesses conflict of interest with its instructors, faculty, planners, and other individuals who are in a position to control the content of CME activities. All relevant conflicts of interest that are identified are thoroughly vetted by EOCME for fair balance, scientific objectivity, and patient care recommendations. EOCME is committed to providing its learners with CME activities that promote improvements or quality in healthcare and not a specific proprietary business or a commercial interest.

The planning committee, staff, authors and editors listed below have identified no financial relationships or relationships to products or devices they or their spouse/life partner have with commercial interest related to the content of this CME activity:
Stacy P. Ardoin, MD, MS; Sharon Bout-Tabaku, MD, MSCE; Courtney B. Crayne, MD; Polly J. Ferguson, MD; Kathleen A. Haines, MD; Gloria C. Higgins, MD, PhD; Kerry Holland; Adam M. Huber, MSc, MD; Alison Kemp; Jennifer J.Y. Lee, MD; Rajkumar Mayakrishnan; Kathleen M. O'Neil, MD; Casey Potter; Bonita F. Stanton, MD; Jennifer N. Stinson, RN, PhD; Kathleen E. Sullivan, MD, PhD; Stacey E. Tarvin, MD, MS; Jennifer E. Weiss, MD; Pamela F. Weiss, MD, MSCE.

The planning committee, staff, authors and editors listed below have identified financial relationships or relationships to products or devices they or their spouse/life partner have with commercial interest related to the content of this CME activity:
Timothy Beukelman, MD, MSCE: has received consulting fees from Novartis AG, Genentech, Inc., UCB SA, Bristol-Myers Squibb Company, and Swedish Orphan Biovitrum AB
Robert A. Colbert, MD, PhD: has received consulting fees from Eli Lilly and Company
Suzanne C. Li, MD, PhD: has received consulting fees from Bristol-Myers Squibb Company
Rayfel Schneider, MBBCh: has received consulting fees from Novimmune SA, Novartis AG, and Swedish Orphan Biovitrum AB
Yongdong Zhao, MD, PhD: has received research support from Bristol-Myers Squibb Company

UNAPPROVED/OFF-LABEL USE DISCLOSURE
The EOCME requires CME faculty to disclose to the participants:
1. When products or procedures being discussed are off-label, unlabelled, experimental, and/or investigational (not US Food and Drug Administration [FDA] approved); and
2. Any limitations on the information presented, such as data that are preliminary or that represent ongoing research, interim analyses, and/or unsupported opinions. Faculty may discuss information about pharmaceutical agents that is outside of FDA-approved labelling. This information is intended solely for CME and is not intended to promote off-label use of these medications. If you have any questions, contact the medical affairs department of the manufacturer for the most recent prescribing information.

TO ENROLL

To enroll in the *Pediatric Clinics of North America* Continuing Medical Education program, call customer service at 1-800-654-2452 or sign up online at http://www.theclinics.com/home/cme. The CME program is available to subscribers for an additional annual fee of USD 301.60.

METHOD OF PARTICIPATION

In order to claim credit, participants must complete the following:
1. Complete enrolment as indicated above.
2. Read the activity.
3. Complete the CME Test and Evaluation. Participants must achieve a score of 70% on the test. All CME Tests and Evaluations must be completed online.

CME INQUIRIES/SPECIAL NEEDS

For all CME inquiries or special needs, please contact elsevierCME@elsevier.com.

PEDIATRIC CLINICS OF NORTH AMERICA

Foreword

Pediatric Rheumatology: A Field of Great Progress

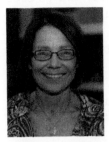

Bonita F. Stanton, MD
Consulting Editor

An estimated 294,000 American children under the age of 18 suffer from arthritis or other rheumatic conditions.[1]

Among the multiple forms of arthritis affecting children, juvenile idiopathic arthritis (JIA; previously called juvenile rheumatoid arthritis in the United States or juvenile chronic arthritis in Europe) is the most common, with an estimated prevalence in the United States of 15,000 to 36,000. Rates are substantially higher among Caucasians compared with African Americans and Asians.[2] Globally, the incidence is estimated to be 1 per 1000 children. Besides the intense pain that can be associated with arthritis in children, it is also true that the prevalence of additional disorders is disproportionately higher among children with arthritis and other rheumatic conditions.[3] As is discussed in this issue, there are several different subtypes. Until the last decade, most of the treatment advances for this disorder were symptomatic. But now with rapidly expanding genome engineering technology, including CRISPR-Cas9, scientist and clinicians have a greatly expanded treatment platform for a range of diseases, including JIA.[4]

In addition to JIA, other arthritic and autoimmune disorders affecting children are covered in this issue, including systemic lupus erythematosus, inflammatory myopathies, scleroderma, and chronic nonbacterial osteomyelitis, juvenile fibromyalgia syndrome, and osteochondrosis. As the authors describe, new treatments have become available and multiple new treatments are being evaluated.

Pediatr Clin N Am 65 (2018) xiii–xiv
https://doi.org/10.1016/j.pcl.2018.05.002
0031-3955/18/© 2018 Published by Elsevier Inc.

pediatric.theclinics.com

An exciting theme emerges from all of these articles: much progress has been made in the last decade regarding both diagnosis and treatment options for pediatric rheumatic diseases, with many more approaches on the horizon.

Bonita F. Stanton, MD
Hackensack Meridian School of Medicine
Seton Hall University
400 South Orange Street
South Orange, NJ 07079, USA

E-mail address:
bonita.stanton@shu.edu

REFERENCES

1. National Institute of Arthritis and Musculoskeletal and Skin Disorders. Available at: https://www.niams.nih.gov/health-topics/juvenile-arthritis#tab-risk. Accessed May 21, 2018.
2. Grom AA. Juvenile idiopathic arthritis: Epidemiology and immunopathogenesis. Up to date. Available at: https://www.uptodate.com/contents/juvenile-idiopathic-arthritis-epidemiology-and-immunopathogenesis#!. Accessed May 21, 2018.
3. Beukelman T, Patkar NM, Saag KG, et al. 2011 American College of Rheumatology recommendations for the treatment of juvenile idiopathic arthritis: initiation and safety monitoring of therapeutic agents for the treatment of arthritis and systemic features. Arthritis Care Res 2011;63(4):465–82.
4. Adkar SS, Brunger JM, Willard VP, et al. Genome engineering for personalized arthritis therapeutics. Trends Mol Med 2017;23(10):917–31.

Preface

Overview of Pediatric Rheumatology for the Primary Care Provider

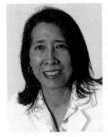 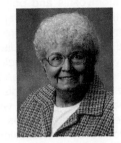

Suzanne C. Li, MD, PhD   Gloria C. Higgins, MD, PhD
Editors

Since the last Rheumatology issue of *Pediatric Clinics of North America* in 2012, there has been an explosion of information, especially on the elucidation of pathways of inflammation and autoimmunity, improving our understanding of old diseases and leading to the discovery of new ones. These scientific accomplishments have resulted in major advances in treatment, especially for the inflammatory arthritides, with new treatments continuing to be introduced. However, cures remain a dream, and many patients continue to have inadequately controlled disease. Given the rarity of pediatric rheumatic diseases, the variety of their presenting features, and disease courses, the diagnosis and management of patients with these diseases remain challenging.

This issue provides an overview of the major pediatric rheumatic diseases to help the primary care provider and other nonrheumatology physicians understand their main disease features and treatment issues. The disease-specific articles are formatted similarly to make it easy for readers to find relevant information. The focus is on providing information that the nonrheumatologist who might be referring, comanaging, or providing other care to children with rheumatic disease needs to know, and how medical care providers and rheumatologists can work together to optimize care for these children. A major aim is to promote early recognition of these diseases, because earlier diagnosis and initiation of appropriate treatment are associated with better long-term outcome. Currently, the time to diagnosis for many patients is often a year or longer, with some studies finding each month's delay reduces the likelihood of a good outcome.

We thank the authors who brought their expertise and experience to their articles to provide both fundamental and new information to the nonrheumatologist. A comprehensive overview on the approach to evaluating a child with joint complaints is

Pediatr Clin N Am 65 (2018) xv–xvi
https://doi.org/10.1016/j.pcl.2018.05.001
0031-3955/18/© 2018 Published by Elsevier Inc.

provided by Kathleen Haines, followed by an overview of autoimmune and autoinflammatory derangements associated with rheumatic diseases by Kathleen Sullivan. Chronic childhood arthritis, which is referred to as juvenile idiopathic arthritis (JIA), has several different subtypes that differ in disease patterns, patient characteristics, and recommended treatments. These subtypes are covered in three articles: oligoarticular and polyarticular JIA by Courtney Crayne and Tim Beukelman, spondyloarthritis by Pamela Weiss and Robert Colbert, and systemic JIA by Jennifer Lee and Rafael Schneider. Stacey Tarvin and Kathleen O'Neil review systemic lupus erythematosus, and two related diseases, mixed connective tissue disease and Sjogren syndrome. Inflammatory myositis, including dermatomyositis and polymyositis, is discussed by Adam Huber, while scleroderma, both localized and systemic forms, are reviewed by Suzanne Li. One of the autoinflammatory diseases, chronic nonbacterial osteomyelitis (aka chronic recurrent multifocal osteomyelitis), is discussed by Dan Zhao and Polly Ferguson, while noninflammatory pain conditions, including juvenile fibromyalgia syndrome and osteochondroses, are reviewed by Jennifer Weiss and Jennifer Stinson. Most of the medications used to treat rheumatic diseases of children and their potential adverse effects are discussed by Gloria Higgins, with recommendations provided for patient immunization. General health concerns for these patients is discussed by Sharon Bout-Tabaku, followed by a discussion of challenges faced by young adults with rheumatic disease, issues associated with transitioning these patients to adult providers, and strategies for successful transition by Stacy Ardoin.

Not included are the vasculitides, immune-mediated diseases of the central nervous system, and many of the autoinflammatory diseases, as they were recently covered in excellent articles in the February 2017 issue of *Pediatric Clinics of North America* (Undiagnosed and Rare Diseases in Children).

We thank Bonita Stanton, the Consulting Editor, and Kerry Holland, the Editor for the *Pediatric Clinics of North America* for their helpful advice and support of this issue. We express our sincere gratitude to Casey Potter, the Senior Developmental Editor, whose excellent guidance and encouragement made our task much easier, and the staff of *Pediatric Clinics of North America* for their help with this issue.

Suzanne C. Li, MD, PhD
Pediatrics
Hackensack Meridian School of Medicine at Seton Hall University
Joseph M. Sanzari Children's Hospital
30 Prospect Avenue
IMUS 348
Hackensack, NJ 07601, USA

Gloria C. Higgins, MD, PhD
Department of Pediatrics
The Ohio State University
Division of Rheumatology
Nationwide Children's Hospital
700 Children's Drive
Columbus, OH 43205, USA

E-mail addresses:
suzanne.li@hackensackmeridian.org (S.C. Li)
gloria.higgins@nationwidechildrens.org (G.C. Higgins)

The Approach to the Child with Joint Complaints

Kathleen A. Haines, MD

KEYWORDS

- Joints • Inflammation • Autoimmunity • Pain • Infection • Trauma • Sports injuries
- Vasculopathy

KEY POINTS

- The care provider should focus on a complete history, including the presence or absence of pain and acuity, the chronicity of the complaint, antecedent events, triggers, and means of relief.
- The care provider should do a complete examination rather than one that focuses on the involved area.
- Laboratory studies should be ordered with a focus on the pertinent points gleaned from the history and physical examination rather than ordering broad antecedent event panels.

INTRODUCTION

Despite the general belief of the public that healthy children do not experience pain, multiple surveys have demonstrated that as many as 50% of children have pain complaints at some time during a single year.[1] Moreover, it has been reported that 6% of visits by children 3 ages to 15 years to a pediatrician's office are due to pain complaints.[2] The problem for the primary care provider is to distinguish between harmless complaints and those indicating pathologic conditions. This article outlines an approach to distinguish pathologic joint conditions in children because, despite the frequency of pain complaints, not all pathologic joint conditions are accompanied by joint discomfort. Similarly, a pathologic joint condition may or may not be accompanied by swelling; it may be associated with local inflammation or be a noninflammatory process. It can be accompanied by a rash or fever. As with all medical complaints, the history is the most important part of the visit for developing a differential diagnosis. (See discussion of widespread extraarticular pain in Jennifer E. Weiss and Jennifer N. Stinson's article, "Pediatric Pain Syndromes and Non-inflammatory Musculoskeletal Pain," in this issue.)

Disclosures: The author has no relevant disclosures.
Pediatric Immunology, Section of Pediatric Rheumatology and Immunology, Department of Pediatrics, Seton Hall-Hackensack Meridian School of Medicine, Hackensack University Medical Center, 30 Prospect Avenue, Room WFAN 360, Hackensack, NJ 07601, USA
E-mail address: Kathleen.Haines@HackensackMeridian.org

Pediatr Clin N Am 65 (2018) 623–638
https://doi.org/10.1016/j.pcl.2018.03.003
0031-3955/18/© 2018 Elsevier Inc. All rights reserved.

pediatric.theclinics.com

Approach to Taking the History

Pain or not?

Among the first considerations is whether the observed joint problem is painful or pain-less (**Box 1**). Rather than pain, the chief complaint may be swelling or impairment in func-tion, such as a limp or difficulty with flexion or extension of the joint. Critical to establishing the diagnosis is the ascertainment of pain characteristics. Has the pain or dysfunction been present for days, weeks, or months? Was there a known precipitating factor or did it begin insidiously and worsen? Is there pain at rest? Do they have pain, swelling, or dysfunction throughout the day, or is it intermittent? If intermittent, does it occur daily or less frequently? Is it most painful or dysfunctional after a period of rest, with activity improving the sense of wellbeing, or is it the opposite, worsening with increasing activity? Is the joint swollen or does the pain seem to be primarily inside the joint? This phrase, inside the joint, is chosen deliberately to permit the parent or patient to describe pain in a normal appearing joint rather than fear the complaint will not be taken seriously in the absence of perceived swelling. Pain quality (sharp, dull, burning, twisting, aching) can be helpful but children most often find pain very difficult to describe (**Table 1**).

One joint or more?

Next, is it localized to a single joint or less focused and involving the whole limb? Does it involve many joints or is it felt diffusely throughout the body. Severe pain in a single joint, particularly with acute onset, is most likely to be associated with trauma or infection. (See discussion of diffuse, generalized pain in the absence of systemic features in Jennifer E. Weiss and Jennifer N. Stinson's article, "Pediatric Pain Syndromes and Non-inflammatory Musculoskeletal Pain," in this issue.) Much to the surprise of many, auto-immune arthritides can be painless or can be associated with only mild pain.[3]

Box 1
Factors in taking a history

- Painful versus painless

- Location
  - Single joint versus multiple joints
  - Large joint versus small joint

- Onset
  - Acute versus chronic
  - Constant versus intermittent

- Potential precipitating factors of antecedent trauma
  - Antecedent infection

- Accompanying signs and/or symptoms
  - Rash
  - Fever
  - Swelling
  - Bowel complaints

- Triggers
  - Time of day
  - Physical position
  - Physical activities

- Ameliorating therapy
  - Physical agents
  - Medication
  - Degree of relief

Table 1
Typical pain severity

Mild to None	Moderate	Severe
Lyme arthritis	Trauma	Trauma
Juvenile idiopathic arthritis (JIA)	Reactive arthritis	Septic joint
Henoch-Schönlein purpura (HSP)	HSP	Bony infarct
Legg-Calvé-Perthes (LCP) syndrome	Autoimmune diseases or JIA	Leukemia
	Viral-associated arthritis	Metastatic disease
	Biomechanical	Pain amplification
	Osteoid osteoma	
	Slipped capital femoral epiphysis (SCFE)	

In the absence of a traumatic cause, the history of an antecedent infection should be addressed and put in a temporal context, along with associated symptoms and signs. Has the child been ill within the last month? The care provider should specifically inquire about fevers, rashes, respiratory infections, gastroenteritis, or urinary symptoms. Recent or concurrent infection with the articular pain can be a clue to an infected joint or bone, or a reactive synovitis (**Box 2**).

How long has it been going on?
Whether the onset of pain is recent or longstanding is important in organizing and prioritizing a differential diagnosis. However, the provider must always keep in mind that a child may present early with the pain complaints of what will prove to be a chronic disease. Thus, diagnoses of pain complaints of rapid or recent onset should

Box 2
Fever

None
- Juvenile idiopathic arthritis (JIA)
- Trauma
- Biomechanical
- Metastatic disease
- Chondrodysplasia
- Other autoimmune

Moderate
- JIA (systemic)
- Leukemia
- Other autoimmune
- Autoinflammatory
- Osteomyelitis
- Acute rheumatic fever (ARF) or poststreptococcal arthritis

High
- Septic arthritis
- Autoinflammatory

be pursued (including consideration of those more typically presenting after a more extended time frame) until resolution or a diagnoses is reached (**Boxes 3** and **4**).

Selected Causes of Pain with Recent Onset, Typically Short (<6 Weeks) Time to Presentation

Trauma

The onset of trauma is precipitous with significant pain, it is localized to a single site, and the causal event can most often be immediately identified. However, sports participation can be an exception to that rule. Not infrequently, parents and children will deny any possibility of injury but when asked directly they report the child belongs to football, soccer, lacrosse, gymnastics, competitive cheerleading, or other sports teams in which contact injuries are dismissed as being part of the game. A forgotten injury may reveal the cause of a painful joint. A swollen joint with a rapid onset of effusion immediately after significant trauma to the joint might suggest a hemarthrosis and associated damage to joint structures, such as ligament or meniscal tears. Although sports-related trauma is the most common cause of a hemarthrosis, in the absence of this history a bleeding diathesis is suggested. Both hemophilia and von Willebrand disease vary in their severity and can, therefore, present later in childhood.[4,5] Sports injuries can also include a traction injury at an apophysis. The apophyses are growth plates, or ossification centers, which are extraarticular and, as such, do not add length to a growing bone. Close to the various apophyses are the bony attachment sites of tendons and ligaments (entheses). In the growing child, the muscles and tendons can be stronger than the growth plate at the apophysis and a sudden strong force can cause an avulsion injury with associated acute pain. Common sites for such injuries are the anterior iliac crest and more rarely in the ischial tuberosity.[6] (See discussion of this type of injury in Jennifer E. Weiss and Jennifer N. Stinson's article, "Pediatric Pain Syndromes and Non-inflammatory Musculoskeletal Pain," in this issue.)

Septic arthritis

Intraarticular infection presents acutely and must be diagnosed with some urgency because delay in diagnosis can lead to destruction of joint cartilage.[7] Children with septic arthritis most commonly appear ill with significant fever. There may be a history of a purulent infection (otitis, cellulitis) before the onset of joint pain but this is often not elicited. They may experience only moderate pain and limping initially but within the first day their pain will crescendo and they will usually refuse to bear weight or allow any range of motion of the affected joint. Most patients with septic arthritis are younger than 5 years of age.

Toxic synovitis

Toxic, or transient, synovitis is the most common cause of hip pain in young children between ages 4 and 10 years but may occur in other large joints. It is of acute

---

Box 3
Pain of recent onset

- Traumatic
  - Fracture or sprain
  - Apophyseal evulsion
- Septic arthritis with or without osteomyelitis
- Acute infarct (SS or SC disease)
- Toxic synovitis or reactive arthritis

Box 4
Pain of prolonged duration

Intermittent

- Biomechanical or overuse
- Hypermobility or lax ligaments
- Benign limb pain of childhood
- Autoinflammatory disease (excluding NOMID-CINCA)

Persistent

- Slipped capital femoral epiphysis
- Legg-Calvé-Perthes syndrome
- Osteochondral dysplasias
- Osteoid osteoma
- JIA/Autoimmune
- Autoinflammatory (NOMID-CINCA)

onset and often, though not invariably, associated with a prior upper respiratory infection. It is rarely associated with low-grade fever. The pain of toxic synovitis varies from moderate to quite severe and, occasionally, the child will refuse to bear weight. More often than not they will stand and limp with ambulation. The pain is daily and persistent, although it lessens with analgesic agents. Pain and stiffness after inactivity (greatest pain on arising in the morning, after napping, or after prolonged sitting) is seen. Toxic synovitis may be bilateral but, if so, usually 1 hip is significantly more affected than the other. The recent history should be that of an otherwise well child. It has been associated with development of avascular necrosis of the femoral head (Legg-Calvé-Perthes [LCP]) disease months later in less than 5% of patients.[8,9]

Reactive arthritis or postviral arthritis

Reactive arthritis has been described as main cause of hip pain in young children, between ages 4 and 10 years but may occur in other areas of the body. Some investigators limit the term reactive to arthritides associated with bacterial infections.[10,11] Infections, as the distinction between truly reactive versus infective arthritis when virus infections trigger arthritis is unclear. Viruses have been isolated from the synovial fluid of patients in some cases. Arthritis associated with a viral disease has been reported after infection with essentially all viruses, and particularly parvovirus B19, the causative virus of erythema infectiosum or fifth disease. Viral-associated arthritis may involve either large or small joints. Since the advent of rubella vaccine, its associated arthritis is rare but should be considered when joint pain and swelling develops after receiving a booster vaccine, particularly in adolescents. Viral or bacterial gastroenteritides are also well-described triggers of postinfectious arthritis. The most commonly associated bacteria are *Salmonella*, *Shigella*, *Yersinia*, and *Campylobacter*, although *Mycoplasma* has also been reported. The arthritis usually occurs 1 to 4 weeks after an infection and is an oligoarthritis (4 joints or fewer) most often affecting joints below the waist. Weight loss or anemia in a patient with gastrointestinal symptoms should always increase concern for arthritis associated with inflammatory bowel disease.

Lyme arthritis

Lyme arthritis is caused by infection with the spirochete *Borrelia burgdorferi*, transmitted by the black-legged or deer tick. The initial symptoms, within the first month, are a flu-like illness with fever, headache, and polyarthralgias. A rash called erythema migrans can develop within 30 days at the site of the tick bite. However, recall of either bite or rash is low.[12] The subsequent arthritis develops on average 6 months after the erythema migrans rash is seen.[13,14] It is most frequent in large joints, is often a monoarthritis, and can be migratory. It is not particularly painful but the associated effusion can be quite large, causing discomfort. In the United States, Lyme disease or arthritis is most common in the northeastern states from Maine to Virginia, and in the midwestern states of Wisconsin and Minnesota. In Canada, Lyme disease is most common in the regions contiguous to those in the United States (in southeastern Ontario and southwestern Quebec bordering the Great Lakes and St. Lawrence River, and in Southern Manitoba), as well as in Nova Scotia and southwestern British Columbia. Its geographic distribution in North America is increasing. A travel history, including day trips to the endemic areas, should always be documented.[14]

Streptococcal-associated arthritis

The association of group A β-hemolytic streptococcal pharyngitis and arthritis has been known for longer than a century; however, the distinction between acute rheumatic fever (ARF) and poststreptococcal arthritis (PSA) remains problematic (**Table 2**). It remains a clinical diagnosis. Both conditions should demonstrate evidence of a prior streptococcal pharyngitis via a positive throat culture or rapid strep test or changing antibody titers. The patterns of onset are somewhat different. PSA begins approximately 1 to 2 weeks after the infection, whereas ARF does not begin for at least 2 weeks. The arthritis in PSA is fixed, and can involve large and small joints, as well as entheses and the axial skeleton. Arthritis in ARF is migratory, additive, and quite painful, primarily affecting large to intermediate joints. The age distribution of both diseases overlaps with a broad peak from 8 to 12 years for PSA and from 5 to 15 years for ARF.[15]

Henoch-Schönlein purpura

Anaphylactoid purpura, more commonly known as Henoch-Schönlein purpura (HSP), is an immunoglobulin (Ig)A-mediated vasculitis. It is associated with a classic rash occurring primarily on the feet and legs, and extending up onto the buttocks. It can extend to the face and arms but the number of lesions is far fewer than that on the legs. The typical palpable purpura is often preceded for a day or 2 by an urticarial

Table 2
Differences between acute rheumatic fever and poststreptococcal arthritis

	PSA	ARF
Arthritis	Fixed	Migratory, painful
Joints	Large and small Entheses and axial	Large Knees, ankles, wrists
Response to nonsteroidal antiinflammatory drugs	Moderate and slow	Rapid
Inflammatory markers (C-reactive protein, erythrocyte sedimentation rate)	Low to moderate	Very elevated
Other	None	Carditis, subcutaneous nodules, erythema marginatum

rash and angioedema of the legs and feet. Abdominal pain and renal involvement complete the triad of HSP symptoms. Arthritis associated with HSP is primarily in the large joints of knees and ankles. It can be essentially painless or associated with significant pain. Low-grade fever and malaise is common. In most cases, HSP is a self-limited disease that resolves in 6 to 8 weeks, although more persistent symptoms are not rare. The signs and symptoms come in waves, with the rash and arthritis appearing to wane over 1 to 2 weeks, then recur, and again wane and recur. The major concerns are gastrointestinal involvement with intussusception and renal disease, which typically appear after the rash has begun.[16]

Sickle cell disease

Sickle cell disease (ie, hemoglobin SS [SS] or hemoglobin SC [SC] disease) is a well-known cause of bone and joint pain, with the acute onset of bony infarct. Presentation in infants is the classic hand-foot syndrome with acute pain and swelling of the fingers and toes (dactylitis). Older children can get periarticular infarcts with pain. It will be of acute onset.[17] Currently, all 50 states in the United States and the District of Columbia have mandatory neonatal screening for hemoglobinopathies, which should make a diagnosis of SS or SC disease-associated pain less onerous than in past decades. Although the greatest prevalence of SS disease is in sub-Saharan Africa, its distribution is worldwide. Moreover, children born outside of the United States do not always have neonatal screening available; therefore, SS disease should remain in the differential diagnosis of acute bone and joint pain.

Malignancy-associated symptoms

Although articular or periarticular pain as the presenting sign of malignancy is uncommon, it should always be included in the differential diagnosis, particularly if the pain is severe. Although there are isolated case reports of intermittent pain, it is more frequently experienced as a constant pain throughout the day and night and can be severe enough to wake the patient from sleep.[18–20] The arthritis can involve any number of joints, which most commonly are the large joints; that is, knee, ankle, shoulder, and elbow. The vertebral bodies can also be involved. The patients may have only joint complaints but more often they are associated with other signs and symptoms, such as anemia, fatigue, loss of appetite, weight loss, and fever. None of these symptoms are specific and can be seen in rheumatic diseases, particularly systemic onset juvenile idiopathic arthritis, lupus, and juvenile dermatomyositis. Morning stiffness, a typical complaint of an inflammatory arthritis, is unusual. Significant pain relief with nonsteroidal antiinflammatory drugs (NSAIDs) should not reassure the physician that the process is benign if other signs are of concern. However, response to NSAIDs rarely lasts more than several weeks in children with neoplasms and, therefore, should not significantly prolong the path to diagnosis[21] (the author's personal observation).

Selected Causes of Persistent Pain of Insidious Onset

Slipped capital femoral epiphysis

Slipped capital femoral epiphysis (SCFE) is described as a boring pain localized to the groin or buttocks, which is where true hip pain is felt, rather than the area of the trochanter. The incidence varies markedly internationally and even regionally in the United States. Bilateral disease has been reported in 6% to 50% of cases, with slips occurring either simultaneously or sequentially. Reported male/female range ratios range from 3:1 in Japan to approximately 1.2:1 in the United States. Chronic SCFE (pain for longer than 3 weeks duration) make up 85% of cases.[22] SCFE is seen in preadolescents and early adolescents before the proximal femoral growth plate is closed. Obesity is a known risk factor. However, endocrinopathies involving delay of closure of physes, such as hypothyroidism, are less well known risk factors.[22,23] (See discussion of SCFE in Jennifer E. Weiss and Jennifer N. Stinson's article, "Pediatric Pain Syndromes and Non-inflammatory Musculoskeletal Pain," in this issue.)

Aseptic necrosis of the femoral head or Legg-Calvé-Perthes disease

Named after the 3 orthopedic surgeons who independently described it in 1910, LCP is a destructive lesion of the epiphysis of the femur due to loss of blood supply and resulting necrosis. It is most often seen in children ages 5 to 8 years and has a male/female preponderance of 5:1. The onset is most often insidious with the development of a limp as the presenting sign.[24] It has been reported as a sequela of toxic synovitis. (See discussion of LCP in Jennifer E. Weiss and Jennifer N. Stinson's article, "Pediatric Pain Syndromes and Non-inflammatory Musculoskeletal Pain," in this issue.)

Osteoid osteoma

Osteoid osteoma is the third most common benign bone tumor. Its peak incidence is between the ages of 10 and 20 years and is reported to be 1.6 to 4 times more common in boys.[25] Its most common location is the femoral head or neck but it has been reported in many sites, including the spine. The pain is localized, insidious, and worsens over time. The patient experiences daily pain that peaks at night, occasionally causing nighttime awakenings. It is very responsive to the analgesia provided by NSAIDs.

Osteochondral dysplasias

Osteochondral dysplasias are bone abnormalities due to genetic disorders of collagen structure that lead to short stature, abnormal joint development, pain, and early onset osteoarthritis. The 2 most common types are pseudoachondroplasia (PSACH) and multiple epiphyseal dysplasia (MED). PSACH is inherited in an autosomal dominant (AD) manner with mutations in the collagen oligomeric matrix protein (COMP) gene. Approximately 50% of patients with AD-MED have COMP mutations, generally in different domains than that seen in PSACH. Another approximately 25% of AD-MED patients have mutations in other collagen genes. Autosomal recessive MED is caused by mutations in a sulfate transporter. Patients with PSACH are usually diagnosed by age 2 years because they are more severely affected with its phenotype of short limbs as compared with trunk length becoming noticeable by that time. The phenotype of patients with MED is usually less obvious and, indeed, the diagnosis may come from other signs and symptoms instead of short stature. Complaints of early fatigue with activities, significant joint pain, and loss of motion around the affected joints should increase suspicion for MED. There may be hypotonia or frank myopathy. The skeletal maturation is delayed. Most patients with MED are shorter than the midparental height would predict. Its prevalence has been estimated at 1 per 20,000, although the accuracy of this estimate is questioned because an index case has led to its discovery in family members previously undiagnosed.[26]

Autoimmune arthropathies

All autoimmune diseases are clinical diagnoses that can only be arrived at after other causes of disease are sought and eliminated.[27] (See discussion of juvenile idiopathic arthritis and other disorders in Courtney B. Crayne and Timothy Beukelman's article, "Juvenile Idiopathic Arthritis: Oligoarthritis and Polyarthritis," and Pamela F. Weiss and Robert A. Colbert's article, "Juvenile Spondyloarthritis: A Distinct Form of Juvenile Arthritis," and Jennifer J.Y. Lee and Rayfel Schneider's article, "Systemic Juvenile Idiopathic Arthritis (JIA)," in this issue) These arthritides can only be diagnosed after 6 weeks of at least some of the hallmark signs of inflammation (pain or tenderness, swelling, heat, redness, and loss of function) affecting 1 or more joints. Although many children have significant pain, it often can be a surprisingly minor complaint, with functional problems (eg, stiffness in the morning and after periods of inactivity, limp, writing difficulty) bringing the patient to medical attention.[3] Other autoimmune disorders, such as systemic lupus erythematosus (see Stacey E. Tarvin and Kathleen M. O'Neil's article, "Systemic Lupus Erythematosus, Sjögren Syndrome, and MCTD in Children and Adolescents, in this issue), juvenile dermatomyositis (see Adam M. Huber's article, "Juvenile Idiopathic Inflammatory Myopathies," in this issue; see Suzanne C. Li's article, "Scleroderma in Children and Adolescents: localized scleroderma and systemic sclerosis" in this issue), and the systemic vasculitides (granulomatous with polyangiitis, microscopic polyangiitis, Takayasu arteritis), can have associated arthritis but most often other hallmark symptoms, such as fever, fatigue, rash, or weakness, are the signs and symptoms that prompt a visit to the physician.[16,28,29] (See discussions of other autoimmune disorders, in this issue.)

Selected Examples of Intermittent Longstanding Pain

Biomechanical or overuse syndromes or repetitive motion injuries
Most sports-related injuries in the United States are overuse or repetitive stress injuries ("microtrauma") rather than what has been called "macrotrauma"[30] (see Box 4). (See discussion of these conditions in Jennifer E. Weiss and Jennifer N. Stinson's article, "Pediatric Pain Syndromes and Non-inflammatory Musculoskeletal Pain," in this issue.) Many of these injuries are due to apophysitis, the most common of which is Osgood-Schlatter syndrome, with pain at the apophysis of the tibial tubercle. Patellofemoral syndrome, also called idiopathic anterior knee pain, is common in runners and soccer players. Sever disease is an apophysitis at the calcaneus. Gymnast wrist is a repetitive trauma injury of the physeal plate due to the high impact experienced in floor exercise and vault of gymnasts, and similar tumbling and repetitive impacts in cheerleading.[31] Shoulder pain is common among swimmers and baseball players. Factors associated with these injuries include sudden increase in intensity of sports participation, along with insufficient and inappropriate training on a background of poor conditioning.[30] In these conditions, the pain is at first associated solely with the sports activity. If it is not treated, the pain can be brought on by daily activities and, finally, remaining inadequately treated, become constant. Non-sports repetitive-use injuries have also been reported with excessive video gaming and texting being culprits. Such injuries may not be trivial; tendon ruptures have resulted.[32–34]

Hypermobility or lax ligaments
Hypermobility of joints is a relatively common finding in children. It is unclear whether benign familial hypermobility and Ehlers Danlos syndrome are distinct syndromes because there are many overlapping features.[35–37] However, it is agreed that these children have a greater incidence of generalized pain sensitivity[38,39] and can suffer from joint dislocations due to lax ligaments. The mechanism of hyperalgesia is not understood but it is not associated with an underlying inflammatory process. (See discussion of benign joint hypermobility syndrome in Jennifer E. Weiss and Jennifer N. Stinson's article, "Pediatric Pain Syndromes and Non-inflammatory Musculoskeletal Pain," in this issue.)

Benign limb pain of childhood
This disorder, also called benign nocturnal limb pain and growing pains (despite not being related to growth) is a common cause of pain in children, with estimates of prevalence ranging from 2.6% to 49.9%.[40] Growing pains usually begin at some time between the ages of 3 and 6 years.[41] The pain is not localized to a joint but rather the calves, shins, and/or popliteal fossae. Rarely does it involve an upper limb. The pain is intermittent with approximately 50% of affected children having pains at least monthly and 50% less frequently.[42,43] Bilateral pain is the norm, with some investigators reporting greater than 80%.[43] However, the child may report pain that alternates sites from episode to

episode. The pain begins late in the day to nighttime and can be quite severe, waking a child from sleep. It is most often completely resolved by the time the child awakens in the morning. Pain that is not resolved by morning and/or always localized to the same site should trigger consideration of another cause for the pain. (See discussion of benign limb pain of childhood in Jennifer E. Weiss and Jennifer N. Stinson's article, "Pediatric Pain Syndromes and Non-inflammatory Musculoskeletal Pain," in this issue.)

Autoinflammatory disease

Autoinflammatory disease was recently discussed in the February 2017 volume of *Pediatric Clinics of North America*,[44] so is only briefly mentioned here. Familial Mediterranean fever, mevalonate kinase deficiency (hyper-IgD syndrome), tumor necrosis factor receptor–associated periodic syndrome, and cryopyrin-associated periodic syndromes (eg, familial cold autoinflammatory syndrome, Muckle Wells, and Neonatal Onset Multisystem Inflammatory Disease-Chronic Infantile Neurological Cutaneous Articular Syndrome [NOMDI-CINCA]) are the most well-known of the inherited disorders associated with fevers, some of which have a periodicity. They usually have distinct dermatologic findings, as well as arthralgia and arthritis. With the exception of NOMID-CINCA, the patients are relatively well between episodes.[45,46] (See further features of these and many other autoinflammatory diseases in Table 4 of Kathleen E. Sullivan's article, "Pathogenesis of Pediatric Rheumatologic Diseases," in this issue.)

Physical Examination

A full physical examination should be performed looking for signs of common infections suggestive of a viral-associated arthritis. Skin findings (**Box 5**) should be

---

Box 5
Skin findings

Generalized rash

- Viral exanthems

- Parvovirus: slapped face and lacy rash on limbs or torso

- HSP: palpable purpura lower limbs greater than on upper limbs

- *Streptococcus pyogenes*: erythema marginatum with AR, scarlet fever, red face, maculopapular sandpaper rash on trunk and limbs

- Systemic onset JIA: salmon-colored rash, pronounced with fever, can resemble urticarial

Localized rashes or lesions

- Systemic lupus erythematosus: malar rash, discoid rash, photosensitive rashes in sun exposed areas

- Juvenile dermatomyositis: heliotrope rash on cheeks, eyelids; dry, overgrown cuticles; Gottron rashes on elbows, knees, knuckles

- Psoriatic arthritis: psoriasis patches, pitted fingernails

- Scleroderma
  - Localized scleroderma: linear or circumscribed lesions usually adjacent to or overlying joint but can be remote from joint
  - Systemic sclerosis: early diffuse swelling of fingers and hands, later skin thickening and dyspigmentation spreading proximally from fingers

- Monogenic fever syndromes (familial Mediterranean fever, tumor necrosis factor receptor–associated periodic syndrome, mevalonate kinase deficiency, and cryopyrin-associated periodic syndrome): urticarial, cellulitic, and polymorphous

noted as clues to viral-associated, autoimmune, and autoinflammatory diseases, as well as redness and warmth, which may indicate underlying infection.

Despite the child and parent reporting localized pain, the joint examination should not be limited to the concerning joint. In inflammatory arthropathies it is not uncommon to find more than 1 joint involved, with the patient or parent only reporting the most painful joint. A rapid generalized joint examination, such as the pediatric gait, arms, legs, and spine (pGALS),[47] should be done, followed by a more detailed assessment of the identified areas of pain complaints, the contralateral joint, and any new pathologic condition noted via the pGALS examination (**Fig. 1**).

Arthritis is more than joint pain. It must demonstrate at least some of the hallmarks of inflammation. Thus, the joints should be inspected for warmth, swelling, and redness. Palpation of the area to elicit any point tenderness suggestive of bone infection or fracture should be performed. The involved joints, as well as the contralateral joints, should be compared because discordance in size and shape will reveal swelling. Similarly, the affected and contralateral joint must be manipulated through range of motion. Special note should be made symmetry in joint motion. For example, a child with

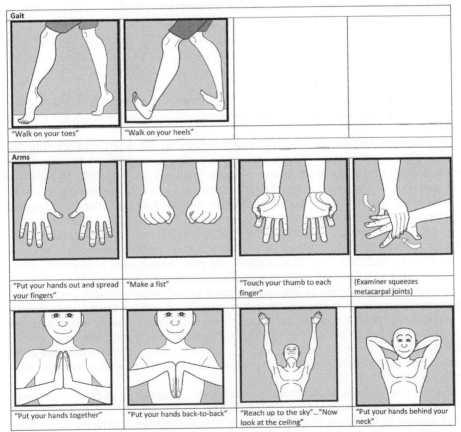

Fig. 1. pGALS examination. (*Adapted from* Foster HE, Kay LJ, Friswell M, et al. Musculoskeletal screening examination (pGALS) for school-age children based on the adult GALS screen. Arthritis Rheum 2006;55(5):713; with permission.)

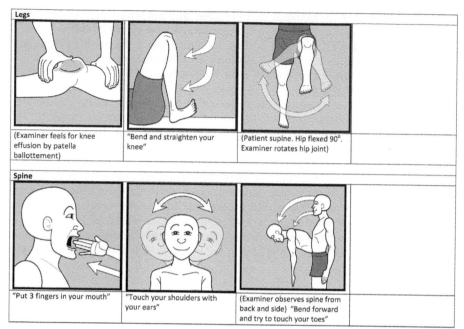

Legs			
(Examiner feels for knee effusion by patella ballottement)	"Bend and straighten your knee"	(Patient supine. Hip flexed 90°. Examiner rotates hip joint)	
Spine			
"Put 3 fingers in your mouth"	"Touch your shoulders with your ears"	(Examiner observes spine from back and side) "Bend forward and try to touch your toes"	

Fig. 1. (*continued*).

0° extension of the knee or elbow on the right but with 5° of hyperextension on the left, does not have a normal examination despite joint motion on each side falling within the normal range (**Box 6**).

Physical examination of any inflammatory arthritis will often demonstrate the involved joint held in partial flexion; hip involvement is suggested when the leg is preferentially held in external rotation. These positions are assumed to minimize compression of the joint capsule by an associated effusion, which, if small, may not be easily appreciated on examination. Pain is elicited with an attempt to achieve full range of motion. With regard to hip motion, pain is also elicited with internal rotation the hip, compressing the capsule. SCFE has similar limitations but less pain on motion. The affected leg may be shorter, depending on the amount of slip. LCP demonstrates marked diminution of abduction with pain. Apophyseal tenderness, which may be bilateral, indicates the aforementioned inflammatory apophysitis syndromes; pain at multiple apophyses or entheses suggests spondyloarthropathy and/or an inflammatory process in the bowel. (See discussion of spondyloarthropathy in Pamela F. Weiss and Robert A. Colbert's article, "Juvenile Spondyloarthritis: A Distinct Form of Juvenile Arthritis," in this issue.) Finally, if the presenting joint has a completely normal examination in the presence of a suspicious pGALS examination, the joints above and below warrant a careful examination so as not to ignore the possibility of referred pain.

Benign hypermobility is assessed by application of the Beighton criteria for hypermobility.[36] (See discussion of Beighton criteria for hypermobility in Jennifer E. Weiss and Jennifer N. Stinson's article, "Pediatric Pain Syndromes and Non-inflammatory Musculoskeletal Pain," in this issue.) In the presence of arthralgia in 4 or more joints, for more than 3 months, a score of greater than or equal to 4 meets the criteria for benign hypermobility.

Box 6
Normal ranges of motion of large joints

Shoulder
- Abduction (up and away): 180°
- Adduction (across chest): 45°
- Flexion (forward): 90°
- Extension (backward): 45°
- Internal rotation: 55°
- External rotation: 45°

Elbows
- Flexion: 135°
- Extension: 0° to -5°
- Supination (palm up): 90°
- Pronation (palm down): 90°

Hips
- Flexion: 120°
- Extension: 30°
- Abduction – 45° to 50°
- Adduction – 20° to 30°
- Internal rotation: 35°
- External rotation: 45°

Knee
- Flexion: 135°
- Extension: 0°
- Internal rotation: 10°
- External rotation: 10°

Ankle
- Ankle dorsiflexion: 20°
- Ankle plantar flexion: 50°
- Subtalar inversion: 5°
- Subtalar eversion: 5°
- Forefoot adduction: 20°
- Forefoot abduction: 10°

Laboratory studies

Laboratory studies should be chosen with discretion. Rheumatic disorders are not diagnosed by laboratory results alone but require specific physical findings plus the exclusion of nonrheumatic conditions that can mimic them. Using antinuclear antibody (ANA) tests or panels containing ANA and rheumatoid factor as screens is not useful because these tests are not at all specific for any rheumatologic disorder. Even in systemic lupus erythematosus, in which essentially all patients have positive ANA titers, a positive ANA does not establish the diagnosis in the absence of physical signs included in lupus criteria.[48,49] (See further discussion in Stacey E. Tarvin and Kathleen M. O'Neil's article, "Systemic Lupus Erythematosus, Sjögren Syndrome, and MCTD in Children and Adolescents, in this issue.) Complete blood count (CBC) and the acute phase reactants (APRs) most often reflect high levels of inflammation in children with septic joints but can be equally abnormal in systemic onset juvenile idiopathic arthritis, inflammatory bowel disease–associated arthritis, ARF, and other diseases. Patients with joint pain due to malignant disease can have elevated APR with a normal CBC.[20,50] APRs are usually normal or only mildly elevated in toxic synovitis, postviral arthritis, and the other juvenile idiopathic arthritides, despite the inflammatory process in the joint. Normal APRs would be expected in trauma, overuse, hypermobility, and osteochondroses. Testing for Lyme arthritis should be done as a 2-step process, with IgG and IgM titers done as the first step, followed by immunoblot if titers are high.[13]

Imaging studies

Imaging studies to be considered include radiograph, ultrasound, and MRI. Radiograph of the affected area is most often the initial image to be obtained. It is useful to obtain an image of the contralateral (nonaffected) side for comparison because bilateral symmetry of an unusual finding can help distinguish a normal from a pathologic variant. Fractures, avulsion injuries, bone infections, and microtrauma, such as gymnast's wrist, can be identified by plain film. Lucent metaphyseal lines suggestive of leukemias can be observed. Moderate to large effusions of the involved joint can often be identified. Musculoskeletal ultrasound has become more generally available and a skilled ultrasonographer can pick up effusions, increased blood flow suggestive of an inflammatory process, and synovial thickening consistent with synovitis. MRI is usually reserved for suspicion of soft tissue injuries but is also useful to image bone edema, osteomyelitis, and tumors. To define an inflammatory process, imaging with and without contrast is most useful.

ACKNOWLEDGMENTS

Original artwork by Jim Haines https://www.behance.net/Jim_Haines.

REFERENCES

1. Mikkelsson M, Salminen JJ, Kautiainen H. Non-specific musculoskeletal pain in preadolescents. Prevalence and 1-year persistence. Pain 1997;73(1):29–35.
2. de Inocencio J. Musculoskeletal pain in primary pediatric care: analysis of 1000 consecutive general pediatric clinic visits. Pediatrics 1998;102(6):E63.
3. McGhee JL, Burks FN, Sheckels JL, et al. Identifying children with chronic arthritis based on chief complaints: absence of predictive value for musculoskeletal pain as an indicator of rheumatic disease in children. Pediatrics 2002;110(2 Pt 1):354–9.
4. Leebeek FW, Eikenboom JC. von Willebrand's disease. N Engl J Med 2016; 375(21):2067–80.
5. Carcao MD. The diagnosis and management of congenital hemophilia. Semin Thromb Hemost 2012;38(07):727–34.
6. Singer G, Eberl R, Wegmann H, et al. Diagnosis and treatment of apophyseal injuries of the pelvis in adolescents. Semin Musculoskelet Radiol 2014;18(5): 498–504.
7. Dodwell ER. Osteomyelitis and septic arthritis in children: current concepts. Curr Opin Pediatr 2013;25(1):58–63.

8. Landin LA, Danielsson LG, Wattsgard C. Transient synovitis of the hip. Its incidence, epidemiology and relation to Perthes' disease. J Bone Joint Surg Br 1987;69(2):238–42.

9. Cook PC. Transient synovitis, septic hip, and Legg-Calvé-Perthes disease: an approach to the correct diagnosis. Pediatr Clin North Am 2014;61(6):1109–18.

10. Laxer RM, Wright J, Lindsley CB. Infectious arthritis and osteomyelitis. In: Petty RE, Laxer RM, Lindsley CB, et al, editors. Textbook of pediatric rheumatology. 7th edition. Philadelphia: Elsevier; 2016. p. 533–50.

11. Petty RE, Tingle AJ. Arthritis and viral infection. J Pediatr 1988;113(5):948–9.

12. Brettschneider S, Bruckbauer H, Klugbauer N, et al. Diagnostic value of PCR for detection of Borrelia burgdorferi in skin biopsy and urine samples from patients with skin borreliosis. J Clin Microbiol 1998;36(9):2658–65.

13. Arvikar SL, Steere AC. 5. Diagnosis and treatment of Lyme arthritis. Infect Dis Clin North Am 2015;29(2):269–80.

14. Steere AC, Strle F, Wormser GP, et al. Lyme borreliosis. Nat Rev Dis Primers 2016; 2:16090.

15. Barash J. Rheumatic Fever and post-group a streptococcal arthritis in children. Curr Infect Dis Rep 2013;15(3):263–8.

16. Eleftheriou D, Batu ED, Ozen S, et al. Vasculitis in children. Nephrol Dial Transplant 2015;30(Suppl 1):i94–103.

17. Almeida A, Roberts I. Bone involvement in sickle cell disease. Br J Haematol 2005;129(4):482–90.

18. Riccio I, Marcarelli M, Del Regno N, et al. Musculoskeletal problems in pediatric acute leukemia. J Pediatr Orthop B 2013;22(3):264–9.

19. Trapani S, Grisolia F, Simonini G, et al. Incidence of occult cancer in children presenting with musculoskeletal symptoms: a 10-year survey in a pediatric rheumatology unit. Semin Arthritis Rheum 2000;29(6):348–59.

20. Ostrov BE, Goldsmith DP, Athreya BH. Differentiation of systemic juvenile rheumatoid arthritis from acute leukemia near the onset of disease. J Pediatr 1993; 122(4):595–8.

21. Shiner EK, McLean T, Pang CS, et al. A 9-year-old girl with ankle, knee, and shoulder pain. Arthritis Care Res (Hoboken) 2012;64(1):149–56.

22. Loder RT, Skopelja EN. The epidemiology and demographics of slipped capital femoral epiphysis. ISRN Orthop 2011;2011:19.

23. Kadowaki S, Hori T, Matsumoto H, et al. Prepubertal onset of slipped capital femoral epiphysis associated with hypothyroidism: a case report and literature review. BMC Endocr Disord 2017;17(1):59.

24. Kim HKW. Legg-Calvé-Perthes disease. J Am Acad Orthop Surg 2010;18:10.

25. Boscainos PJ, Cousins GR, Kulshreshtha R, et al. Osteoid osteoma. Orthopedics 2013;36(10):792–800.

26. Unger S, Bonafe L, Superti-Furga A. Multiple epiphyseal dysplasia: clinical and radiographic features, differential diagnosis and molecular basis. Best Pract Res Clin Rheumatol 2008;22(1):19–32.

27. Petty RE, Southwood TR, Manners P, et al. International League of Associations for Rheumatology classification of juvenile idiopathic arthritis: second revision, Edmonton, 2001. J Rheumatol 2004;31(2):390–2.

28. Wedderburn LR, Rider LG. Juvenile dermatomyositis: new developments in pathogenesis, assessment and treatment. Best Pract Res Clin Rheumatol 2009;23(5):665–78.

29. Hochberg MC. Updating the American College of Rheumatology revised criteria for the classification of systemic lupus erythematosus. Arthritis Rheum 1997;40(9):1725.

30. Patel DR, Yamasaki A, Brown K. Epidemiology of sports-related musculoskeletal injuries in young athletes in United States. Transl Pediatr 2017;6(3):160–6.
31. Chawla A, Wiesler ER. Nonspecific wrist pain in gymnasts and cheerleaders. Clin Sports Med 2015;34(1):143–9.
32. Gilman L, Cage DN, Horn A, et al. Tendon rupture associated with excessive smartphone gaming. JAMA Intern Med 2015;175(6):1048–9.
33. Singh R, Manoharan G, Moores TS, et al. Nintendo Wii related Achilles tendon rupture: first reported case and literature review of motion sensing video game injuries. BMJ Case Rep 2014;2014 [pii:bcr2013202657].
34. Fernandez-Guerrero IM. WhatsAppitis. Lancet 2014;383(9922):1040.
35. Beighton P, De Paepe A, Steinmann B, et al. Ehlers-Danlos syndromes: revised nosology, Villefranche, 1997. Ehlers-Danlos National Foundation (USA) and Ehlers-Danlos Support Group (UK). Am J Med Genet 1998;77(1):31–7.
36. Grahame R, Bird HA, Child A. The revised (Brighton 1998) criteria for the diagnosis of benign joint hypermobility syndrome (BJHS). J Rheumatol 2000;27(7):1777–9.
37. Tinkle BT, Bird HA, Grahame R, et al. The lack of clinical distinction between the hypermobility type of Ehlers-Danlos syndrome and the joint hypermobility syndrome (a.k.a. hypermobility syndrome). Am J Med Genet A 2009;149A(11): 2368–70.
38. Rombaut L, Scheper M, De Wandele I, et al. Chronic pain in patients with the hypermobility type of Ehlers–Danlos syndrome: evidence for generalized hyperalgesia. Clin Rheumatol 2015;34(6):1121.
39. Scheper MC, Pacey V, Rombaut L, et al. Generalized hyperalgesia in children and adults diagnosed with hypermobility syndrome and Ehlers-Danlos syndrome hypermobility type: a discriminative analysis. Arthritis Care Res (Hoboken) 2017; 69(3):421–9.
40. Lehman PJ, Carl RL. Growing pains. Sports Health 2017;9(2):132–8.
41. Kaspiris A, Chronopoulos E, Vasiliadis E. Perinatal risk factors and genu valgum conducive to the onset of growing pains in early childhood. Children (Basel) 2016;3(4) [pii:E34].
42. Kaspiris A, Zafiropoulou C. Growing pains in children: epidemiological analysis in a Mediterranean population. Joint Bone Spine 2009;76(5):486–90.
43. Pavone V, Lionetti E, Gargano V, et al. Growing pains: a study of 30 cases and a review of the literature. J Pediatr Orthop 2011;31(5):606–9.
44. Verbsky JW. When to suspect autoinflammatory/recurrent fever syndromes. Pediatric Clinics 2017;64(1):111–25.
45. Goldbach-Mansky R, Dailey NJ, Canna SW, et al. Neonatal-onset multisystem inflammatory disease responsive to interleukin-1beta inhibition. N Engl J Med 2006; 355(6):581–92.
46. Kastner DL, Aksentijevich I, Goldbach-Mansky R. Autoinflammatory disease reloaded: a clinical perspective. Cell 2010;140(6):784–90.
47. Foster HE, Kay LJ, Friswell M, et al. Musculoskeletal screening examination (pGALS) for school-age children based on the adult GALS screen. Arthritis Rheum 2006;55(5):709–16.
48. Malleson PN, Mackinnon MJ, Sailer-Hoeck M, et al. Review for the generalist: the antinuclear antibody test in children - when to use it and what to do with a positive titer. Pediatr Rheumatol Online J 2010;8:27.
49. McGhee JL, Kickingbird LM, Jarvis JN. Clinical utility of antinuclear antibody tests in children. BMC Pediatr 2004;4:13.
50. Cabral D, Tucker L. Malignancies in children who initially present with rheumatic complaints. J Pediatr 1999;134(1):53–7.

Pathogenesis of Pediatric Rheumatologic Diseases

Kathleen E. Sullivan, MD, PhD

KEYWORDS

• Inflammation • Autoimmunity • Tolerance • Rheumatic diseases

KEY POINTS

• Inflammation is due primarily to changes in microcirculation.
• Autoimmunity implies that the normal tolerance checkpoints have been breached.
• Autoinflammation can promote autoimmunity.
• Therapeutic advances depend on knowledge of pathogenesis of the rheumatic diseases.

INTRODUCTION

Inflammation is inherently understood by anyone who has burned their hand, had a localized infection, or suffered a large cut. The skin becomes red, there is swelling, and the site is tender. These are the hallmarks of inflammation. At a cellular level, inflammation is well understood to reflect activation of pain fibers, vasodilation, and increased vascular permeability. This article also describes the current understanding of loss of tolerance and the evolution of autoimmunity, as well as autoinflammation and the consequences of elevated cytokine expression. In many cases, current understanding is incomplete and there have been great advances coupled with increasingly perplexing questions. As anticipated, the improved understanding of pathogenesis has translated, in some cases, to improvements in therapeutics.

HISTORICAL UNDERSTANDING OF ARTHRITIS

Arthritis clearly affected ancient civilizations (**Table 1**); however, a medical appreciation of pediatric arthritis did not occur until 1545. The first inklings that inflammation was part of a pathologic process occurred after microscopy was developed and invading white cells could be observed. Dutrochet identified white cells that accumulate in inflammation in 1824. Currently, the character of the invading cells is still used to define the type of inflammation requiring treatment. Pathologists reference the cell types in

Disclosure: The author has no relevant disclosures.
Department of Pediatrics, Division of Allergy Immunology, The Children's Hospital of Philadelphia, University of Pennsylvania Perelman School of Medicine, 3615 Civic Center Boulevard, Philadelphia, PA 19104, USA
E-mail address: sullivank@email.chop.edu

Pediatr Clin N Am 65 (2018) 639–655
https://doi.org/10.1016/j.pcl.2018.03.004
0031-3955/18/© 2018 Elsevier Inc. All rights reserved.

Table 1
Rheumatic diseases in the ancient era

Findings	Therapy	Key People	Time
Earliest skeletal findings of rheumatoid arthritis (RA)		Native Americans, Tennessee River	4500 BCE
Gout (podagra) described; Mummies with spondyloarthropathy (SpA) and osteoarthritis (OA) found from this era.	Water therapy, willow extracts	Egyptian hieroglyphs	3000–2000 BCE
Gout recognized as related to gender, affluence	Diet therapy	Hippocrates	400 BCE
Charaka Samhita text describes an entity resembling RA	Diet, lifestyle, and herbal remedies	Ayurvedic texts Greek physician Dioscorides	200 CE
First use of term "rheumatismos" meaning "to flow" and associating respiratory disease with painful maladies	Colchicine used for gout	Galen Alexander of Trailes	200 CE 600 CE
Madhav Nidan describes amavata: rheumatic fever	Diet, lifestyle, and herbal remedies	Ayurvedic texts	700 CE
Earliest skeletal findings of psoriatic arthritis PsoA		Saxon village	1200 CE
Pediatric arthritis described as "stiffness of lymmes" and thought to be due to cold exposure		Thomas Phaer	1545 CE
Recognition that gout, RA, and rheumatic fever are distinct entities		Guillaume do Baillou	1600 CE
"Inflammation of the lymphatic arteries" described as the cause of rheumatic fever Chronic rheumatism recognized as a distinct entity		Thomas Sydenham	1666 CE

their descriptions. Synovial fluid neutrophil count, lymphocytic infiltration into muscle, and granulomas in skin are revealed by pathologic evaluation and are used diagnostically and to determine therapy in some circumstances. The migration of cells has proven to be a pivotal facet that has been mined therapeutically (see later discussion).

If inflammation represents an ancient concept that has been refined over the years, autoimmunity represents a much more recent concept. The overall concept of immunity sputtered through history, beginning with Thucydides' description of the plague of Athens, which rendered sufferers immune to a second attack.[1] Autoimmunity as a concept was not recognized until quite recently. In 1900, Paul Ehrlich stated flatly that antibodies could not be generated to self but in the 1950s autoantibodies were clearly demonstrated in human disease states.[2] In the intervening time, it has become understood that T cells also can be autoreactive. As the understanding of host defense and immunity has improved, the ability to manipulate the immune system has also improved (**Table 2**). This rapid evolution in immunology has translated into improved therapeutics specifically for pediatric rheumatology. Perhaps the best argument for pursuing studies on pathogenesis is to develop new and better therapeutics that lessen the burden of disease, improve outcomes, and allow children to live the life they envision for themselves. It is in this spirit that this article reviews pathogenesis.

Table 2
Rheumatic diseases in the therapeutic era

Findings	Therapy	Key People	Time
	Willow bark for agues	Rev. Edward Stone	1763
	Salicin purified	Henri Leroux	1829
Lupus erythematosus described: patches of skin with red, raised edges		Pierre Louis Alphée Cazenave	1833
RA distinguished from gout The thread test on synovial fluid, first clinical chemical test		Sir Alfred Garrod	1897
X-rays developed		Wilhelm Roentgen	1895
	Glucocorticoids used for RA	Philip Hench	1947
Anti-nuclear antibodies ANA and Rheumatoid factor RF identified			1948
	Methotrexate MTX used for dermatomyositis		1968
	TNF inhibitors developed for RA	Marc Feldmann, Ravinder Maini	1993

MICROCIRCULATION IN INFLAMMATION

Microcirculation regulates cellular influx into inflammatory sites. Any type of injury, including infection, reveals collagen on the luminal side of the vessel, which activates Hageman factor (factor XII) of the clotting cascade. Activated Hageman factor activates the kinin system, which causes smooth muscle contraction, arteriolar dilatation,

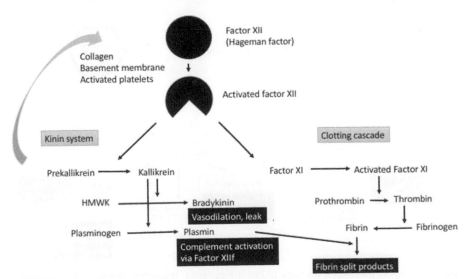

Fig. 1. Microcirculatory changes in inflammation. Factor XII (Hageman factor) is activated by damaged endothelium and the exposure of collagen. Once activated, Factor XII can directly activate the complement cascade (not shown), activate the kinin pathway with the ultimate result of bradykinin production, and activate the clotting cascade. Complement is also activated by plasmin. Bradykinin is the major mediator of vascular leak and vasodilatation. HMWK, high molecular weight kininogen.

increased permeability of venules, and pain (**Fig. 1**).[3] The kinin pathway also activates the complement system and the clotting cascade. The clotting cascade is relevant in injury by staunching the flow of blood. Thus, within a few minutes of injury, blood flow is increased to the area, vascular permeability is increased, and neutrophil passage is slowed within the blood vessel.[4] Therefore, the erythema, swelling, and pain can occur in the absence of infection, and can occur quite rapidly. In the setting of rheumatologic conditions, the cause of injury and the induction of inflammation can be rapid or slow, and the mechanisms of injury are varied. Nevertheless, this simple process reflects most of what the ancients observed as inflammation and physicians still observe during physical examination.

Many inflammatory prostaglandins are targeted therapeutically.[5] Leukotriene B4 is activated by tissue injury; it is released from damaged cell membranes and also produced by neutrophils, amplifying the inflammatory process (**Fig. 2**) through increased chemotaxis. Physicians routinely exploit current understanding of this pathway in the use of nonsteroidal antiinflammatory drugs (NSAIDs) and corticosteroids.[6] Phospholipids in the cell membrane can be converted to arachidonic acid. Arachidonic acid is in turn a substrate for 5-lipoxygenase or cyclooxygenase enzymes, leading to the production of leukotrienes or prostaglandins, respectively. Aspirin and NSAIDs inhibit cyclooxygenase but not lipoxygenase. Corticosteroids inhibit both pathways. Prostaglandins are, therefore, amplifiers of the critical processes of inflammation and are intimately related to the sensation of pain. Although inflammation is often considered pathologic, from the perspective of injury or infection, the process can be seen as protective in infectious settings:

- Increased blood flow delivers cells and proteins to the affected area
- Increased vascular permeability allows leakage of antibody and complement proteins to the affected tissue

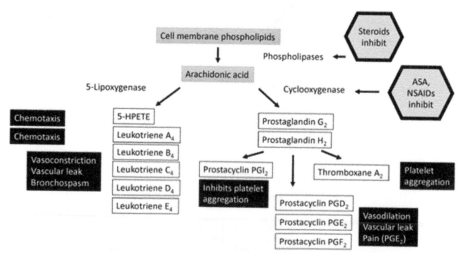

Fig. 2. Eicosanoid pathways. Damage to cell membranes, thrombin, bradykinin, and angiotensin activate arachidonic acid. Cyclooxygenase and 5-lipoxygenase convert arachidonic acid into prostaglandins and leukotrienes, respectively. These eicosanoids, oxidized fatty acid mediators, have diverse functions in the regulation of inflammation. Several medications used in rheumatology target this pathway. Steroids, aspirin, and nonsteroidal antiinflammatory drugs act early in the pathway (octagons). ASA, aspirin; NSAID, non-steroidal anti-inflammatory drugs. HPETE, hydroperoxyeicosatetraenoic acid; PG, prostaglandin.

- Clots allow improved adhesion of neutrophils to the vascular endothelium
- Pain and limitation of use minimizes the opportunity for bacteria to become systemic.

Pain is the most common symptom of inflammation and control of pain by treating the inflammation is an overall goal. Sometimes, directing efforts specifically to control pain can be beneficial. Capsaicin is used clinically to desensitize sensory C-fibers and can be a valuable adjunct to treatment.

When inflammation becomes systemic, the process is less favorable. The components that provided protection against local infection or injury now become wholly deleterious. Fibrin split products appear in the circulation as systemic activation of the clotting system occurs. Cytokine production, which is valuable in local tissues, can cause a storm effect when systemically activated. Tumor necrosis factor (TNF) and interleukin (IL)-1β are the major cytokines driving fever and systemic inflammation. Systemic effects include the well-known constitutional symptoms of fever, increased sleep, poor appetite, hypotension, leukocytosis, and acute phase response in the liver with increased fibrinogen (the high erythrocyte sedimentation rate), C-reactive protein, and complement components. The vascular endothelium increases its synthesis of adhesion molecules, causing sludging of cells and increasing the platelet adherence.[7] Additional cytokines and chemokines can become activated, leading to a cascade effect and a sepsis-like picture. Facets of this cytokine storm are apparent in systemic juvenile idiopathic arthritis (JIA), which evolves into a macrophage activation syndrome. Therapeutic efforts target the suppression of inflammatory cytokine production (**Table 3**).

COMPLEMENT

The complement system is a group of proteins produced primarily in the liver that interact to control B-cell production of antibodies, chemotaxis of neutrophils, and microcirculatory changes in inflammation. Early classic pathway complement proteins play an important role in clearance of apoptotic cells and immune complexes.[8] Complement is a familiar facet of the immune system in rheumatology because complement components (C)3 and C4 have been monitored and used as surrogates for immune complex production for many years.[9,10] Complement is traditionally thought of having 3 activation arms: classical pathway activation is most often driven by immune complexes, lectin pathway activation is driven by oligosaccharides on the surface against microorganisms, and alternative pathway activation is driven by surface charges most often encountered on microorganisms. Complement is involved primarily in the defense against bacteria and plays a much reduced role in the defense against viruses and fungi. The hallmark of this evolutionarily ancient facet of the immune system is that as proteins become activated, they are consumed. Thus, a falling C3 and C4 signal complement activation is usually taken as evidence that immune complexes have formed.

INFLAMMATORY CELLS AND THEIR MIGRATION

The first English language treatise on pediatrics by Thomas Phaer in 1545 recognized that arthritis could occur in children.[11] Using their eyes, hands, and ears (to take a history), early physicians described the key features of disease: swelling, pain, and loss of function. It was the "father of British paediatrics", George Frederic Still,[12] who noted that chronic arthritis in children could affect different joints and had different patterns. He clearly described the inflammatory nature by stating, "The

Table 3
Therapeutics targeting specific immunologic pathways in rheumatic diseases

Immune Target	Drugs in Category	Mechanism of Action	Rheumatologic Conditions
TNFα	Etanercept Adalimumab Infliximab Golimumab Certolizumab	Reduced endothelial cell activation Decreased neutrophil migration	Poly-JIA, RA Psoriasis, psoriatic arthritis Spondyloarthropathies Uveitis Inflammatory bowel disease Sarcoidosis Autoinflammatory diseases
IL-6	Tocilizumab Sarilumab	Reduced endothelial activation	Poly- and systemic JIA, RA Giant cell arteritis
IL-1β	Anakinra Canakinumab Rilonacept	Reduced endothelial activation Decreased neutrophil activation	Systemic JIA, RA Gout Behçet disease Autoinflammatory diseases
T-cell costimulation	Abatacept	Reduced T cell activation Reduced antigen presentation	JIA, RA
B cells	Rituximab Belimumab	Depletion of CD20 B cells Altered antigen presentation	Systemic lupus erythematosus (only indication for belimumab) Vasculitis Autoimmune cytopenias RA
Janus kinase	Tofacitinib	Signaling molecules downstream of several cytokines are inhibited	RA Interferonopathies (autoinflammatory)
IL-12 or IL-23	Ustekinumab	Inhibition of T-cell activation	Psoriasis and psoriatic arthritis Autoinflammatory diseases
IL-17	Secukinumab	Inhibition of the T cell cytokine IL-17	Psoriasis and psoriatic arthritis Spondyloarthropathies Autoinflammatory diseases

synovial membrane showed active proliferation and fibrosis spreading to cartilage." From this seminal observation, pediatricians, pathologists, and immunologists proceeded to vigorously analyze inflammatory cells in nearly all of the pediatric rheumatologic conditions. Synovial fluid analysis, pathologic description, and flow cytometry are currently central to the clinical understanding of the cells that participate in inflammation. The following section describes the regulation of migration of cells contributing to inflammation.

In JIA, the synovial fluid leukocyte count is typically 15,000 to 20,000 per mm³ with a neutrophil predominance. What drives these neutrophils into the joint space? As is true for all neutrophilic infiltrates, the migration is governed mainly by chemokines and adhesion molecules. Neutrophils circulate in the blood and survey the vascular endothelium in their transit through the bloodstream. The initial interaction is governed by the upregulation of adhesion molecules on the surface of vascular endothelial cells.[13] Specifically, selectins are upregulated by thrombin, TNF, IL-4, C5a, histamine, and reactive oxygen species. Selectins on postcapillary venules engage the ligand

PSGL-1 on neutrophils to induce rolling behavior. The selectin-mediated rolling of neutrophils is followed by their firm adhesion to the endothelium. This step depends on β2 integrins, which are activated by chemokines.[14,15] The final stage of migrating across the endothelium is regulated by the adhesion molecules PECAM and CD99, which are expressed at the junction of endothelial cells.[14] The neutrophil, arriving into the tissue space, then marches up the chemotactic gradient to its final location. This entire process further activates the neutrophil.

The mechanisms regulating neutrophil recruitment are similar across all anatomic locations, and neutrophil recruitment is among the most common features of inflammatory diseases. Neutrophil production of enzymes, reactive oxygen species, and other agents designed to kill pathogens can be detrimental to host tissues.[16] One of the byproducts, proline-glycine-proline peptide, can trigger additional neutrophil influx, amplifying the inflammatory process.[17] One of the most successful biologic therapies of all time is TNF inhibition. One of their pivotal functions is to diminish activation of the vascular endothelial cells and expression of adhesion molecules, thereby limiting neutrophil recruitment. This effect is also responsible for the most frequent adverse event: increased susceptibility to infection.

Monocytes represent another myeloid cell important in inflammatory settings. One subset of circulating monocytes patrols the vascular endothelial cells.[18] These cells seek out tissue damage and are poised to repair it. The other subset is induced by inflammation and plays an important role in host defense.

Many types of organ-specific autoimmunity are characterized by lymphocytic infiltrates; however, even in disorders in which neutrophil predominate, lymphocytes are usually observed. A strong rationale for the integral role of the lymphocytes is suggested by the strong association of most rheumatologic conditions with certain major histocompatibility (MHC) haplotypes.[19] These molecules are usually the strongest genetic susceptibility factor for autoimmune diseases. Proteins encoded by the MHC present antigen to T cells. Thus, the strong genetic association is thought to support a T-cell–centric process. When lymphocytes arrive in tissues, they are out of their element, so to speak. Whereas neutrophils and monocytes will normally enter into tissues as part of host defense, it is not typical for conventional T cells and B cells to be anywhere other than blood, lymph, or lymphatic tissues.

Lymphocytes enter tissues under the same conceptual stimuli as monocytes and neutrophils. That is to say, they use a combination of adhesion molecules and chemokines to direct their migration. Lymphocytes are so accustomed to forming structures in lymphoid organs that they often do so in tissues. Pathologic assessment reports often describe these structures as lymphoid follicles. B cells form germinal center follicular structures in patients with Sjögren syndrome, rheumatoid arthritis, myasthenia gravis, and multiple sclerosis have characteristics of antigen-driven clonal expansion.[20–22] In JIA, lymphoid structures correlate with autoantibodies and plasma cell infiltration.[23] These data suggest that the B cells are producing autoantibodies at these sites and may be participating directly in the autoimmune process. Studies of T cells from the synovial fluid of patients with JIA have similarly shown evidence of activation, also supporting the concept that these processes are driven by antigens, likely self-antigens. The antigens themselves, however, remain elusive. Nevertheless, in recent years there has been an expansion of therapeutics directed at lymphoid cells. This includes medications such as rituximab, which depletes B cells; abatacept, which interferes with T cell activation; and new biological treatments for psoriatic arthritis, which focus on inhibiting T-cell cytokines (ustekinumab and secukinumab) (see **Table 3**).

THE BASIS OF RHEUMATOLOGIC CONDITIONS

The ancient description of inflammation was limited to what physicians in antiquity could observe with a physical examination and a history. In the modern era, physicians are similarly limited by their tools. Gene expression changes, cell changes, and what can be seen under the microscope have been defined. Yet, for many rheumatologic conditions, there remains an incomplete understanding of who gets the condition, why they get it, what is the trigger, and how the condition evolves. The immune system may be broadly thought of as 2 facets related to host defense (**Fig. 3**). The adaptive immune system comprises T-cell and B-cell responses. These cells require training to distinguish self-tissues from foreign invaders. T cells are educated in the thymus, where autoreactive cells are programmed to die off. This process is referred to as central tolerance and is highly but imperfectly effective.[24] A small number of autoreactive T cells escape the thymus and circulate in the peripheral blood. A second layer of control is imposed on these T cells to prevent autoimmune responses, referred to as peripheral tolerance. Peripheral tolerance is mediated by 2 entirely separate strategies.[25] Regulatory T cells prevent other T cells from starting an autoreactive response. The second strategy uses the innate immune system to vet foreign invaders by producing a danger signal. In the absence of that danger signal, the T cells will not produce a response. There are examples of autoimmunity due to pure defects in either central tolerance or peripheral tolerance; however, most autoimmune diseases of children are due to subtle dysfunction of both types of tolerance alongside the misfortune of having exposure to triggers.

B cells similarly require education and their education occurs in the bone marrow. Early B cell precursors exposed to self-antigens die in the bone marrow. B cells also have a form of peripheral tolerance.[26] Regulatory T cells monitor B-cell autoreactivity and provide the most important facet of peripheral tolerance.[27] B cells also use vetting of responses by the innate immune system to ensure they make productive responses preferentially to foreign pathogens. Antigens tagged with complement are more stimulatory to B cells than nontagged antigens.[28] In addition, B cells require

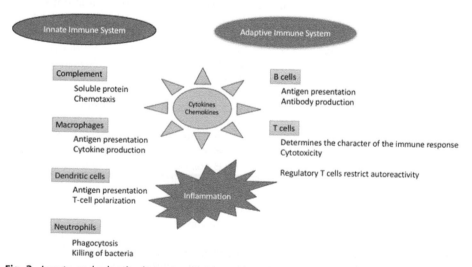

Fig. 3. Innate and adaptive immune responses. The adaptive immune response is mediated by classic T cells and B cells. Diverse cell types mediate innate responses and communication between the 2 compartments relies on both cell–cell communication and soluble mediators.

help from T cells focused on the same antigen; a second layer of protection to ensure that only responses to true threats are produced. This multilayered protection to prevent autoreactivity testifies to the high priority human bodies place on its prevention.

Autoimmunity is contrasted with autoinflammation, which refers to dysfunction of control mechanisms of the innate immune system.[29,30] This type of inflammation is not associated with loss of tolerance but rather dysregulated inflammation. These types of processes are driven most often by myeloid (neutrophils, monocytes) or somatic cells rather than lymphocytes. Nevertheless, chronic inflammation can drive loss of tolerance.

An example of inflammation driving autoimmunity relates to interferon (IFN). Many autoimmune diseases, such as systemic lupus erythematosus (SLE), dermatomyositis, and Sjögren syndrome, have what is termed a type I IFN signature.[31] Signature is a term typically referencing a set of genes with altered expression in a characteristic manner. In studies of subjects receiving α-IFN therapeutically, 2% developed thyroid disease, 5% developed sarcoidosis, 1% developed SLE, and less than 1% developed rheumatoid arthritis.[32] The mechanism by which type I IFNs promote autoimmunity includes activation of B-cell differentiation and increased antigen presentation. As another example, lung inflammation is known to more generally break tolerance with cystic fibrosis and with prolonged inhalation of particulates, predisposing to arthritis.[33,34] The exposure to chronic inflammation serves as a danger signal and allows presentation of self-antigens. Cytokines can also promote activation of lymphocytes such that checkpoints may be bypassed.[35] Thus, an inflammatory milieu can promote autoimmunity. In summary, multiple cytokines and inflammatory processes are capable of promoting autoimmunity and this concept of the inflammatory milieu underlies current thinking about the gradual development of most rheumatologic conditions (**Fig. 4**).

HALLMARKS OF AUTOIMMUNITY

In a given patient with an ongoing rheumatologic disease, it is not always clear on clinical grounds whether the process is autoimmune or autoinflammatory. The distinction is quite useful because autoimmune diseases benefit from treatments directed at lymphocyte function, whereas autoinflammatory diseases benefit from treatment

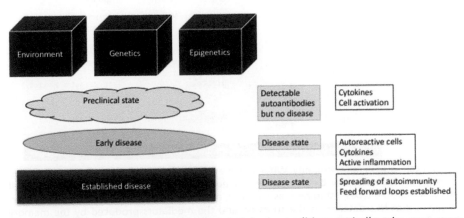

Fig. 4. Progression of autoimmunity. Rheumatologic conditions typically arise over years with autoantibodies detectable long before overt disease. A characteristic of progression is the acquisition of antibodies to new specificities.

directed at the myeloid cell compartment. The distinction is not absolute and JIA, usually considered an autoimmune disease, is treated with TNF inhibitors. This is because both types of settings converge at the tissue level as inflammation. Nevertheless, it is important to ask how an autoimmune disease can be identified. Autoimmunity can usually be identified clinically by the production of autoantibodies. These autoantibodies need not be directly pathologic but serve as a marker that tolerance has been broken. The pathologic processes of tissue damage and inflammation can be driven by T cells through direct cytotoxicity, elaboration of cytokines that influence neutrophil production, induction of autoantibodies by B cells, and modulation of other cells' cytokine production (**Fig. 5**). T cells are seen in many tissues involved in rheumatologic conditions of childhood. They are most prominently seen in dermatomyositis, systemic sclerosis, and lupus nephritis. Although T cells are not prominent in some autoimmune conditions, they are thought to play a significant role in most autoimmune diseases for 5 reasons[36]:

1. Most autoimmune diseases are associated with specific MHC risk alleles, implying that T cells are involved because they require antigen presentation on MHC
2. T cells are important for autoantibody production
3. Loss of tolerance implies imperfect regulatory T cell function
4. T cells can be observed, even if not prominent, in most autoimmune diseases
5. T-cell production of IL-17 and TNF can regulate the innate cell infiltrate.

A significant technical limitation has been that clinical assessment of T cells in autoimmunity is far more limited than that of B cells, in which autoantibodies can be easily measured. Therefore, operationally, a condition is usually thought to be autoimmune based on autoantibody production; however, most disorders have at least a component that is mechanistically associated with T-cell–mediated pathologic processes.

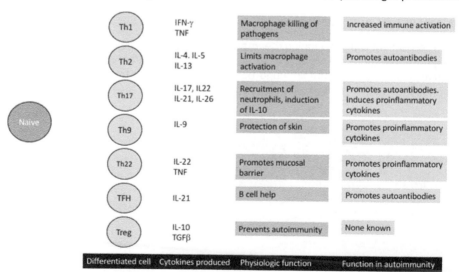

Fig. 5. T cell roles in autoimmunity. When a naïve T cell encounters antigen, the character of the response is determined by the cytokine milieu. The cytokines polarize the memory T cell into 1 of multiple types, listed here as Th1, Th2, and so forth. The importance of the polarization is that this determines the function and the mediators produced by the memory T cell. The physiologic function is shown to the right of each polarized T-cell type and the proposed role in autoimmunity is shown in the far right column. TFH, follicular helper T cell; TGF, transforming growth factor; Th, T helper; Treg, regulatory T cell.

T-cell–directed therapy is now available for JIA (abatacept), and depletion of B cells is a common therapeutic strategy in SLE (rituximab and belimumab) and vasculitis (rituximab) (see **Table 3**).

HALLMARKS OF AUTOINFLAMMATION

Autoimmunity can be recognized as associated with the production of characteristic autoantibodies in most patients. In contrast to that feature, most patients with autoinflammatory diseases do not have specific autoantibodies. Characteristics of autoinflammation are fevers with or without triggers that are most often episodic but can be persistent. End organ involvement is diverse and specific for each type of autoinflammatory disorder. These are most often conditions that manifest in childhood and are due to mutations in genes that regulate immune function. Autoinflammatory conditions were recently reviewed in this series (February 2017).[37,38] They are typically divided into 3 categories based on the mechanism, which in turn predicts the therapeutic response:

1. Inflammasome-mediated autoinflammatory conditions
2. Interferonopathies
3. Noninflammasome-mediated autoinflammatory conditions.

Table 4 lists the disorders and some of their key clinical features for reference, with each of the 3 categories displayed separately. The inflammasome is a cellular structure that exists to provide protection from invading bacterial pathogens. In contrast, the IFN pathway exists to protect from invading viral pathogens. The third group of autoinflammatory disorders has dysfunction of waste removal as its core feature.

Inflammasome structures assemble after sensing pathogens or cell damage proteins. There are different types of inflammasomes, named for the scaffold protein that supports the assembly. Three main types are known: AIM2, NLRP3, and NLRC4.[39] NLRP3 inflammasomes are initially primed by exposure to a bacterial pathogen and sensing through the toll-like receptors. Activation of primed NLRP3 inflammasomes can be through pathogens or by crystals such as found in gout. The assembled inflammasome structure cleaves pro-IL-1β and pro-IL-18 into their active cytokine molecules. The roles of these 2 cytokines are different but related. IL-1 induces a fever, upregulates endothelial adhesion molecules to recruit neutrophils, and induces cyclooxygenase type 2.[40] IL-18 activates T cells and can produce fever.[41]

The interferonopathies are a group of disorders that clinically can overlap with features of SLE.[42] Most frequently, they mimic features of in utero infections. They differ in several important ways from the inflammasome disorders. For example, the central cytokines in the inflammasome disorders are IL-1β and IL-18. In the interferonopathies, the central cytokines are the type I IFNs: IFNα and IFNβ. Clinically, the 2 categories can be contrasted as well. The inflammasome disorders tend to be episodic, whereas the interferonopathies tend to exhibit chronic unrelenting inflammation. Additionally, the inflammasome disorders often affect skin, joints, and muscle. The interferonopathies often affect the central nervous system and skin. Finally, the inflammasome disorders are associated with inflammatory diseases, including arthritis, inflammatory bowel disease, and vasculitis, all conditions in which autoantibodies are not prominent. In contrast, the interferonopathies are associated with autoantibody-driven cytopenias and lupus-like autoimmunity[43,44] (see **Table 4**).

The last category of autoinflammatory disorders represents a clinically heterogeneous group. Many of these disorders are associated with compromise in waste disposal, a recent concept in the understanding of autoimmunity and inflammation.

Table 4
Some autoinflammatory diseases

Mechanism or Common Name	Gene	Inheritance	Fever Pattern	Selected Clinical Findings	Treatment
Inflammasome-related					
Familial Mediterranean fever (pyrin inflammasome activation)	MEFV (Pyrin)	Autosomal recessive AR	Episodes 1–3 d, variable frequency	Erysipeloid erythema, arthritis, serositis, Henoch Shonlein purpura HSP (infrequent)	Colchicine IL-1 inhibition
Mevalonate kinase deficiency (hyper IgD syndrome HIDS) (affects pyrin inflammasome)	MVK	AR	Episodic (induced by stress, infections, injury, vaccinations)	Lymphadenopathy, rash, diarrhea, stomatitis	IL-1 inhibition
Familial cold autoinflammatory syndrome (FCAS)	NLRP3	Autosomal dominant AD	Onset 1–3 h after systemic cold exposure	Urticarial rash	Cold avoidance IL-1 inhibition
Muckle-Wells syndrome	NLRP3	AD	Random	Frequent rash, hearing loss	IL-1 inhibition
Neonatal onset multisystem inflammatory disease (NOMID)	NLRP3	AD	Continuous	Chronic rash, central nervous system abnormalities, sterile meningitis, joint inflammation, bony overgrowth	IL-1 inhibition
NLRC4 syndrome	NLRC4	AD	Continuous or stress-induced	Macrophage activation syndrome, neonatal enterocolitis, rash	IL-18 and IL-1 inhibition?
NLRP-1 syndrome	NLRP	AD	None	Arthritis, dyskeratosis, autoinflammation	?
WDR1 deficiency (actin-depolymerizing cofactor deficiency)	WDR1	AR	Episodic	Recurrent infections, stomatitis, poor wound healing, thrombocytopenia	? IL-18 inhibition

Interferonopathies					
Aicardi-Goutières syndrome (AGS)			Variable	Intracranial calcifications, cerebral atrophy, developmental delay or regression, seizures, eye movement abnormalities, and chilblains can occur in all types. Other manifestations vary, some depending on genotype	JAK inhibition?
Type 1	TREX1	AR and AD			
Type 2	RNASEH2B	AR			
Type 3	RNASEH2C	AR			
Type 4	RNASEH2A	AR			
Type 5	SAMHD1	AR			
Type 6	ADAR1	AR and AD			
Type 7	IFIH1	AD			
Spondyloenchondrodysplasia (SPENCD)	ACP5	AR	Variable	Immune deficiency, bone defects	JAK inhibition?
STING-associated vasculopathy with onset in infancy (SAVI)	TMEM173	AD	Variable	Cutaneous vasculopathy, pulmonary inflammation, systemic inflammation	JAK inhibition?
Chronic atypical neutrophilic dermatitis with lipodystrophy (CANDLE)	PSMA3; PSMB8; PSMB4; POMP	AR, digenic?; AR, digenic?; AR, digenic?; AD	Frequent	Annular cutaneous plaques, aseptic meningitis, episcleritis, periorbital edema, chondritis	JAK inhibition?
ISG15 deficiency	ISG15	AR		Brain calcifications, seizures, susceptibility to mycobacteria	JAK inhibition?
Singleton-Merten syndrome (SMS)	IFIH1, not same as AGS7	AD	None	Calcifications in blood vessels, dental dysplasia, skeletal abnormalities, psoriasis	JAK inhibition?
Atypical SMS	DDX58	AD	None	As SMS above, but without dental dysplasia	JAK inhibition?
Others					
TNF-receptor associated periodic syndrome (TRAPS)	TNFRSF1	AD	Episodic	Serositis, arthralgia or arthritis, rash, conjunctivitis	TNF inhibition
Blau syndrome	NOD2	AD	Episodic	Granulomatous arthritis, uveitis, and rash	Steroids? TNF inhibition?
Pyogenic sterile arthritis, pyoderma gangrenosum, acne (PAPA) syndrome	PSTPIP1	AD	Episodic	Pyogenic sterile arthritis, acne, pyoderma gangrenosum, acne, myositis	TNF or IL-1 inhibition

(continued on next page)

Table 4
(continued)

Mechanism or Common Name	Gene	Inheritance	Fever Pattern	Selected Clinical Findings	Treatment
Majeed syndrome	LPIN2	AR	Episodic high	Chronic sterile osteomyelitis, dyserythropoietic anemia, Sweet syndrome	NSAIDs, steroids?
Deficiency of IL-1 receptor antagonist (DIRA)	IL-1RN	AR	Low-grade	Sterile multifocal osteomyelitis, pustulosis, mucosal ulcers, arthritis	Recombinant IL-1 receptor antagonist
Deficiency of IL-36 receptor antagonist (DITRA)	IL36RN	AR	Episodic high	Pustular psoriasis, cardiomyopathy, nausea	IL-1 or IL-17 inhibition?
Adenosine deaminase 2 deficiency	CECR1	AR	Episodic	Polyarteritis nodosa lesions, stroke, B-cell dysfunction	TNF inhibition, transplant?
CARD14 mediated psoriasis (CAMPS)	CARD14	AD	None	Psoriasis, arthritis	TNF, IL-17 or IL-23 inhibition
Cherubism	SH3BP2	AD	None	Bony deformity of jaw	Surgery, calcitonin
Otulipenia	OTULIN	AR	Episodic	Rash, diarrhea, arthritis	TNF inhibition
Haploinsufficiency of A20	TNFAIP3	AD	Episodic	Mucosal ulcers, arthralgia, ocular lesions	TNF inhibition, colchicine
PLCG2-associated antibody deficiency and immune dysregulation (PLAID or APLAID)	PLCG2	AD	None	Evaporative cold urticaria, nasal lesions, GI inflammation, infections	Cold avoidance
SLC29A3 spectrum disorder	SLC29A3	AR	None	Hyperpigmentation, hypertrichosis, IDDM, histiocytosis, adenopathy	?
X-linked reticular pigmentary disorder (XLPDR)	POLA1	X-linked	None	Hyperpigmentation, dysmorphism, lung and gastrointestinal inflammation	?
ADAM17 deficiency	ADAM17	AR	None	Neonatal inflammatory skin and bowel disease, recurrent sepsis	?

Recognition of cellar debris as nonthreatening and in need of disposal is a silent but important function of the immune system. Complement, macrophages, and various serum proteins regulate this unglamorous role. Lacking adequate disposal, autoreactive responses can develop and, in some cases, the waste products are themselves inflammatory.

SUMMARY

The intricate choreography of the immune system is elegantly regulated and supremely successful in defending against infections, which is its primary purpose. Autoimmunity occurs when breaks occur in central tolerance or peripheral tolerance and can be promoted by the presence of inflammatory mediators that encourage antigen presentation and activation of lymphocytes. As appreciation of the details increases, specific cellular pathways are being targeted to great effect.[45] Thousands of years ago, recognition that the site was inflamed and that aspirin (willow bark) could be beneficial was among the first recognized medical treatments. Today, precision medicine with targeting of single pivotal mediators has become a reality.

REFERENCES

1. Littman RJ. The plague of Athens: epidemiology and paleopathology. Mt Sinai J Med 2009;76(5):456–67.
2. Witebsky E, Rose NR, Terplan K, et al. Chronic thyroiditis and autoimmunization. J Am Med Assoc 1957;164(13):1439–47.
3. Calixto JB, Cabrini DA, Ferreira J, et al. Kinins in pain and inflammation. Pain 2000;87(1):1–5.
4. Vanhoutte PM. Endothelium and control of vascular function. State of the Art lecture. Hypertension 1989;13(6 Pt 2):658–67.
5. Serhan CN, Savill J. Resolution of inflammation: the beginning programs the end. Nat Immunol 2005;6(12):1191–7.
6. Hata AN, Breyer RM. Pharmacology and signaling of prostaglandin receptors: multiple roles in inflammation and immune modulation. Pharmacol Ther 2004; 103(2):147–66.
7. D'Elia RV, Harrison K, Oyston PC, et al. Targeting the "cytokine storm" for therapeutic benefit. Clin Vaccine Immunol 2013;20(3):319–27.
8. Botto M, Dell'Agnola C, Pandolfi PP, et al. Homozygous C1q deficiency: a cause of systemic lupus erythematosus in humans and mice. Arthritis Rheum 1997; 40(supplement):S122.
9. Sullivan KE, Wisnieski JJ, Winkelstein JA, et al. Serum complement determinations in patients with quiescent systemic lupus erythematosus. J Rheumatol 1996;23:2063–7.
10. Noris M, Remuzzi G. Overview of complement activation and regulation. Semin Nephrol 2013;33(6):479–92.
11. Bywaters EG. The history of pediatric rheumatology. Arthritis Rheum 1977;20:145–52.
12. Still G. On a form of chronic joint disease in children. Am J Dis Child 1978;132:195–200.
13. de Oliveira S, Rosowski EE, Huttenlocher A. Neutrophil migration in infection and wound repair: going forward in reverse. Nat Rev Immunol 2016;16(6):378–91.
14. Vestweber D. How leukocytes cross the vascular endothelium. Nat Rev Immunol 2015;15(11):692–704.

15. Muller WA. Getting leukocytes to the site of inflammation. Vet Pathol 2013;50(1): 7–22.
16. Kruger P, Saffarzadeh M, Weber AN, et al. Neutrophils: between host defence, immune modulation, and tissue injury. PLoS Pathog 2015;11(3):e1004651.
17. Weathington NM, van Houwelingen AH, Noerager BD, et al. A novel peptide CXCR ligand derived from extracellular matrix degradation during airway inflammation. Nat Med 2006;12(3):317–23.
18. Geissmann F, Manz MG, Jung S, et al. Development of monocytes, macrophages, and dendritic cells. Science 2010;327(5966):656–61.
19. Lettre G, Rioux JD. Autoimmune diseases: insights from genome-wide association studies. Hum Mol Genet 2008;17(R2):R116–21.
20. Armengol MP, Juan M, Lucas-Martin A, et al. Thyroid autoimmune disease: demonstration of thyroid antigen-specific B cells and recombination-activating gene expression in chemokine-containing active intrathyroidal germinal centers. Am J Pathol 2001;159(3):861–73.
21. Salomonsson S, Jonsson MV, Skarstein K, et al. Cellular basis of ectopic germinal center formation and autoantibody production in the target organ of patients with Sjögren's syndrome. Arthritis Rheum 2003;48(11):3187–201.
22. Manzo A, Paoletti S, Carulli M, et al. Systematic microanatomical analysis of CXCL13 and CCL21 in situ production and progressive lymphoid organization in rheumatoid synovitis. Eur J Immunol 2005;35(5):1347–59.
23. Gregorio A, Gambini C, Gerloni V, et al. Lymphoid neogenesis in juvenile idiopathic arthritis correlates with ANA positivity and plasma cells infiltration. Rheumatology (Oxford) 2007;46(2):308–13.
24. Sprent J, Kishimoto H. The thymus and central tolerance. Philos Trans R Soc Lond B Biol Sci 2001;356(1409):609–16.
25. Xing Y, Hogquist KA. T-cell tolerance: central and peripheral. Cold Spring Harb Perspect Biol 2012;4(6):1–15.
26. Meffre E, Wardemann H. B-cell tolerance checkpoints in health and autoimmunity. Curr Opin Immunol 2008;20(6):632–8.
27. Meffre E. The establishment of early B cell tolerance in humans: lessons from primary immunodeficiency diseases. Ann N Y Acad Sci 2011;1246:1–10.
28. Carroll MC. CD21/CD35 in B cell activation. Semin Immunol 1998;10(4):279–86.
29. Ciccarelli F, De Martinis M, Ginaldi L. An update on autoinflammatory diseases. Curr Med Chem 2014;21(3):261–9.
30. van Kempen TS, Wenink MH, Leijten EF, et al. Perception of self: distinguishing autoimmunity from autoinflammation. Nat Rev Rheumatol 2015;11(8): 483–92.
31. Banchereau J, Pascual V. Type I interferon in systemic lupus erythematosus and other autoimmune diseases. Immunity 2006;25(3):383–92.
32. Gota C, Calabrese L. Induction of clinical autoimmune disease by therapeutic interferon-alpha. Autoimmunity 2003;36(8):511–8.
33. Dixey J, Redington AN, Butler RC, et al. The arthropathy of cystic fibrosis. Ann Rheum Dis 1988;47(3):218–23.
34. Joshua V, Chatzidionisyou K, Catrina AI. Role of the lung in individuals at risk of rheumatoid arthritis. Best Pract Res Clin Rheumatol 2017;31(1):31–41.
35. Tsubata T. B-cell tolerance and autoimmunity. F1000Res 2017;6:391.
36. Bluestone JA, Bour-Jordan H, Cheng M, et al. T cells in the control of organ-specific autoimmunity. J Clin Invest 2015;125(6):2250–60.
37. Verbsky JW. When to suspect autoinflammatory/recurrent fever syndromes. Pediatr Clin North Am 2017;64(1):111–25.

38. Co DO, Bordini BJ, Meyers AB, et al. Immune-mediated diseases of the central nervous system: a specificity-focused diagnostic paradigm. Pediatr Clin North Am 2017;64(1):57–90.
39. Guo H, Callaway JB, Ting JP. Inflammasomes: mechanism of action, role in disease, and therapeutics. Nat Med 2015;21(7):677–87.
40. Dinarello CA. Immunological and inflammatory functions of the interleukin-1 family. Annu Rev Immunol 2009;27:519–50.
41. Dinarello CA, Novick D, Kim S, et al. Interleukin-18 and IL-18 binding protein. Front Immunol 2013;4:289.
42. Crow YJ. Type I interferonopathies: a novel set of inborn errors of immunity. Ann N Y Acad Sci 2011;1238:91–8.
43. Canna SW, Goldbach-Mansky R. New monogenic autoinflammatory diseases–a clinical overview. Semin Immunopathol 2015;37(4):387–94.
44. de Jesus AA, Canna SW, Liu Y, et al. Molecular mechanisms in genetically defined autoinflammatory diseases: disorders of amplified danger signaling. Annu Rev Immunol 2015;33:823–74.
45. Furst DE, Keystone EC, So AK, et al. Updated consensus statement on biological agents for the treatment of rheumatic diseases, 2012. Ann Rheum Dis 2013; 72(Suppl 2):ii2–34.

Juvenile Idiopathic Arthritis
Oligoarthritis and Polyarthritis

Courtney B. Crayne, MD, Timothy Beukelman, MD, MSCE*

KEYWORDS

- Juvenile idiopathic arthritis • Oligoarthritis • Polyarthritis • Classification • Diagnosis
- Treatment

KEY POINTS

- Juvenile idiopathic arthritis (JIA) is defined as arthritis of 6 weeks' or more duration in a child 16 years of age or younger with an unknown cause. It is a clinical diagnosis based on history and physical examination.
- Different categories of JIA have different arthritis patterns and demographics. Arthritis is divided into oligoarthritis (<5 joints) and polyarthritis, each composed of 2 subtypes.
- There is no specific diagnostic laboratory test or image, although the presence of antinuclear antibody and rheumatoid factor can help classify JIA and better guide prognosis and therapy.
- Early aggressive therapy leads to improved outcomes and prevents potential disease complications (eg, growth disturbances, joint contractures, vision loss).
- Patients should be followed by a pediatric rheumatologist for careful monitoring of medication toxicity, adverse events, and infection in all patients receiving systemic immunomodulatory medications.

INTRODUCTION

Juvenile idiopathic arthritis (JIA) broadly refers to a group of heterogeneous diseases that share the common feature of chronic inflammatory arthritis of unknown cause lasting longer than 6 weeks with onset before 16 years of age. Historically, the terms *juvenile rheumatoid arthritis* (JRA) and *juvenile chronic arthritis* were used by clinicians in accordance with the publication of classification criteria as proposed by the American College of Rheumatology (ACR) and the European League Against Rheumatism (EULAR), respectively.[1] The preferred term, *JIA*, was first introduced in 1995 by the International League of Associations for Rheumatology (ILAR) as part of the classification criteria aimed at unifying the ACR and EULAR's criteria and eliminating confusion while being

Dr C.B. Crayne has no financial disclosures. Dr T. Beukelman has received consulting fees from Novartis, Genentech/Roche, UCB, Bristol-Myers Squibb, and Sobi.
Department of Pediatrics, Division of Rheumatology, University of Alabama at Birmingham, 1600 7th Avenue South, CPPN G10, Birmingham, AL 35233, USA
* Corresponding author.
E-mail address: tbeukelman@peds.uab.edu

Pediatr Clin N Am 65 (2018) 657–674
https://doi.org/10.1016/j.pcl.2018.03.005
0031-3955/18/© 2018 Elsevier Inc. All rights reserved.

pediatric.theclinics.com

more broadly inclusive of all forms of chronic childhood arthritis. Although the ILAR's criteria originally served to standardize research, they have been adopted by rheumatologists as a clinical diagnostic approach toward children with chronic arthritis.[1,2]

The ILAR's criteria further divide JIA into 7 relatively homogenous categories: oligoarthritis, rheumatoid factor (RF)–negative polyarthritis, RF-positive polyarthritis, systemic arthritis, psoriatic arthritis, enthesitis-related arthritis, and undifferentiated arthritis (Table 1). Each category differs with respect to clinical presentation and anticipated disease course. Classification is based on several factors, including the number of joints affected with arthritis, RF and HLA-B27 positivity, medical and family history, and associated extra-articular manifestations. Unlike previous classification systems, the ILAR's classification set includes exclusion criteria in an attempt to prevent overlap between categories.[1] This article focuses on oligoarthritis and polyarthritis (RF-negative and

Table 1
International League of Associations for Rheumatology's classification

ILAR Category	Definition
Oligoarthritis	Arthritis affecting 1–4 joints during the first 6 mo of disease Persistent: affecting 4 or fewer during disease course Extended: affecting more than 4 joints after first 6 mo *Exclusions: a, b, c, d, e*
RF-negative polyarthritis	Arthritis affecting 5 or more joints during the first 6 mo of disease plus a negative RF *Exclusions: a, b, c, d, e*
RF-positive polyarthritis	Arthritis affecting 5 or more joints during the first 6 mo of disease plus 2 or more positive RF tests at least 3 mo apart *Exclusions: a, b, c, e*
Systemic arthritis	Arthritis in one or more joints with or preceded by fever of at least 2-wk duration documented to be daily quotidian for at least 3 d and accompanied by at least one of the following: evanescent erythematous rash, generalized lymphadenopathy, hepatomegaly and/or splenomegaly, serositis *Exclusions: a, b, c, d*
Psoriatic arthritis	Arthritis and psoriasis OR arthritis and at least 2 of the following: dactylitis, nail pitting or onycholysis, psoriasis in a first-degree relative *Exclusions: b, c, d, e*
Enthesitis-related arthritis	Arthritis and enthesitis OR arthritis or enthesitis and at least 2 of the following: sacroiliac joint tenderness (present or historical) and/or inflammatory lumbosacral pain; presence of HLA-B27 antigen; onset of arthritis in a boy older than 6 y; acute symptomatic anterior uveitis; history of ankylosing spondylitis, enthesitis-related arthritis, sacroiliitis with inflammatory bowel disease, Reiter syndrome, or acute anterior uveitis in a first-degree relative *Exclusions: a, d, e*
Undifferentiated arthritis	Arthritis that fulfils criteria in no category or in more than 1 of the above categories

Exclusions: a: Psoriasis or a history of psoriasis in patients or first-degree relative; b: Arthritis in an HLA-B27–positive boy beginning after the 6th birthday; c: History of or a first-degree relative with ankylosing spondylitis, enthesitis-related arthritis, sacroiliitis with inflammatory bowel disease, Reiter syndrome, or acute anterior uveitis in a first-degree relative; d: Presence of immunoglobulin M RF on at least 2 occasions at least 3 months apart; e: Presence of systemic JIA.

From Petty RE, Southwood TR, Manners P, et al. International League of Associations for Rheumatology classification of juvenile idiopathic arthritis: second revision, Edmonton, 2001. J Rheumatol 2004;31(2):390–2; with permission.

RF-positive) with the remaining JIA categories discussed in Pamela F. Weiss and Robert A. Colbert's article, "Juvenile Spondyloarthritis: A Distinct Form of Juvenile Arthritis," and Jennifer J.Y. Lee and Rayfel Schneider's article, "Systemic Juvenile Idiopathic Arthritis (JIA)," in this issue.

INCIDENCE

JIA, including all categories, occurs in approximately 1 in 1000 children. The incidence of oligoarthritis is approximately 1 in 10,000 children annually. Population studies vary widely given the inconsistent diagnostic criteria and nomenclature. It is estimated RF negative polyarticular JIA affects 1 to 4 per 100,000 children annually. Less commonly, RF-positive polyarticular JIA occurs in an estimated 0.3 to 0.7 per 100,000 children each year.[2]

DEMOGRAPHICS

Demographics vary with respect to category, with a female predominance for both oligoarthritis and polyarthritis. The age, gender ratio, and race predominance for oligoarticular and polyarthritis are shown in **Table 2**.

MAJOR DIFFERENCES FROM ADULT IDIOPATHIC INFLAMMATORY ARTHRITIS

The pattern of idiopathic inflammatory arthritis differs with RF-positive polyarthritis and spondyloarthritis, the predominant subtypes in adults. In contrast, 5% or less of patients with JIA have RF-positive polyarthritis.

HOW TO DIAGNOSE JUVENILE IDIOPATHIC ARTHRITIS

The diagnosis of JIA is typically made from the history and physical examination **(Table 3)**. The most specific symptom, joint stiffness, worsens with inactivity, such as sleeping or long periods of sitting; however, stiffness may be difficult to assess in young children, particularly toddlers with limited expressive skills. Joint stiffness is most pronounced in the morning, usually described by parents as an abnormal gait or walking like an old person. Parents may report increased use of a stroller or decreased activity or play. Stiffness usually improves throughout the day with increased activity or with warm showers.

Swelling is another complaint specific to arthritis but is often not correctly identified by children and families. Joint pain is often present but is usually not severe, especially at rest. Joint pain may be absent, especially in younger children; pain need not be present to diagnose JIA. In fact, if joint pain is the sole complaint in the absence of stiffness, swelling, or limitations of activity, then the likelihood of arthritis is low.

On physical examination, active arthritis is characterized by joint effusion (ie, swelling), joint warmth, decreased range of motion, tenderness, and pain with range of motion. Chronic arthritis very rarely results in erythematous joints; this is more commonly seen in septic joints or rheumatic fever. Pain at rest is uncommonly associated with arthritis, particularly if it is severe.[2] Prompt referral of suspected or suspicious arthritis to a pediatric rheumatologist is crucial to prevent a delay in diagnosis and treatment.

OLIGOARTHRITIS

Oligoarthritis is the most common category of JIA, accounting for 40% to 50% of children with JIA in most published cohorts (see **Table 2**). Oligoarthritis by definition

Table 2
Characteristics of oligoarthritis and polyarthritis

	Proportion of Children with JIA (%)	Typical Age of Onset	Sex Predominance	Race	Number of Affected Joints	Joint Distribution	Joint Pattern	Associated Features
Oligoarthritis	40–50	1–3 y	3:1 F> M	Caucasian	Persistent <4; extended ≥5 (6 mo after onset)	Large joints (eg, knees, ankles, wrists)	Asymmetric	ANA + increases risk of uveitis
RF-negative polyarthritis	20	1–3 y; early adolescents	3:1 F> M	No racial predominance	≥5	Large and small joints (eg, knees, ankles, hands)	Symmetric	ANA + increases risk of uveitis; high risk of TMJ and cervical spine involvement
RF-positive polyarthritis	5	9–11 y	F >>M	Nonwhite >Caucasians	≥5	Large and small joints (eg, knees, ankles, hands)	Symmetric	RF + polyarthritis often equivalent to adult RF + RA

Abbreviations: ANA, antinuclear antibody; RA, rheumatoid arthritis; TMJ, temporomandibular joint.

Table 3
Clinical highlights of oligoarthritis and polyarthritis

Common Features	Uncommon Features
Joint stiffness	Joint erythema
• Most pronounced in mornings	Significant pain at rest
• Worse with prolonged inactivity	Rash
• Improves throughout the day	Systemic features (eg, fever, weight loss)
Joint swelling	Bone pain
Joint warmth	Acute onset
Decreased range of motion	
Pain with range of motion	

affects 4 or fewer cumulative unique joints during the first 6 months of disease, similar to the pauciarticular designation in the prior JRA classification system. Oligoarthritis is further classified as being either persistent (ie, affecting 4 or fewer cumulative unique joints throughout the disease course) or extended (ie, affecting 5 or more cumulative unique joints after 6 months from disease onset). Children who develop arthritis affecting 5 or more cumulative unique joints within the first 6 months of disease onset are excluded from the oligoarthritis category (**Box 1**; see **Table 1**).[1,2]

When to Consider Oligoarthritis

A typical scenario is a 3-year-old Caucasian girl presenting with a persistently swollen right knee after falling on the playground several weeks prior. Parents have noticed a limp that is worse in the morning or after nap time. The child is otherwise well and does not seem to be in pain. Suspicion for JIA should be high.

How Oligoarthritis Presents

Large joints, such as the knees, elbows, wrists, and ankles, are most commonly affected, although small joints of the hand may also be affected. Oligoarthritis classically presents with arthritis in the lower extremities, especially the knee (**Fig. 1**). Involvement of the wrists and ankles may be a risk factor for progression to polyarthritis in patients initially presenting with oligoarthritis. Extra-articular manifestations are rare with the exception of chronic anterior uveitis, which can occur in about 20% to 30% of children with oligoarthritis. Children with a positive antinuclear antibody (ANA) titer are at greater risk for the development of uveitis (see Disease-related complications).[2,3]

Disease onset peaks between 1 and 3 years of age; although onset can occur after the toddler years, it should raise suspicion for the possibility of other categories of JIA or other rheumatic diseases. Oligoarthritis predominantly affects girls (3:1 female to male ratio), and the prevalence is higher among children of European decent compared with those of other populations (ie, East Indian, Native American, and Asian).[2,4]

Box 1
Oligoarthritis

- Affects 4 or fewer cumulative joints during the first 6 months of disease
- Persistent: affects 4 or fewer cumulative unique joints throughout disease course
- Extended: affects 5 or more cumulative unique joints after 6 months from disease onset

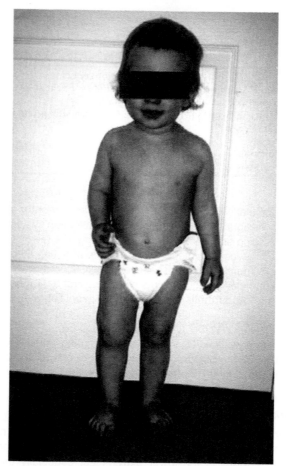

Fig. 1. Patient with oligoarthritis with swollen knee and limited extension. (*From* Gowdie PJ, Tse SM. Juvenile idiopathic arthritis. Pediatr Clin North Am 2012;59:305; with permission.)

POLYARTHRITIS

Polyarthritis accounts for approximately 25% of all JIA diagnoses, and roughly 85% of these patients are RF negative (see **Table 2**).[5] Polyarthritis is defined as arthritis in 5 or more joints during the first 6 months of disease. Per the ILAR's criteria, polyarthritis is divided into 2 distinct categories based on the presence or absence of RF, because RF can be associated with important differences in disease manifestations and response to therapy. Exclusion criteria are the same as for oligoarthritis, with the obvious exception of RF positivity (see **Table 1**). Unlike oligoarthritis, systemic symptoms, including fatigue and weight loss, can be present with active disease[1,2,4,6] (**Box 2**).

Box 2
Polyarthritis

- Affects 5 or more cumulative joints during the first 6 months of disease
- RF-negative: negative RF test
- RF-positive: positive RF test on at least 2 occasions, with testing at least 3 months apart

---

When to Consider Rheumatoid Factor–Negative Polyarthritis

A typical scenario is a 14-year-old Caucasian girl presenting with swelling of bilateral knees, several proximal interphalangeal joints bilaterally, and bilateral wrists and ankles. She reports stiffness for about 1 hour every morning, improved with a long hot shower. She also reports difficulty opening jars and doing push-ups during physical education class. Suspicion for polyarthritis should be very high.

How Rheumatoid Factor–Negative Polyarthritis Presents

RF-negative polyarthritis tends to be limited to articular involvement; however, chronic anterior uveitis occurs in approximately 14%. RF-negative polyarthritis can be associated with a positive ANA, and this may impart a higher risk of uveitis. Involvement of the large joints is most common; however, patients can have arthritis in the small joints of the hands and feet[2,3](**Fig. 2**). The temporomandibular joint (TMJ) is commonly affected in patients with polyarthritis, and the risk seems to be higher in the RF-negative category[2,7] (**Fig. 3**).

Onset of RF-negative polyarthritis can occur at any age before 16 years; however, it typically presents early between 1 and 3 years of age or later during adolescence. Like oligoarthritis, RF-negative polyarthritis predominantly affects females, particularly those who present as teenagers.[2]

When to Consider Rheumatoid Factor–Positive Polyarthritis

A typical scenario is a 15-year-old African American girl presenting with several swollen joints, including numerous proximal and distal interphalangeal joints. She has difficulty extending her neck to look up during upward facing dog in yoga class. She has stiffness for several hours that improves throughout the day. She also notices her fingers do not fully extend and struggles with daily tasks, including writing and opening toothpaste.

How Rheumatoid Factor–Positive Polyarthritis Presents

This category is often equivalent to typical adult-onset rheumatoid arthritis (RA) with respect to clinical presentation, autoantibody production, and prognosis. It is perhaps

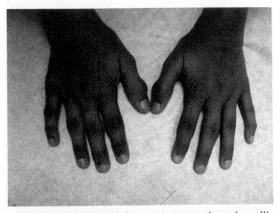

Fig. 2. Patient with polyarticular JIA with bony overgrowth and swelling of several joints, including wrists, metacarpophalangeal, proximal interphalangeal, and distal interphalangeal joints of fingers on both hands. (*Courtesy of* Gloria Higgins, MD, Nationwide Children's Hospital, Columbus, OH, USA.)

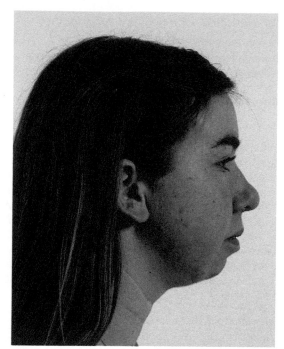

Fig. 3. Chronic arthritis of the TMJ resulting in micrognathia. (*From* Gowdie PJ, Tse SM. Juvenile idiopathic arthritis. Pediatr Clin North Am 2012;59:312; with permission.)

the least common of all categories, occurring in fewer than 5% of patients with JIA in most published cohorts (see **Table 2**).

Large and small joints are affected, usually in a symmetric pattern. Joint disease tends to cause erosions of the surrounding bone, leading to significant morbidity if left untreated. Like RF-negative polyarthritis, the TMJ and cervical spine can be involved and be important causes of morbidity.[2,3]

A positive ANA may be present in a high percentage of RF-positive patients; however, uveitis is rarely seen in this JIA category.[5] The most common extra-articular complication is subcutaneous nodules, usually found on pressure points.[2] Other complications of adult-onset RA, such as rheumatoid lung and Felty syndrome, are very rare in children.

It presents most commonly in girls, with an average age of onset of 9 to 11 years of age. RF-positive polyarthritis more frequently affects children of nonwhite races (ie, African Americans, those of Asian descent), and those of Hispanic background.[2,3,5,6]

DISEASE-RELATED COMPLICATIONS
Uveitis

One of the most significant complications associated with JIA is chronic anterior uveitis. JIA-associated uveitis is manifested by inflammation of the iris and ciliary body and is, therefore, sometimes referred to as iritis or iridocyclitis.[8] The severity and disease course of uveitis may not parallel that of the arthritis. Uveitis may develop in the absence of active arthritis or even before its initial clinical presentation (ie, before the diagnosis of JIA). The onset of uveitis is insidious and frequently initially asymptomatic, necessitating regular eye evaluations for early recognition to prevent debilitating sequelae. Chronic inflammation of the anterior chamber can lead to synechiae (inflammatory adhesions), band keratopathy (calcium depositions in the cornea), and ultimately blindness.[8]

Table 4
Modified ophthalmologic screening recommendations

JIA Category	ANA Status	Age (y) of Onset	Disease Duration (y)	Frequency of Eye Examination
Oligoarthritis/RF− polyarthritis/psoriatic arthritis	+	≤6	≤4	3 mo
	+	≤6	>4	6 mo
	+	≤6	≥7	12 mo
	+	>6	≤2	6 mo
	+	>6	>2	12 mo
	−	≤6	≤4	6 mo
	−	≤6	>4	12 mo
	−	>6	N/A	12 mo
RF + polyarthritis	+/−	N/A	N/A	12 mo
Systemic arthritis	+/−	N/A	N/A	12 mo
Enthesitis-related arthritis	+/−	N/A	N/A	12 mo

Abbreviations: ANA, antinuclear antibody; N/A, not applicable.
Adapted from Heiligenhaus A, Niewerth M, Ganser G, et al, German Uveitis in Childhood Study Group. Prevalence and complications of uveitis in juvenile idiopathic arthritis in a population-based nation-wide study in Germany: suggested modification of the current screening guidelines. Rheumatology (Oxford) 2007;46(6):1018; with permission.

Slit-lamp examinations should be performed at the time of diagnosis of JIA and then at regular intervals depending on risk stratification to identify uveitis before the development of complications (**Table 4**). A younger age at disease onset, a positive ANA, and a shorter disease duration indicate a higher risk for asymptomatic anterior uveitis in children with oligoarthritis and RF-negative polyarthritis categories of JIA. RF-positive polyarthritis is much less frequently complicated by anterior uveitis.[8,9] Uveitis can occur during any disease state, including remission; uveitis screening examinations should continue indefinitely.

Initial treatment of uveitis typically includes topical glucocorticoid eye drops (eg, prednisolone). Often a topical mydriatic agent is added to dilate the pupil and prevent synechiae development as well as decrease any associated pain from ciliary muscle spasm. Chronic use of topical glucocorticoids, however, may lead to cataracts and increased intraocular pressure. Therefore, second-line therapy with methotrexate or monoclonal antibody tumor necrosis factor (TNF) inhibitors (eg, adalimumab) is often initiated to control uveitis and permit discontinuation of glucocorticoid eye drops.[8,10,11]

Growth Abnormalities

Growth disturbances are a well-known complication of JIA and can be both generalized and localized. Both proinflammatory cytokines (eg, TNF, interleukin [IL]-1, and IL-6) and systemic glucocorticoids occasionally used for treatment of arthritis interfere with insulinlike growth factor, resulting in overall growth restriction and reduced height. With the advent of more effective immunomodulatory therapies, generalized growth abnormalities, such as short stature, are far less frequent.[12] Localized growth disturbances can result from chronic inflammation of a single joint. Inflammation at the growth plate can lead to overstimulation of the ossification center, resulting in increased growth of the affected limb. Conversely, chronic inflammation may alternatively cause premature closure of the epiphyseal plate, resulting in a shorter limb.[13] The most common localized growth abnormality is a leg-length discrepancy caused by increased growth from arthritis of the knee (**Fig. 4**), but occasionally arthritis of the ankle or wrist can cause localized growth abnormalities too.

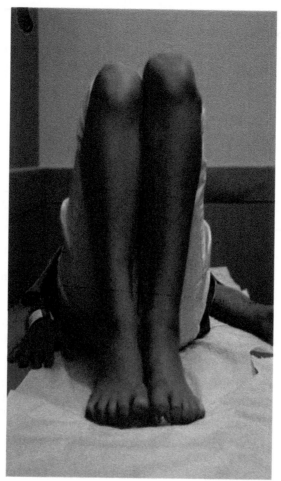

Fig. 4. Leg-length discrepancy resulting from chronic left knee arthritis in a child with JIA.

Joint Destruction and Disability

Uncontrolled arthritis can progress to contractures, limited range of motion, and bony deformities, ultimately causing significant disability, particularly if the wrists, small joints of the hands, and ankles are affected. Chronic joint inflammation can lead to bone erosions and joint space narrowing from loss of cartilage. Joint damage in TMJ arthritis may manifest as micrognathia (see **Fig. 3**), retrognathia, asymmetry, and jaw deviation.[7,14] Cervical spine arthritis may result in atlantoaxial subluxation, erosions, and spinal fusion.[15] Joint destruction is far less common in patients with oligoarthritis compared with the polyarticular categories.

Differential Diagnosis or Mimics

Many potential diagnoses should be considered in the evaluation of children with recent-onset arthritis (**Box 3** and see Kathleen A. Haines' article, "The Approach to the Child with Joint Complaints," in this issue). An acutely warm and exquisitely tender joint, bone pain, fever, or weight loss should raise concern for infection and malignancy. Fever and rash should raise concern for other causes, as these signs are rare in

---

Box 3
Differential diagnoses in patients presenting with monoarthritis

Monoarthritis Differential

Rheumatic disease
  JIA (oligoarthritis, enthesitis related, psoriatic)
  Inflammatory bowel disease—related arthropathy
  Systemic lupus erythematosus
  Sarcoidosis
  Sjögren syndrome
  Vasculitis (including Henoch-Schönlein purpura)

Malignancy
  Leukemia
  Sarcoma
  Pigmented villonodular synovitis

Trauma

Infection
  Septic arthritis
  Tuberculosis
  Osteomyelitis

Infection associated
  Reactive arthritis

Blood disorders
  Sickle cell disease
  Hemophilia

Fever syndromes
  Neonatal onset multisystem inflammatory disease
  Familial Mediterranean fever

---

oligoarticular and polyarticular JIA. Systemic infections and other rheumatic diseases, including but not limited to systemic onset JIA, systemic lupus erythematosus and related connective tissue diseases, vasculitis, and sarcoidosis, should be considered in the differential.

LABORATORY AND IMAGING STUDIES FOR DIAGNOSIS AND CARE

JIA is a clinical diagnosis; however, various laboratory tests can aid in the diagnosis of JIA as well as determination of the disease category and guidance of treatment. Inflammatory markers, such as elevated white blood cell count, platelet count, erythrocyte sedimentation rate, and C-reactive protein, may be present, especially in patients with polyarthritis. Other signs of chronic inflammation, such as anemia and hypoalbuminemia, may be present, again, more commonly in polyarthritis. The absence of laboratory signs of inflammation does not exclude the diagnosis of oligoarthritis or polyarthritis.[2] Appropriate laboratory surveillance for medication side effects is discussed in Gloria C. Higgins' article, "Complications of Treatments for Pediatric Rheumatic Diseases," in this issue.

Autoantibodies

Antinuclear antibody
In JIA, the ANA test is most useful for determining the risk of development of anterior uveitis and consequently the frequency of recommended ophthalmologic screening examinations. Importantly, a positive ANA can be found in approximately 10% to 20% of all healthy children; thus, a positive result is not diagnostic of JIA.

Nevertheless, approximately two-thirds of children with oligoarthritis are ANA positive and are at higher risk for asymptomatic anterior uveitis.

Rheumatoid factor

A positive RF is neither necessary nor sufficient for the diagnosis of JIA. More children with JIA will be RF negative. Nevertheless, RF is useful for identifying children with known JIA who fit the RF-positive polyarthritis category with its associated more severe arthritis and potential for worse disease outcomes.[1,2] RF-positive polyarthritis requires repeat testing to confirm a positive RF, with tests done on 2 or more occasions at least 3 months apart. This repeat testing is required because the RF test can be transiently positive or spuriously elevated, particularly if only to a modest degree, as an epiphenomenon of the immune system response to infection.

Anticitrullinated protein antibodies

Similar to adults with RA, children with RF-positive polyarthritis can also develop anticitrullinated protein antibodies (ACPAs). Studies of ACPA in children are limited, but it is presumed that the presence of ACPA is associated with more severe disease, similar to adults with RA.[16,17]

Imaging

Radiographic images may be helpful to exclude alternative diagnoses, but radiographs are rarely useful in establishing the diagnosis of JIA. In children with long-standing inadequately controlled JIA, radiographic changes may show periarticular osteopenia, joint space narrowing, premature maturation, and erosions (**Fig. 5**), with joint space narrowing and erosions associated with a poor prognosis.[18] Bony overgrowth may occur earlier in the disease. Likewise on radiographs, the presence of growth lines, or rather transverse lines migrating away from the growth plate, may suggest underlying chronic inflammation, although these are not specific to inflammation and may be evident in malnutrition, endocrinopathies, or fractures.

MRI without contrast can show signs of synovitis, including synovial thickening, increased intraarticular fluid, and bone marrow edema, while also excluding signs of

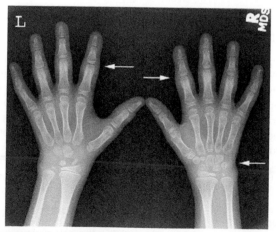

Fig. 5. Radiographs of hands and wrists of a patient with RF-negative polyarticular JIA. Note the soft tissue swelling around proximal interphalangeal and wrist joints (*arrows*), periarticular osteopenia, joint space narrowing, and premature maturation of carpal bones. (*From* Gowdie PJ, Tse SM. Juvenile idiopathic arthritis. Pediatr Clin North Am 2012;59:306; with permission.)

traumatic insult. The addition of contrast may highlight areas of synovial enhancement indicating active inflammation. Some joints, such as the TMJ, are difficult to reliably assess clinically; MRI may be beneficial to monitor disease progression and treatment response.[15] Ultrasound is a relatively inexpensive and noninvasive means of diagnosing and monitoring chronic arthritis. However, the interpretation of ultrasound images in children is different than in adults; additional evidence is needed in this area.[19]

HOW JUVENILE IDIOPATHIC ARTHRITIS IS TREATED

Historically, treatment emphasis was placed on nonsteroidal antiinflammatory drugs (NSAIDs). Given the significant disability inflicted if JIA is not properly treated, rheumatologists are shifting toward more aggressive therapy with disease-modifying antirheumatic drugs (DMARDs) as the first-line therapy, particularly in polyarthritis. This treat-to-target approach sets a primary goal of disease remission and aims to maximize therapy. The current generally accepted treatment goal is clinically inactive disease.[20] The ACR's 2011 published recommendations on the treatment of JIA use risk stratification to guide the escalation of therapy.[18]

Nonsteroidal Antiinflammatory Drugs

Once a mainstay therapy, NSAIDs are no longer commonly used as monotherapy for durations longer than 1 to 2 months, as there is no long-term disease-modifying effect.[18] NSAIDs are an appropriate first-choice therapy in patients without a confirmed diagnosis of JIA and may be used in selected patients with oligoarthritis if disease activity is sufficiently low. NSAIDs remain an important adjunct therapy and may be used in combination with immunosuppressive medications. Chronic NSAID use is not without risk, especially to the kidneys and gastrointestinal (GI) tract; periodic laboratory monitoring should be performed (see Gloria C. Higgins' article, "Complications of Treatments for Pediatric Rheumatic Diseases," in this issue).

Glucocorticoids

Systemic glucocorticoids are effective for the treatment of arthritis, but their clinical utility is markedly limited by adverse effects (see Gloria C. Higgins' article, "Complications of Treatments for Pediatric Rheumatic Diseases," in this issue). Systemic glucocorticoids are most appropriately used as a means to quiet inflammation while other systemic therapies are initiated (ie, as a bridge to therapy) or infrequently during times of disease flare despite other systemic immunosuppression.

In contrast, intra-articular glucocorticoids typically do not cause significant adverse effects and are routinely recommended as a treatment of JIA, particularly in patients with a single active joint and irrespective of other current therapies.[18]

Conventional Disease-Modifying Antirheumatic Drugs

Methotrexate continues to be the most used DMARD in the management of JIA. Methotrexate is often initiated after failure of a NSAID trial or intra-articular glucocorticoid injection. In patients with oligoarthritis or polyarthritis who have a high disease activity and/or poor prognostic features, it should be used as the first-line therapy.[18,21] Methotrexate is a folic acid analogue that competitively inhibits dihydrofolate reductase and subsequently blocks purine synthesis and DNA production, although its exact mechanism of action in JIA has yet to be fully elucidated.[22]

The safety and efficacy of methotrexate in JIA were first reported more than 25 years ago.[23] Methotrexate can be administered either orally or as a subcutaneous injection. The current literature does not strongly support a difference in adverse events, including GI upset; however, recent studies have shown increased bioavailability and improved joint responses with the use of subcutaneous methotrexate compared with oral methotrexate.[21],[24] These responses were not dose dependent and did not change with dose escalation.[21]

Methotrexate has several common adverse effects, including nausea and fatigue. Less commonly, methotrexate can cause hematologic or liver toxicity. Methotrexate is a known teratogen and should not be taken during pregnancy, and females should receive appropriate contraceptive counseling. Routine laboratory studies are recommended while receiving methotrexate, with monitoring recommended to be performed every 12 weeks[18] (see Gloria C. Higgins' article, "Complications of Treatments for Pediatric Rheumatic Diseases," in this issue).

Leflunomide inhibits pyrimidine synthesis and alters cytokine production. In a head-to-head randomized controlled trial, leflunomide was found to be slightly less effective than methotrexate for the treatment of JIA.[25] Leflunomide is less commonly associated with nausea compared with methotrexate.[26]

Sulfasalazine is more frequently used in enthesitis-related arthritis and inflammatory bowel disease; however, studies have shown a benefit in both oligoarthritis and polyarthritis.[27] Adverse events occur in approximately 30% of children with JIA, with the most common being rash and GI upset (see Gloria C. Higgins' article, "Complications of Treatments for Pediatric Rheumatic Diseases," in this issue). Sulfasalazine is contraindicated in any patient with a known hypersensitivity to sulfa drugs, including patients with G6PD deficiency.

Biological Disease-Modifying Antirheumatic Drugs

Biological DMARDs (also known as biologics) differ from conventional DMARDs in that they target specific biological molecules and require a living organism for their synthesis. With respect to oligoarticular and polyarticular JIA, the major biologic classes include TNF inhibitors, IL-6 inhibitors, and T-cell costimulator inhibitors.

Tumor Necrosis Factor Inhibitors

The proinflammatory cytokine TNF has long since been linked to the pathogenesis of RA.[21] Several TNF inhibitors (TNFi) have been shown to be effective for the treatment of RA and subsequently JIA as well.[21] At present, TNFi are recommended by the ACR for use in patients with polyarticular JIA with moderate to high disease activity who have not responded to 3 months of methotrexate.[18]

Etanercept is a fully humanized soluble TNF receptor and is administered by subcutaneous injection. Approved by the US Food and Drug Administration (FDA) and Health Canada in 1999 for use in children, it was the first TNFi studied in JIA. Lovell and colleagues[28] published the first randomized controlled trial comparing etanercept with placebo. Disease control was found to be durable in a follow-up report.[29] In contrast to adalimumab and infliximab, etanercept is not very effective in treating JIA-associated uveitis.[10]

Adalimumab is a fully humanized recombinant immunoglobulin G monoclonal antibody that directly binds to TNF and is administered by subcutaneous injection. It is approved for the treatment of polyarticular JIA by the FDA and Health Canada. In a randomized controlled trial, Lovell and colleagues[30] found adalimumab to be both safe and effective both as monotherapy and in combination with methotrexate in patients with polyarticular JIA; a subsequent study demonstrated the safety and effectiveness down to 2 years of age. Adalimumab has been shown to be effective for the treatment of anterior uveitis in children and has been approved for similar conditions in adults.[11]

Infliximab is a chimeric murine-human monoclonal antibody against TNF, and it is administered by intravenous infusion. Although infliximab has not been approved by the FDA, Health Canada, and the European Medicines Agency (EMA) for the treatment of JIA, it is nevertheless used off label, particularly for the treatment of children with uveitis.[10]

Other Tumor Necrosis Factor Inhibitors

Golimumab is a fully human, TNF monoclonal antibody administered as either an intravenous infusion or subcutaneous injection and currently approved for use in Europe for children with polyarticular JIA.[31] Certolizumab is a TNFi, approved for use in adults, that is pegylated: modified by the addition of polyethylene glycol chains to extend the half-life. It is currently in the clinical trial phase for JIA.

Tumor necrosis factor inhibitor safety profile

Although the immunosuppressive effects of biological response modifiers are more targeted than those of DMARDS, there is still an increased risk for infection and possibly for malignancy (see Gloria C. Higgins' article, "Complications of Treatments for Pediatric Rheumatic Diseases," in this issue).

Interleukin-6 Inhibitor

Tocilizumab is an anti–IL-6 receptor monoclonal antibody and can be administered intravenously or subcutaneously. Tocilizumab has been shown to be effective for the treatment of both systemic JIA and polyarticular JIA.[32,33] Given the established practice of TNFi use as the first biologic agent, the most appropriate use of tocilizumab in the treatment approach for polyarticular JIA is yet to be determined.

T-cell Costimulation Inhibitor

Abatacept is a soluble CTLA4-IgFcγ fusion protein binding to CD80/CD86 and subsequently inhibiting the T-cell costimulatory pathway. It is FDA and Health Canada approved for use in children 6 years and older with moderate to severe polyarticular JIA and can be administered intravenously or subcutaneously.[34] Abatacept is generally used in cases of ineffectiveness or intolerance of TNFi, although determination of the most appropriate use is not yet established.

The Future Treatment of Oligoarthritis and Polyarthritis

Treatment advances continue for chronic inflammatory arthritis. Newer therapies that have demonstrated effectiveness in adults with RA are currently being studied in children with JIA. Tofacitinib is a Janus kinase inhibitor approved for use in adults with RA. Unlike the aforementioned biologics, it is a small molecule and can, therefore, be administered orally.

As the patents of the earliest biologics begin to expire, biosimilars are emerging on the market. Biosimilars are akin to generic medications; but unlike generics, they may not have the precise chemical structure of the original therapeutic agent because of the slight differences in their manufacture. Nevertheless, according to the FDA and EMA, available biosimilars have demonstrated sufficiently similar effectiveness and safety compared with the original biologic reference drug. Biosimilars should help lower the economic costs of biologics, although perhaps not as significantly as was once anticipated.[35]

WHAT IS THE PROGNOSIS FOR JUVENILE IDIOPATHIC ARTHRITIS?

The disease prognosis varies with respect to the JIA category. About 50% of patients with persistent oligoarthritis achieve remission, strictly defined as the absence of active disease while off medication for 12 or more months. On the other hand, a significant proportion of children with oligoarthritis at onset will develop extended oligoarthritis, with active polyarthritis persisting into adulthood.[36] There is no consensus with respect to therapy discontinuation, and disease flares are not uncommon. It is important to encourage continued monitoring by a pediatric rheumatologist as well as scheduled uveitis screenings.

In the Research in Arthritis in Canadian Children Emphasizing Outcomes (ReACCh-Out) cohort of 1104 patients with JIA, Guzman and colleagues[37] found the probability of attaining an active joint count of zero within 2 years exceeded 78% on contemporary therapy. Patients with RF-positive polyarthritis had the worst outcomes; still, the probability of achieving inactive disease within 5 years was 90%. Within 5 years, 57% of patients with oligoarthritis were in remission off medication, compared with 0% of the patients with RF-positive polyarthritis who were able to discontinue therapy.

Poor prognostic features include arthritis of the hip, cervical spine, ankles, or wrists; prolonged elevation of inflammatory markers; and radiographic joint damage, such as erosions or joint space narrowing. Additionally, a positive RF and/or ACPA suggests more aggressive disease and subsequently poorer outcomes. Patients with RF-positive polyarthritis have the lowest rates of remission and often require lifelong medication for maintenance.[2,18]

SUMMARY

JIA comprises a group of heterogeneous diseases further divided into various categories based on shared clinical presentation, laboratory markers, and disease prognosis. The disease course and prognosis vary with respect to each JIA category. Early recognition of arthritis and prompt referral to a qualified rheumatologist is necessary to prevent disease sequelae. Over the past few decades, considerable treatment advances have significantly reduced the morbidity associated with childhood arthritis. Despite the use of immunomodulatory medications, more than half of the children continue to have active disease into adulthood. Emphasis is placed on the initiation of early aggressive therapy in hopes of delaying disease progression and inducing remission.

REFERENCES

1. Petty RE, Southwood TR, Manners P, et al. International League of Associations for Rheumatology classification of juvenile idiopathic arthritis: second revision, Edmonton, 2001. J Rheumatol 2004;31(2):390–2.
2. Petty RE, Laxer RM, Lindsley CB, et al. Textbook of pediatric rheumatology. 7th edition. Philadelphia: Elsevier; 2016.
3. Gowdie PJ, Tse SM. Juvenile idiopathic arthritis. Pediatr Clin North Am 2012; 59(2):301–27.
4. Eisenstein EM, Berkun Y. Diagnosis and classification of juvenile idiopathic arthritis. J Autoimmun 2014;48-49:31–3.
5. Saurenmann RK, Rose JB, Tyrrell P, et al. Epidemiology of juvenile idiopathic arthritis in a multiethnic cohort: ethnicity as a risk factor. Arthritis Rheum 2007; 56(6):1974–84.
6. Oberle EJ, Harris JG, Verbsky JW. Polyarticular juvenile idiopathic arthritis - epidemiology and management approaches. Clin Epidemiol 2014;6:379–93.
7. Stoll ML, Sharpe T, Beukelman T, et al. Risk factors for temporomandibular joint arthritis in children with juvenile idiopathic arthritis. J Rheumatol 2012;39(9): 1880–7.

8. Angeles-Han ST, Rabinovich CE. Uveitis in children. Curr Opin Rheumatol 2016; 28(5):544–9.
9. Heiligenhaus A, Niewerth M, Ganser G, et al, German Uveitis in Childhood Study Group. Prevalence and complications of uveitis in juvenile idiopathic arthritis in a population-based nation-wide study in Germany: suggested modification of the current screening guidelines. Rheumatology (Oxford) 2007;46(6):1015–9.
10. Cordero-Coma M, Sobrin L. Anti-tumor necrosis factor-alpha therapy in uveitis. Surv Ophthalmol 2015;60(6):575–89.
11. Ramanan AV, Dick AD, Jones AP, et al. Adalimumab plus methotrexate for uveitis in juvenile idiopathic arthritis. N Engl J Med 2017;376(17):1637–46.
12. Bechtold S, Simon D. Growth abnormalities in children and adolescents with juvenile idiopathic arthritis. Rheumatol Int 2014;34(11):1483–8.
13. Packham JC, Hall MA. Long-term follow-up of 246 adults with juvenile idiopathic arthritis: functional outcome. Rheumatology (Oxford) 2002;41(12):1428–35.
14. El Assar de la Fuente S, Angenete O, Jellestad S, et al. Juvenile idiopathic arthritis and the temporomandibular joint: a comprehensive review. J Craniomaxillofac Surg 2016;44(5):597–607.
15. Colebatch-Bourn AN, Edwards CJ, Collado P, et al. EULAR-PReS points to consider for the use of imaging in the diagnosis and management of juvenile idiopathic arthritis in clinical practice. Ann Rheum Dis 2015;74(11):1946–57.
16. Omar A, Abo-Elyoun I, Hussein H, et al. Anti-cyclic citrullinated peptide (anti-CCP) antibody in juvenile idiopathic arthritis (JIA): correlations with disease activity and severity of joint damage (a multicenter trial). Joint Bone Spine 2013;80(1): 38–43.
17. Tebo AE, Jaskowski T, Davis KW, et al. Profiling anti-cyclic citrullinated peptide antibodies in patients with juvenile idiopathic arthritis. Pediatr Rheumatol Online J 2012;10(1):29.
18. Beukelman T, Patkar NM, Saag KG, et al. 2011 American College of Rheumatology recommendations for the treatment of juvenile idiopathic arthritis: initiation and safety monitoring of therapeutic agents for the treatment of arthritis and systemic features. Arthritis Care Res (Hoboken) 2011;63(4):465–82.
19. Magni-Manzoni S, Scire CA, Ravelli A, et al. Ultrasound-detected synovial abnormalities are frequent in clinically inactive juvenile idiopathic arthritis, but do not predict a flare of synovitis. Ann Rheum Dis 2013;72(2):223–8.
20. Wallace CA, Giannini EH, Huang B, et al. American College of Rheumatology provisional criteria for defining clinical inactive disease in select categories of juvenile idiopathic arthritis. Arthritis Care Res (Hoboken) 2011;63(7):929–36.
21. Stoll ML, Cron RQ. Treatment of juvenile idiopathic arthritis: a revolution in care. Pediatr Rheumatol Online J 2014;12:13.
22. Cronstein BN, Sitkovsky M. Adenosine and adenosine receptors in the pathogenesis and treatment of rheumatic diseases. Nat Rev Rheumatol 2017;13(1):41–51.
23. Giannini EH, Brewer EJ, Kuzmina N, et al. Methotrexate in resistant juvenile rheumatoid arthritis. Results of the U.S.A.-U.S.S.R. double-blind, placebo-controlled trial. The Pediatric Rheumatology Collaborative Study Group and The Cooperative Children's Study Group. N Engl J Med 1992;326(16):1043–9.
24. Falvey S, Shipman L, Ilowite N, et al. Methotrexate-induced nausea in the treatment of juvenile idiopathic arthritis. Pediatr Rheumatol Online J 2017;15(1):52.
25. Silverman E, Mouy R, Spiegel L, et al. Leflunomide or methotrexate for juvenile rheumatoid arthritis. N Engl J Med 2005;352(16):1655–66.
26. Stoll ML, Cron RQ. Treatment of juvenile idiopathic arthritis in the biologic age. Rheum Dis Clin North Am 2013;39(4):751–66.

27. van Rossum MA, Fiselier TJ, Franssen MJ, et al. Sulfasalazine in the treatment of juvenile chronic arthritis: a randomized, double-blind, placebo-controlled, multi-center study. Dutch Juvenile Chronic Arthritis Study Group. Arthritis Rheum 1998;41(5):808–16.

28. Lovell DJ, Giannini EH, Reiff A, et al. Etanercept in children with polyarticular juvenile rheumatoid arthritis. Pediatric Rheumatology Collaborative Study Group. N Engl J Med 2000;342(11):763–9.

29. Lovell DJ, Reiff A, Ilowite NT, et al. Safety and efficacy of up to eight years of continuous etanercept therapy in patients with juvenile rheumatoid arthritis. Arthritis Rheum 2008;58(5):1496–504.

30. Lovell DJ, Ruperto N, Goodman S, et al. Adalimumab with or without methotrexate in juvenile rheumatoid arthritis. N Engl J Med 2008;359(8):810–20.

31. Brunner HI, Ruperto N, Tzaribachev N, et al. Subcutaneous golimumab for children with active polyarticular-course juvenile idiopathic arthritis: results of a multicentre, double-blind, randomised-withdrawal trial. Ann Rheum Dis 2018;77(1):21–9.

32. Brunner HI, Ruperto N, Zuber Z, et al. Efficacy and safety of tocilizumab in patients with polyarticular-course juvenile idiopathic arthritis: results from a phase 3, randomised, double-blind withdrawal trial. Ann Rheum Dis 2015;74(6):1110–7.

33. De Benedetti F, Brunner HI, Ruperto N, et al. Randomized trial of tocilizumab in systemic juvenile idiopathic arthritis. N Engl J Med 2012;367(25):2385–95.

34. Ruperto N, Lovell DJ, Quartier P, et al. Abatacept in children with juvenile idiopathic arthritis: a randomised, double-blind, placebo-controlled withdrawal trial. Lancet 2008;372(9636):383–91.

35. Mehr SR, Brook RA. Factors influencing the economics of biosimilars in the US. J Med Econ 2017;20(12):1268–71.

36. Shoop-Worrall SJW, Kearsley-Fleet L, Thomson W, et al. How common is remission in juvenile idiopathic arthritis: a systematic review. Semin Arthritis Rheum 2017;47(3):331–7.

37. Guzman J, Oen K, Tucker LB, et al. The outcomes of juvenile idiopathic arthritis in children managed with contemporary treatments: results from the ReACCh-Out cohort. Ann Rheum Dis 2015;74(10):1854–60.

Juvenile Spondyloarthritis
A Distinct Form of Juvenile Arthritis

Pamela F. Weiss, MD, MSCE[a],*, Robert A. Colbert, MD, PhD[b]

KEYWORDS

- Juvenile • SpA • Juvenile idiopathic arthritis • Ankylosing spondylitis
- Enthesitis-related arthritis • Psoriatic arthritis

KEY POINTS

- Juvenile spondyloarthritis (SpA) is distinct from other forms of childhood arthritis because of the male predominance, later age of onset, and involvement of the entheses and axial skeleton.
- Some forms of juvenile SpA are associated with psoriasis or bowel inflammation.
- Juvenile SpA is an immune-mediated inflammatory disease strongly linked to HLA-B27.
- The microbial environment is believed to play a role in SpA pathogenesis.
- Most children do not achieve remission off medication within 5 years of diagnosis.

INTRODUCTION

Spondyloarthritis (SpA) is an umbrella term for a group of heterogeneous conditions occurring in adults and children, which differ from other types of inflammatory arthritis in genetic predisposition, pathogenesis, and outcome. SpA is characterized by enthesitis and other features listed in **Box 1**. These conditions are not associated with rheumatoid factor (RF), the marker associated with adult rheumatoid arthritis and the RF-positive polyarticular juvenile idiopathic arthritis (JIA) subset. Instead, they are strongly associated with the presence of HLA-B27. SpA can involve the axial skeleton, which can lead to abnormal bone formation with eventual ankylosis of the spine, resulting in substantial disability.

Nomenclature and classification for juvenile SpA is problematic for several reasons. The current International League of Associations for Rheumatology (ILAR) classification criteria of JIA does not recognize SpA as a distinct entity. Most childhood SpA in the ILAR

Disclosure Statements: Dr P.F. Weiss has served as a consultant for Lilly (<$10,000). Dr R.A. Colbert has no financial conflict of interest.
[a] Department of Pediatrics, Division of Rheumatology, Children's Hospital of Philadelphia, Center for Clinical Epidemiology and Biostatistics, Perelman School of Medicine, University of Pennsylvania, 2716 South Street, Floor 11, Philadelphia, PA 19146, USA; [b] Pediatric Translational Research Branch, National Institute of Arthritis, Musculoskeletal and Skin Diseases, National Institutes of Health, Bethesda, MD, USA
* Corresponding author.
E-mail address: weissspa@email.chop.edu

Pediatr Clin N Am 65 (2018) 675–690
https://doi.org/10.1016/j.pcl.2018.03.006
0031-3955/18/© 2018 Elsevier Inc. All rights reserved.

Box 1
Features of juvenile spondyloarthritis

- Male predominance
- Lower extremity arthritis
- Tenderness at the insertion sites of tendons and ligaments into bone (enthesitis)
- Bowel inflammation
- Spine and sacroiliac joint inflammation
- Symptomatic anterior uveitis
- Psoriasis
- Dactylitis (sausage digits)
- HLA-B27 allele

---

criteria is classified as enthesitis-related arthritis (ERA), with other SpA patients falling under the categories of psoriatic arthritis (PsA) and undifferentiated arthritis (**Box 2**). A major limitation of the ILAR criteria is that they do not specifically recognize the presence of axial disease. In addition, ERA and PsA are mutually exclusive; if patients have psoriasis and fulfill criteria for ERA, they are considered to have undifferentiated arthritis.

Other conditions not specifically addressed by the ILAR classification that are considered SpA include

- Inflammatory bowel disease (IBD)-related arthritis
- Reactive arthritis
- Juvenile ankylosing spondylitis (AS)

Box 2
International League of Associations for Rheumatology classification criteria

Enthesitis-related arthritis

Inclusion criteria
    Arthritis and enthesitis, OR arthritis or enthesitis plus ≥2 of the following:
    - Inflammatory lumbosacral pain or sacroiliac joint tenderness
    - HLA-B27 positivity
    - Onset of arthritis in a male patient older than 6 years
    - Acute anterior uveitis
    - First-degree relative with HLA-B27–associated disease

Exclusion criteria
- RF positivity ≥2 occasions at least 3 months apart
- Systemic JIA
- Personal history of or first-degree relative with psoriasis

Psoriatic arthritis

Inclusion criteria
    Arthritis and psoriasis, OR arthritis and ≥2 of the following:
    - Dactylitis (sausage digit [**Fig. 1**])
    - Nail pitting or onycholysis (**Fig. 2**)
    - First-degree relative with psoriasis

Exclusion criteria
- Arthritis in an HLA-B27–positive male patient hat started after age 6
- Personal or family history of HLA-B27–associated disease
- RF positivity ≥2 occasions at least 3 months apart

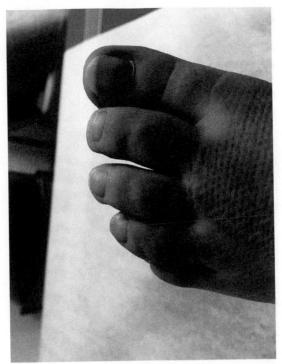

Fig. 1. Dactylitis of the left second and third digits in a child with PsA. (*Courtesy of* J. Mehta, MD, Children's Hospital of Philadelphia, Philadelphia, PA.)

PREVALENCE

The relative frequency of the various JIA categories varies by geographic region (**Fig. 3**). In large parts of eastern and southern Asia,[1,2] and in many indigenous North American populations,[3,4] SpA represents the most common form of childhood arthritis and accounts for as many as one-third of JIA cases.

In 2 large North American JIA cohorts, ERA comprised 10% to 11%, PsA 6% to 11%, and undifferentiated JIA 1% to 2% of the total JIA patients.[5,6]

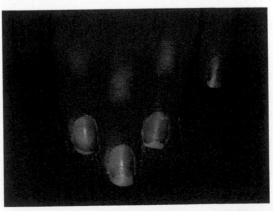

Fig. 2. Onycholysis. (*Courtesy of* Wikimedia commons. Available at: https://commons. wikimedia.org/wiki/Category:Onycholysis#/media/File:Onycholysis.jpg.)

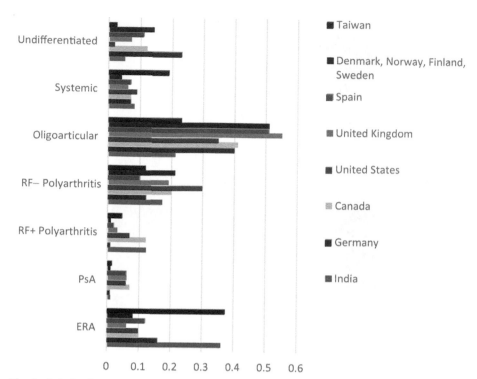

Fig. 3. Relative frequency of JIA categories across geographic region. (*Data from* Refs.[1,2,6,53–57])

DEMOGRAPHICS
Age

Most SpA patients present in early adolescence, but this disease can be seen in children as young as 5 years old. The mean age for ERA is 11.7 years and for PsA 8.9 years.[5]

Gender

Juvenile Spondyloarthritis is the only form of JIA that is male predominant.

Race and Ethnicity

There are few data on racial and ethnic differences for SpA.

MAJOR DIFFERENCES FROM ADULT SPONDYLOARTHRITIS

Unlike in adults with spondyloarthritis, axial involvement in jSpA is uncommon early in the disease course, whereas peripheral disease is more common. Cardiovascular disease is less common than for adult-onset AS and is rarely severe. A minority of juvenile AS patients have been found to have asymptomatic aortic regurgitation.[7,8]

WHEN TO CONSIDER JUVENILE SPONDYLOARTHRITIS

Juvenile SpA should be considered in adolescents with lower extremity arthritis and enthesitis (tenderness at the insertion sites of tendons and ligaments) or inflammatory back pain, in particular boys.

HOW JUVENILE SPONDYLOARTHRITIS PRESENTS

The presentation of juvenile SpA is variable, often insidious, and may consist of combinations of the features listed in **Box 1**. Common presenting symptoms include a sausage toe (dactylitis), swollen ankle, and/or enthesitis, and morning stiffness in the lower back or affected joint(s).

Articular Manifestations

The most common arthritis pattern is asymmetric involvement of the joints of the lower extremities, typically in an oligoarticular pattern (<5 joints). Ankle involvement is common. In some patients, foot pain is common, with 1 study from India reporting that half the children presented with foot pain; another 25% developed it later in the disease course.[9] Foot arthritis most commonly involves the midfoot and tibiotalar joints, followed by metatarsal and subtalar joints.

Axial involvement, primarily sacroilitis, has been found in 28% to 37% of children.[7,10] Features that should raise suspicion of sacroiliitis include

- Chronic back pain
- Morning stiffness in the back
- Back pain that improves with activity, does not improve with rest
- Back pain that causes nighttime awakening
- Alternating buttock pain
- Hip pain
- HLA-B27 positivity with elevated inflammatory markers
- Tenderness to palpation over the sacroiliac joints
- Positive flexion abduction and external rotation (FABER) test

In comparison with adults, children who eventually develop AS are much less likely to have back pain and stiffness at presentation.[11] In 1 study, back pain, the FABER test, and buttock pain all had low positive predictive values for sacroiliitis using edema on MRI fluid-sensitive sequences as the reference standard.[12] Higher active joint and tender enthesis counts at diagnosis,[13] hip arthritis,[10] elevated C-reactive protein, and HLA-B27 positivity[12] all have reported associations with sacroiliitis. How best to diagnosis sacroiliitis remains controversial, with some physicians relying purely on physical examination whereas others believing that periarticular bone marrow edema on MRI (noncontrast) is important to confirm the diagnosis.

Enthesitis

Inflammation where tendons and ligaments insert into bone is called enthesitis. It can be observed in multiple categories of JIA (16% overall) but is most frequent in SpA, where it occurs in 66% or more of patients[7,14] (**Fig. 4**). Patients may have pain and tenderness at the affected sites, sometimes with associated soft tissue swelling. **Fig. 5** shows some of the commonly examined entheses. To evaluate for enthesitis, the examiner should press at the insertion site of the tendon or ligament with a thumb to a pressure at which the nailbed blanches. Which entheses are examined and the threshold for calling an enthesis tender tend to vary between physicians and institutions. Sometimes localized swelling over the insertion site is notable on physical examination and can be misinterpreted as recurrent tendonitis (**Fig. 6**). Inflammation at the entheses can sometimes be visualized using ultrasound with Power Doppler, targeted MRI, or whole-body MRI (**Fig. 7**). In the Canadian ReACCh-Out (The Research In Arthritis In Canadian Children Emphasizing Outcomes) cohort, 16% of patients had

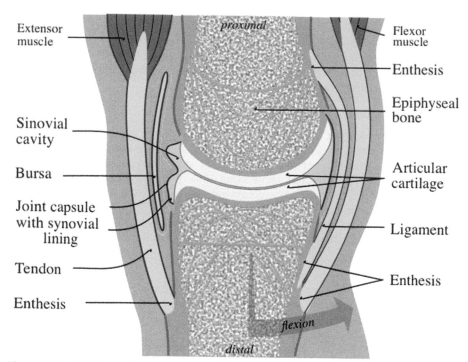

Fig. 4. Enthesitis is tenderness or inflammation at the insertion sites of tendons and ligaments. (*From* Wikimedia commons. Available at: https://en.wikipedia.org/wiki/Enthesitis#/media/File:Joint.svg.)

entheseal tenderness at more than 1 location or on more than 1 occasion; approximately two-thirds of those patients had SpA.[14] Accurate identification of enthesitis is important because it has implications for JIA classification, which in turn has an impact on treatment decisions and monitoring for comorbidities. In a multicenter inception cohort, the proportion of children with enthesitis at diagnosis varied significantly between 5 institutions; this finding is likely secondary to the lack of a standard pediatric enthesitis examination.[15] Enthesitis can be caused by injury or overuse in addition to SpA, underscoring the importance of taking a complete history.

Common features of enthesitis in juvenile SpA[7]:
- Symmetric
- Persistent
- Multifocal, with 25% of subjects exhibiting 3 or more sites
- Involvement of multiple sites is associated with persistence
- May parallel peripheral arthritis disease activity[5]
- Most commonly involves Achilles tendon attachment, superior patella quadriceps attachment, and lateral epicondyle of humerus

Extra-articular Manifestations

Several types of extra-articular manifestations occur in SpA, including anterior uveitis, various skin manifestations, and bowel inflammation. The uveitis differs from that associated with oligoarticular JIA or polyarticular JIA in that it typically has an acute, painful onset associated with conjunctival injection and photophobia. It is usually unilateral and nonscarring.

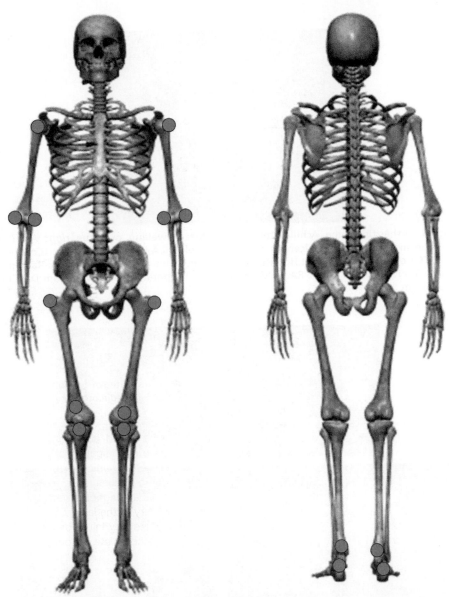

Fig. 5. Entheses commonly examined by pediatric rheumatologists. Sites include insertions of the following: supraspinatus on greater tuberosity of humerus, common extensor tendon on the lateral epicondyle of humerus, common flexor tendon on medial epicondyle of humerus, greater trochanter quadriceps at superior patella, patellar ligament at inferior patella, Achilles tendon, and plantar fascia at the calcaneus. (*From* Nikita E. Osteoarchaeology: A guide to the macroscopic study of human skeletal remains. 1st edition. Philadelphia: Elsevier; 2017. p. 1–75; with permission.)

Bowel Inflammation

The presence of any of the clinical features listed in **Box 3** should raise suspicion of bowel inflammation. Both overt and subclinical gastrointestinal inflammation are common in juvenile SpA. If bowel disease is suspected, fecal calprotectin, a surrogate marker for intestinal inflammation, is a good screening test.

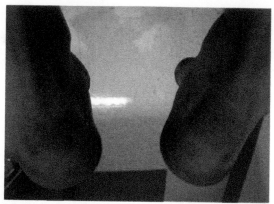

Fig. 6. Enthesitis at the Achilles tendon. Localized swelling over the *right* Achilles tendon insertion on the calcaneus of a 19-year-old HLA-B27–positive man. (*Courtesy of* Dr Carolos Rose, AI DuPont Hopsital for Children, Wilmington, DE; and *From* Ramanathan, Srinivasalu H, Colbert RA. Update on juvenile spondyloarthritis. Rheum Dis Clin North Am 2013;39(4):767.)

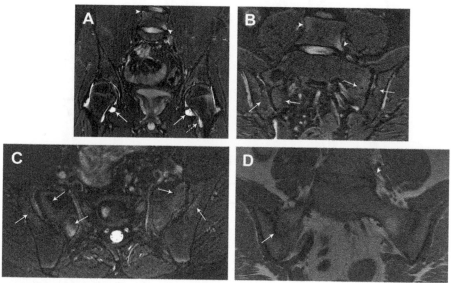

Fig. 7. A 14-year-old boy with lower back pain. (*A*) Coronal T2-weighted fat-saturated image of the pelvis demonstrates bilateral hip effusions (*solid arrows*) with suggestion of synovitis (*dashed arrow*). There is edema within the anterior superior and anterior inferior aspects of the L5 vertebral body indicative of inflammation of the spinal entheses (*arrowheads*). (*B*) Coronal oblique short tau inversion recovery image of the sacroiliac joints demonstrates marrow edema within the subchondral bone in both sacroiliac joints (*arrows*). Marrow edema within the L5 vertebral body is demonstrated (*arrowheads*). (*C*) Axial T2-weighted fat-saturated image of the sacroiliac joints demonstrates subchondral marrow edema (*arrows*). (*D*) Coronal oblique T1-weighted image of the sacroiliac joints demonstrates an erosion within the ilium on the right (*arrow*). There is corresponding decreased T1 signal intensity within the anterior inferior aspect of L5 (*arrowhead*) in the region of edema as depicted in (*A*). (*Courtesy of* Nancy A. Chauvin, MD, Children's Hospital of Philadelphia, Philadelphia, PA.)

Box 3
Features that should raise suspicion of bowel inflammation

- Poor linear growth
- Poor weight gain
- Anemia
- Hypoalbuminemia
- Abdominal pain
- Diarrhea
- Bloody stools
- Family history of IBD

Although the prevalence of subclinical gastrointestinal inflammation is common in adults with SpA, there are no available population-based estimates for this feature in juvenile SpA. In a cross-sectional study of children with SpA, other JIA category controls, and healthy controls, a greater proportion of children with SpA had elevated fecal calprotectin (67% vs 18% and 17%, respectively).[16] Five children with elevated fecal calprotectin (4 of whom had SpA) in that study subsequently underwent magnetic resonance enterography. Three of 5 children had findings highly suggestive of IBD[17] and the incidence of IBD in JIA was 1.31/1000 person years; of the 11 children who developed IBD, 4 had SpA (ERA or PsA).[18]

Skin Involvement

Skin and mucocutaneous manifestations are associated with the following SpA types: reactive arthritis, IBD-associated arthritis, and PsA. SpA-associated reactive arthritis includes those triggered by enteropathic or urogenital infections (*Yersinia, Salmonella, Shigella, Campylobacter*, and *Chlamydia*). Mucocutaneous findings associated with reactive arthritis include oral ulcers, urethritis, cervicitis, circinate balanitis, and keratoderma blennorrhagicum. With IBD-associated SpA, patients can develop oral ulcers, erythema nodosum, and pyoderma gangrenosum; psoriatic lesions can be subtle and be mistaken for eczema, appearing as mild scaling plaques at the hairline, behind the ears, around the umbilicus, and in the intergluteal crease as well as at other sites. Nail changes, including pits, onycholysis, and/or horizontal ridging, are found in most children with PsA. Among children who fulfill criteria for PsA, there are 2 peaks for age of onset, 1 at approximately age 2 years to 4 years and the other in mid to late childhood, with the latter resembling adult PsA.[19] For both groups, joint involvement commonly includes dactylitis and an oligoarthritis pattern. SpA is more commonly associated with the older onset group, which has a lower female predominance (50% vs 76%), lower antinuclear antibody (ANA) positivity, and higher frequency of enthesitis (57% vs 22%) and axial involvement (26% vs 10%).[19]

ATYPICAL PRESENTATIONS OF SPONDYLOARTHRITIS

Although children with IBD-associated SpA can present with arthritis before gastrointestinal symptoms, most have gastrointestinal symptoms months or years before they develop arthritis. Approximately half the children with SpA associated with psoriasis present with skin disease before they develop arthritis.

DIFFERENTIAL DIAGNOSIS OR MIMICS

Because SpA is more common In male adolescents who often participate in sports, some orthopedic conditions, especially osteochondrosis and apophysitis, may be difficult to differentiate from the enthesopathy associated with SpA. These include Sever disease (calcaneus), Osgood-Schlatter disease (tibial tuberosity), and Sinding-Larsen–Johansson syndrome (inferior pole of patella) (all discussed in Jennifer E. Weiss and Jennifer N. Stinson's article, "Pediatric Pain Syndromes and Non-inflammatory Musculoskeletal Pain," in this issue). Exercise-related tendonitis may also resemble the tendinopathy seen in SpA. Persistent symptoms that fail to respond to standard conservative measures may therefore warrant an evaluation by a pediatric rheumatologist.

The pattern of back pain associated with SpA can help with differentiating it from other causes of back pain. Similar to other types of JIA, joint pain typically worsens with rest and is associated with morning stiffness. Other causes of back pain that should be considered, especially in young children, include infection; tumor; other inflammatory problems, such as chronic nonbacterial osteomyelitis (see Yongdong Zhao and Polly J. Ferguson's article, "Chronic Nonbacterial Osteomyelitis and Chronic Recurrent Multifocal Osteomyelitis in Children," in this issue); and overuse, injury, or mechanical problems (see Jennifer E. Weiss and Jennifer N. Stinson's article, "Pediatric Pain Syndromes and Non-inflammatory Musculoskeletal Pain," in this issue). If pain is widespread and disproportionate to examination findings, amplified musculoskeletal pain syndromes should be considered (see Jennifer E. Weiss and Jennifer N. Stinson's article, "Pediatric Pain Syndromes and Non-inflammatory Musculoskeletal Pain," in this issue).

ETIOLOGY AND PATHOGENESIS
Etiology

Juvenile SpA is an immune-mediated inflammatory disease that develops as a consequence of inherited genetic variants combined with environmental exposures. As discussed previously, HLA-B27, encoded in the major histocompatibility complex (MHC), is a strong genetic risk factor for SpA, which is most striking in AS, where the frequency of HLA-B27 is close to 90% compared with 6% to 8% in unaffected individuals. Beyond HLA-B27, understanding of genetic susceptibility relies largely on genome-wide association studies of AS, where more than 110 common genetic variants outside the MHC have been implicated.[20,21] In most cases, the pathogenic variants and how they influence immune or inflammatory pathways remains to be determined. Other forms of SpA, such as PsA. exhibit overlapping risk gene profiles with AS.[22] There is a tendency for sharing of risk loci among seropositive (RF-positive) diseases and among seronegative arthritides but not between the groups.[23]

Studies of known AS risk genes as candidates for susceptibility to ERA are limited. Although HLA-B27 is clearly associated with juvenile SpA, quantitating its relationship with ERA and PsA is confounded by its use as a classification criterion: its presence is either an inclusion criterion (for ERA) or an exclusion criterion (for PsA).

Comparison of the HLA region among the various types of JIA has shown much higher correlations among oligoarticular (persistent and extended) JIA and RF-negative polyarticular JIA than between these types and SpA. These studies support the concept that juvenile SpA is different from other forms of JIA.

Pathogenesis

Understanding the genetic underpinnings of SpA susceptibility has increased the ability to establish links between genetic variants and pathogenic mechanisms. Historically, treatment strategies for AS and related forms of SpA were largely empirical, although there was a strong rationale for the use of a tumor necrosis factor inhibitor (TNFi) based on overexpression of this cytokine in sacroiliac and peripheral joints from subjects with AS[24] and juvenile SpA,[25] respectively. Newer approaches have been developed based on a data emerging from animal models, translational studies, and genetics, including mechanisms that are related to aberrant features of HLA-B27.[26]

The genes encoding HLA antigens are divided into 3 classes (I, II, and III). The main HLA class I genes are further subdivided into HLA-A, HLA-B, and HLA-C, which vary widely among the population. The proteins encoded by these genes are expressed on the surfaces of most human cells, and their function is to bind various small protein fragments (peptides) and present them to receptors on a certain kind of T-lymphocyte (CD8[+]). The peptides usually come from within the cells and may be of foreign origin (for example, from a virus or bacterium) or self-origin (for example, normal proteins that are being broken down). If the CD8[+] T cell recognizes the peptide as foreign, it releases cytotoxins that can kill the infected cell.

It was discovered that different alleles of HLA genes coded for HLA proteins that could bind only certain peptides. This discovery led to the idea that 1 or more HLA-B27-bound peptides might be arthritogenic, resulting in the development of autoreactive CD8[+] T cells. Subsequent discoveries that HLA-B27 can misfold and generate stress responses and form an unusual dimer structure on the cell surface led to novel mechanistic hypotheses.[27] Importantly, these aberrant properties of HLA-B27 are linked to increased production of interleukin (IL)-23 and/or IL-17. Sufficient protein misfolding can cause a stress response, which promotes IL-23 production.[28] This IL-23 production, as well as the cell-surface dimers of HLA-B27 themselves, can in turn activate certain T cells that secrete IL-17 (Th17 T cells). Mouse models of enthesitis and axial arthritis support the participation of IL-17, IL-23, and IL-22 in pathogenesis. Detailed mechanisms of these interactions have not been fully elucidated in experimental models or validated in humans with disease.

A relationship between the microbial environment and SpA has been recognized for some time, based in part on the high frequency of gut inflammation. Development of SpA in HLA-B27 transgenic rats is entirely dependent on commensal gut bacteria,[29,30] suggesting that HLA-B27 might be exerting some of its effect by altering microbiota.[31] The development of culture-independent methods to catalog microbiota has led to a series of studies describing differences in subjects with SpA. In ERA, altered fecal microbiota have been noted.[32] A subsequent study of stool metabolites suggested that reduced metabolic diversity in ERA accompanied loss of bacterial diversity in the disease state. Dysbiosis has also been found in biopsies from the terminal ileum of patients with AS,[33] where species diversity was increased within certain genera, and decreased within others. These studies provide an important proof of concept but need to be replicated in larger populations. Altered gut microbiota have also been reported in adults with PsA[34] and reactive arthritis.[35] Although HLA-B27 can play a role in altering gut microbiota,[36] the relationship is complex and likely depends on existing microbes and other genetic factors.[37]

LABORATORY AND IMAGING STUDIES FOR DIAGNOSIS AND CARE

There are no diagnostic tests for juvenile SpA. Although HLA-B27 is found in 60% to 70% of patients with juvenile SpA,[7,13] and may be even more frequent in those with juvenile AS, it is found in 6% to 8% of unaffected individuals. Markers associated with other types of JIA (RF and ANA) are not helpful in screening for juvenile SpA. Routine screening laboratory studies of CBC, chemistry panel, urinalysis, sedimentation rate, and C-reactive protein are normal in most patients, although some have elevated acute-phase reactants or anemia that may represent chronic disease. If acute-phase reactants are markedly elevated, and/or anemia is persistent, then IBD should be considered, and screening with the fecal calprotectin test should be performed.

Imaging can be helpful for evaluating and monitoring juvenile SpA. Radiographs are often normal initially but can show changes in the sacroiliac and other affected joints, and at entheseal insertion sites, over time with incomplete control of disease. Ultrasound and MRI are more sensitive and can be useful for evaluating enthesitis and peripheral joint involvement. MRI findings include bone marrow and soft tissue edema, synovitis, effusions, and bursitis (see **Fig. 7**). It is important that the radiologist who interprets the scans be familiar with the normal edema-like changes found in the feet of healthy children, which may represent residual hematopoietic marrow.[38] MRI is helpful for evaluating sacroiliac and spine involvement and for differentiating juvenile SpA from infection, malignancy, and orthopedic conditions.

HOW JUVENILE SPONDYLOARTHRITIS IS TREATED

It is not recommended that primary care providers initiate treatment of juvenile SpA, other than with nonsteroidal anti-Inflammatory drugs (NSAIDs), prior to discussion or consultation with a rheumatologist. Current recommendations for the treatment of peripheral arthritis in juvenile SpA are similar to recommendations for other categories of JIA, as established by the American College of Rheumatology.[39] Treatment is primarily determined based on the number of active joints and the presence or absence of sacroiliitis. Treatment options include

- Four or fewer active joints: NSAIDs, glucocorticoid joint injections, and/or methotrexate
- Five or more active joints: NSAIDs and/or methotrexate as initial therapy
- Sacroiliitis: NSAIDs. If patients are symptomatic despite NSAIDs, therapy should be escalated to include a TNFi biologic.[39] First-line therapies for peripheral arthritis, such as methotrexate, are not effective for this particular disease manifestation.[40]

Adalimumab and etanercept have both been evaluated in randomized controlled trials that included children with juvenile SpA.[41,42] These studies also included children with polyarticular or extended oligoarticular JIA and thus are difficult to interpret and generalize to all forms of juvenile SpA. Adalimumab significantly reduced the active joint count at 12 weeks, with sustained improvement through week 52.[41] In the etanercept trial, during the open-label period (phase 1), a significant decrease in all measures of disease activity was observed.[42] In phase 2 (randomized withdrawal), there was a 35% reduction in the risk of flare in the group treated with etanercept versus placebo. In a retrospective comparative effectiveness study of an inception cohort of 217 children with SpA from 5 institutions, over the first year after diagnosis the use of TNFi therapy was associated with decreased disease activity and patient-reported pain compared with no TNFi.[43] The magnitude of estimated effect on all clinical outcomes evaluated, except enthesitis, was greater in those treated with TNFi therapy versus a disease-modifying agent, such as methotrexate.

The American College of Rheumatology also published guidelines for the treatment of adults with AS and nonradiographic axial SpA.[44] Although these recommendations were not intended for children, in certain circumstances (such as for adolescents) they may be helpful. Furthermore, pediatric rheumatologists frequently follow children until age 21. In adults with AS, a TNFi is recommended if symptoms persist despite therapy with an NSAID. Adjunct physical therapy is also recommended. In adults with nonradiographic axial SpA, a TNFi is conditionally recommended if NSAIDs are ineffective.

Given the evidence for involvement of IL-17 in the pathogenesis of SpA, trials of an IL-17 inhibitor secukinumab were conducted in adults,[45–47] resulting in recent regulatory agency approval for treatment of adults with PsA and AS. A study of secukinumab is currently under way in children with PsA and ERA (ClinicalTrials.gov identifier NCT03031782).

WHAT IS THE PROGNOSIS FOR JUVENILE SPONDYLOARTHRITIS?

Recent cross-sectional and longitudinal studies have shown that there is opportunity to improve the care and outcomes of these children.

- Fewer than 20% of children and adolescents with SpA achieve remission within 5 years of diagnosis.[48,49]
- In a study of 118 children followed for 4 years in the German Spondyloarthritis Inception Cohort, 85% of children had at least 1 period of remission off medication, but only 46% achieved remission off medication for longer than 1 year.[50]
  - Of those who attained remission on and off medication at least once, 38% and 32% subsequently flared, respectively.
  - At the end of the 4-year follow-up period, 57% of patients had active disease
- In a retrospective study of 72 Turkish children, higher body mass index (≥85th percentile) and ankle involvement were associated with failure to achieve inactive disease at 1 year.[51]

Several factors have been identified that are associated with poorer prognosis, including increased body mass index, ankle arthritis, hip arthritis, sacroilitis, enthesitis, and HLA-B27.[51,52] It remains unclear which children with SpA will develop severe axial disease leading to abnormal bone formation and ankylosis. Additional long-term outcome studies for this and other complications are needed.

REFERENCES

1. Kunjir V, Venugopalan A, Chopra A. Profile of Indian patients with juvenile onset chronic inflammatory joint disease using the ILAR classification criteria for JIA: a community-based cohort study. J Rheumatol 2010;37(8): 1756–62.
2. Shen CC, Yeh KW, Ou LS, et al. Clinical features of children with juvenile idiopathic arthritis using the ILAR classification criteria: a community-based cohort study in Taiwan. J Microbiol Immunol Infect 2013;46(4):288–94.
3. Rosenberg AM, Petty RE, Oen KG, et al. Rheumatic diseases in Western Canadian Indian children. J Rheumatol 1982;9(4):589–92.
4. Oen K, Schroeder M, Jacobson K, et al. Juvenile rheumatoid arthritis in a Canadian First Nations (aboriginal) population: onset subtypes and HLA associations. J Rheumatol 1998;25(4):783–90.
5. Saurenmann RK, Rose JB, Tyrrell P, et al. Epidemiology of juvenile idiopathic arthritis in a multiethnic cohort: ethnicity as a risk factor. Arthritis Rheum 2007; 56(6):1974–84.
6. Weiss PF, Beukelman T, Schanberg LE, et al. Enthesitis-related arthritis is associated with higher pain intensity and poorer health status in comparison with other categories of juvenile idiopathic arthritis: the childhood arthritis and rheumatology research alliance registry. J Rheumatol 2012;39(12):2341–51.

7. Stamato T, Laxer RM, de Freitas C, et al. Prevalence of cardiac manifestations of juvenile ankylosing spondylitis. Am J Cardiol 1995;75(10):744–6.
8. Huppertz H, Voigt I, Muller-Scholden J, et al. Cardiac manifestations in patients with HLA B27-associated juvenile arthritis. Pediatr Cardiol 2000;21(2):141–7.
9. Phatak S, Mohindra N, Zanwar A, et al. Prominent midfoot involvement in children with enthesitis-related arthritis category of juvenile idiopathic arthritis. Clin Rheumatol 2017;36(8):1737–45.
10. Stoll ML, Bhore R, Dempsey-Robertson M, et al. Spondyloarthritis in a pediatric population: risk factors for sacroiliitis. J Rheumatol 2010;37(11):2402–8.
11. Riley MJ, Ansell BM, Bywaters EG. Radiological manifestations of ankylosing spondylitis according to age at onset. Ann Rheum Dis 1971;30(2):138–48.
12. Weiss PF, Xiao R, Biko DM, et al. Assessment of sacroiliitis at diagnosis of juvenile spondyloarthritis by radiography, magnetic resonance imaging, and clinical examination. Arthritis Care Res (Hoboken) 2016;68(2):187–94.
13. Pagnini I, Savelli S, Matucci-Cerinic M, et al. Early predictors of juvenile sacroiliitis in enthesitis-related arthritis. J Rheumatol 2010;37(11):2395–401.
14. Rumsey DG, Guzman J, Rosenberg AM, et al. Characteristics and course of enthesitis in a juvenile idiopathic arthritis inception cohort. Arthritis Care Res (Hoboken) 2018;70(2):303–8.
15. Gmuca S, Xiao R, Brandon TG, et al. Multicenter inception cohort of enthesitis-related arthritis: variation in disease characteristics and treatment approaches. Arthritis Res Ther 2017;19(1):84.
16. Stoll ML, Punaro M, Patel AS. Fecal calprotectin in children with the enthesitis-related arthritis subtype of juvenile idiopathic arthritis. J Rheumatol 2011; 38(10):2274–5.
17. Stoll ML, Patel AS, Punaro M, et al. MR enterography to evaluate sub-clinical intestinal inflammation in children with spondyloarthritis. Pediatr Rheumatol Online J 2012;10:6.
18. Barthel D, Ganser G, Kuester RM, et al. Inflammatory bowel disease in juvenile idiopathic arthritis patients treated with biologics. J Rheumatol 2015;42(11): 2160–5.
19. Stoll ML, Nigrovic PA. Subpopulations within juvenile psoriatic arthritis: a review of the literature. Clin Dev Immunol 2006;13(2–4):377–80.
20. Ellinghaus D, Jostins L, Spain SL, et al. Analysis of five chronic inflammatory diseases identifies 27 new associations and highlights disease-specific patterns at shared loci. Nat Genet 2016;48(5):510–8.
21. Hanson A, Brown MA. Genetics and the causes of ankylosing spondylitis. Rheum Dis Clin North Am 2017;43(3):401–14.
22. Bowes J, Budu-Aggrey A, Huffmeier U, et al. Dense genotyping of immune-related susceptibility loci reveals new insights into the genetics of psoriatic arthritis. Nat Commun 2015;6:6046.
23. Kirino Y, Remmers EF. Genetic architectures of seropositive and seronegative rheumatic diseases. Nat Rev Rheumatol 2015;11(7):401–14.
24. Braun J, Bollow M, Neure L, et al. Use of immunohistologic and in situ hybridization techniques in the examination of sacroiliac joint biopsy specimens from patients with ankylosing spondylitis. Arthritis Rheum 1995;38(4): 499–505.
25. Grom AA, Murray KJ, Luyrink L, et al. Patterns of expression of tumor necrosis factor alpha, tumor necrosis factor beta, and their receptors in synovia of patients with juvenile rheumatoid arthritis and juvenile spondylarthropathy. Arthritis Rheum 1996;39(10):1703–10.

26. Smith JA, Colbert RA. Review: the interleukin-23/interleukin-17 axis in spondyloarthritis pathogenesis: Th17 and beyond. Arthritis Rheumatol 2014;66(2):231–41.
27. Bowness P. Hla-B27. Annu Rev Immunol 2015;33:29–48.
28. Navid F, Colbert RA. Causes and consequences of endoplasmic reticulum stress in rheumatic disease. Nat Rev Rheumatol 2017;13(1):25–40.
29. Taurog JD, Richardson JA, Croft JT, et al. The germfree state prevents development of gut and joint inflammatory disease in HLA-B27 transgenic rats. J Exp Med 1994;180(6):2359–64.
30. Rath HC, Herfarth HH, Ikeda JS, et al. Normal luminal bacteria, especially Bacteroides species, mediate chronic colitis, gastritis, and arthritis in HLA-B27/human beta2 microglobulin transgenic rats. J Clin Invest 1996;98(4):945–53.
31. Rosenbaum JT, Davey MP. Time for a gut check: evidence for the hypothesis that HLA-B27 predisposes to ankylosing spondylitis by altering the microbiome. Arthritis Rheum 2011;63(11):3195–8.
32. Stoll ML, Kumar R, Morrow CD, et al. Altered microbiota associated with abnormal humoral immune responses to commensal organisms in enthesitis-related arthritis. Arthritis Res Ther 2014;16(6):486.
33. Costello ME, Ciccia F, Willner D, et al. Brief report: intestinal dysbiosis in ankylosing spondylitis. Arthritis Rheumatol 2015;67(3):686–91.
34. Scher JU, Ubeda C, Artacho A, et al. Decreased bacterial diversity characterizes the altered gut microbiota in patients with psoriatic arthritis, resembling dysbiosis in inflammatory bowel disease. Arthritis Rheumatol 2015;67(1):128–39.
35. Manasson J, Shen N, Garcia Ferrer HR, et al. Gut microbiota perturbations in reactive arthritis and postinfectious spondyloarthritis. Arthritis Rheumatol 2018; 70(2):242–54.
36. Lin P, Bach M, Asquith M, et al. HLA-B27 and human beta2-microglobulin affect the gut microbiota of transgenic rats. PLoS One 2014;9(8):e105684.
37. Gill T, Asquith M, Brooks SR, et al. Effects of HLA-B27 on gut microbiota in experimental spondyloarthritis implicate an ecological model of dysbiosis. Arthritis Rheumatol 2018;70(4):555–65.
38. Aquino MR, Tse SM, Gupta S, et al. Whole-body MRI of juvenile spondyloarthritis: protocols and pictorial review of characteristic patterns. Pediatr Radiol 2015; 45(5):754–62.
39. Beukelman T, Patkar NM, Saag KG, et al. 2011 American College of Rheumatology recommendations for the treatment of juvenile idiopathic arthritis: initiation and safety monitoring of therapeutic agents for the treatment of arthritis and systemic features. Arthritis Care Res (Hoboken) 2011;63(4):465–82.
40. Haibel H, Brandt HC, Song IH, et al. No efficacy of subcutaneous methotrexate in active ankylosing spondylitis: a 16-week open-label trial. Ann Rheum Dis 2007; 66(3):419–21.
41. Burgos-Vargas R, Tse SM, Horneff G, et al. A randomized, double-blind, placebo-controlled multicenter study of adalimumab in pediatric patients with enthesitis-related arthritis. Arthritis Care Res (Hoboken) 2015;67(11):1503–12.
42. Horneff G, Foeldvari I, Minden K, et al. Efficacy and safety of etanercept in patients with the enthesitis-related arthritis category of juvenile idiopathic arthritis: results from a phase III randomized, double-blind study. Arthritis Rheumatol 2015;67(8):2240–9.
43. Weiss PF, Xiao R, Brandon TG, et al. Comparative effectiveness of tumor necrosis factor agents and disease-modifying antirheumatic therapy in children with enthesitis-related arthritis: the first year after diagnosis. J Rheumatol 2017; 45(1):107–14.

44. Ward MM, Deodhar A, Akl EA, et al. American College of Rheumatology/Spondylitis Association of America/Spondyloarthritis Research and Treatment Network 2015 recommendations for the treatment of ankylosing spondylitis and nonradiographic axial spondyloarthritis. Arthritis Rheumatol 2016;68(2):282–98.
45. McInnes IB, Mease PJ, Kirkham B, et al. Secukinumab, a human anti-interleukin-17A monoclonal antibody, in patients with psoriatic arthritis (FUTURE 2): a randomised, double-blind, placebo-controlled, phase 3 trial. Lancet 2015;386(9999):1137–46.
46. Mease PJ, McInnes IB, Kirkham B, et al. Secukinumab inhibition of interleukin-17A in patients with psoriatic arthritis. N Engl J Med 2015;373(14):1329–39.
47. Baeten D, Baraliakos X, Braun J, et al. Anti-interleukin-17A monoclonal antibody secukinumab in treatment of ankylosing spondylitis: a randomised, double-blind, placebo-controlled trial. Lancet 2013;382(9906):1705–13.
48. Flato B, Hoffmann-Vold AM, Reiff A, et al. Long-term outcome and prognostic factors in enthesitis-related arthritis: a case-control study. Arthritis Rheum 2006; 54(11):3573–82.
49. Minden K, Niewerth M, Listing J, et al. Long-term outcome in patients with juvenile idiopathic arthritis. Arthritis Rheum 2002;46(9):2392–401.
50. Weiss A, Minden K, Listing J, et al. Course of patients with juvenile spondyloarthritis during 4 years of observation, juvenile part of GESPIC. RMD Open 2017; 3(1):e000366.
51. Makay B, Gucenmez OA, Unsal E. Inactive disease in enthesitis-related arthritis: association of increased body mass index. J Rheumatol 2016;43(5):937–43.
52. Berntson L, Nordal E, Aalto K, et al. HLA-B27 predicts a more chronic disease course in an 8-year followup cohort of patients with juvenile idiopathic arthritis. J Rheumatol 2013;40(5):725–31.
53. Nordal E, Zak M, Aalto K, et al. Ongoing disease activity and changing categories in a long-term nordic cohort study of juvenile idiopathic arthritis. Arthritis Rheum 2011;63(9):2809–18.
54. Modesto C, Anton J, Rodriguez B, et al. Incidence and prevalence of juvenile idiopathic arthritis in Catalonia (Spain). Scand J Rheumatol 2010;39(6):472–9.
55. Davies R, Carrasco R, Foster HE, et al. Treatment prescribing patterns in patients with juvenile idiopathic arthritis (JIA): analysis from the UK Childhood Arthritis Prospective Study (CAPS). Semin Arthritis Rheum 2016;46(2):190–5.
56. Guzman J, Oen K, Tucker LB, et al. The outcomes of juvenile idiopathic arthritis in children managed with contemporary treatments: results from the ReACCh-Out cohort. Ann Rheum Dis 2015;74(10):1854–60.
57. Sengler C, Klotsche J, Niewerth M, et al. The majority of newly diagnosed patients with juvenile idiopathic arthritis reach an inactive disease state within the first year of specialised care: data from a German inception cohort. RMD Open 2015;1(1):e000074.

Systemic Juvenile Idiopathic Arthritis

Jennifer J.Y. Lee, MD, Rayfel Schneider, MBBCh*

KEYWORDS

- Systemic juvenile idiopathic arthritis • Juvenile idiopathic arthritis • Pediatrics
- Rheumatology • Macrophage activation syndrome

KEY POINTS

- The clinical presentation of systemic juvenile idiopathic arthritis (sJIA), often dominated by fever and systemic features, is unique in comparison to the other JIA subtypes.
- sJIA is a diagnosis of exclusion and requires adequate consideration of infectious, oncologic, autoimmune, and autoinflammatory diseases.
- Macrophage activation syndrome is a serious and potentially fatal complication of sJIA, characterized by sustained fever, organomegaly, cytopenias, coagulopathy, and high transaminases. It requires prompt evaluation and treatment.
- Newer biologic agents, particularly interleukin-1 and interleukin-6 inhibitors, are highly effective and have reduced the use of systemic corticosteroids.
- The primary care provider has a crucial role in monitoring children with sJIA for disease-related complications and medication-related adverse events.

INTRODUCTION

Systemic juvenile idiopathic arthritis (sJIA) is a very distinctive subtype of juvenile idiopathic arthritis (JIA) with unique clinical manifestations, associated complications, and therapeutic options. The full expression of sJIA is characterized by fever and arthritis, accompanied by at least one of the following: rash, generalized lymphadenopathy, hepatomegaly and/or splenomegaly, and serositis. However, the classic features are not always present at disease onset. Moreover, the symptoms and signs are nonspecific, overlapping with other inflammatory and non-inflammatory conditions. Therefore, sJIA, a rare cause of fever in children, remains a very challenging condition to diagnose, and pediatric primary care providers require a high index of suspicion to avoid unnecessary delays in establishing the diagnosis. In contrast to other JIA subtypes, children with sJIA often require hospitalization for severe systemic symptoms at onset or during flare-ups, require more intensive systemic treatment, and have higher disease-associated

Disclosure Statement: J.J.Y. Lee has no disclosures; R. Schneider has provided consultation for Novimmune, Novartis, and Sobi.
Department of Paediatrics, Division of Rheumatology, The Hospital for Sick Children, 555 University Avenue, Toronto, Ontario M5G 1X8, Canada
* Corresponding author.
E-mail address: rayfel.schneider@sickkids.ca

morbidity. Providers who comanage sJIA patients need to carefully monitor for associated systemic complications and for treatment-related adverse effects. In this review, the authors discuss primarily the clinical features, the differential diagnosis, complications, and management issues relevant to the pediatric primary care provider.

INCIDENCE OF SYSTEMIC JUVENILE IDIOPATHIC ARTHRITIS

JIA is the most common rheumatic disease in childhood, with an estimated prevalence of 1 to 4 per 1000 children.[1,2] sJIA accounts for approximately 10% to 20% of JIA cases, with incidence rates ranging from 0.4 to 0.8 children per 100,000 children.[3]

DEMOGRAPHICS
Age

Peak age of presentation is 1 to 5 years of age. However, children can present throughout childhood and adolescence.[4]

Gender

Male and female children are affected equally, unlike other JIA subtypes.[4]

Ethnicity

sJIA occurs in children of all ethnic backgrounds.[5] A slightly higher prevalence rate has been reported in Japan and India than in the United States or Canada.[6,7]

WHEN TO CONSIDER SYSTEMIC JUVENILE IDIOPATHIC ARTHRITIS

The diagnosis of sJIA should be considered in children who have unexplained, prolonged fever that spikes once or twice daily, especially when it is associated with intermittent rash, arthralgias, or arthritis.

HOW SYSTEMIC JUVENILE IDIOPATHIC ARTHRITIS PRESENTS
Classification Criteria

Widely accepted classification criteria for sJIA are based on the International League of Associations for Rheumatology (ILAR) classification criteria for JIA, which were revised in 2001 (**Box 1**).[5] These criteria require that the onset of symptoms occurs before the age of 16 years, the duration of arthritis is at least 6 weeks, and that other conditions are excluded. The term adult-onset Still disease may be considered part of the spectrum of sJIA and describes patients whose symptoms begin at the age of 16 years or older.[8] Distinct classification criteria exist for adult-onset Still disease, with the Yamaguchi criteria[9] and Fautrel's criteria[10] being the most well recognized. In contrast to the sJIA classification criteria, these criteria include arthralgia and do not require the presence of frank arthritis.

The ILAR criteria were developed to achieve consensus in identifying relatively homogeneous subgroups of JIA patients, primarily for research studies. Although not developed as diagnostic criteria, many physicians use them for this purpose. Most children with sJIA do not, in fact, meet ILAR classification criteria at initial presentation. Behrens and colleagues[4] found that only 30% met these criteria when they initially presented to a pediatric rheumatologist for assessment. Janow and colleagues[11] found that 71% of sJIA patients will eventually meet ILAR criteria during their disease course. The ILAR criteria may therefore not be sufficiently sensitive for the timely diagnosis and treatment of severe symptoms associated with new-onset sJIA. In practice, a presumptive diagnosis of sJIA is often made without arthritis being present for 6 weeks, if the symptoms

---

Box 1
International League of Associations for Rheumatology classification criteria for systemic juvenile idiopathic arthritis

Definition

Arthritis affecting one or more joints, with or preceded by fever of at least 2 weeks' duration, that is documented to be daily (quotidian) for at least 3 days, and accompanied by one or more of the following:
1. Evanescent (nonfixed) erythematous rash
2. Generalized lymphadenopathy
3. Hepatomegaly and/or splenomegaly
4. Serositis

Exclusions:

- Psoriasis or a history of psoriasis in the patient or first-degree relative

- Arthritis in an HLA-B27-positive male child beginning after the sixth birthday

- Ankylosing spondylitis, enthesitis-related arthritis, sacroiliitis with inflammatory bowel disease, acute anterior uveitis, or history of one of these disorders in a first-degree relative

- Presence of IgM rheumatoid factor on at least 2 occasions, at least 3 months apart

From Petty RE, Southwood TR, Manners P, et al. International League of Associations for Rheumatology classification of juvenile idiopathic arthritis: second revision, Edmonton, 2001. J Rheumatol 2004;31(2):390; with permission.

---

are typical and other diseases have satisfactorily been excluded. North American researchers from the Childhood Arthritis and Rheumatology Research Alliance (CARRA), for example, have developed an operational case definition for sJIA, which allows children with new-onset sJIA to be included in the CARRA consensus treatment protocols after 2 weeks of fever, provided they meet other criteria.[12]

Clinical Features

Fever

The finding of fever at presentation is almost universal in these patients.[4] The classic fever pattern seen in sJIA is distinctive with temperatures that spike above 39°C, once or twice a day, with a rapid return to normal or to below baseline temperatures **(Fig. 1)**.[13] Children may be quite unwell at the peak of fever and then may appear remarkably well when the fever abates.[13–15] Regular monitoring and documentation of the temperature with a fever chart can be very helpful in delineating this striking pattern.[4] Sustained high fevers in a patient with suspected sJIA should alert the clinician to the possibility of macrophage activation syndrome (MAS), which can occur at disease onset.

Cutaneous manifestations

In more than 80% of patients, a transient, salmon-colored macular or maculopapular rash accompanies the fever. Less commonly, the rash is urticarial. Absence of rash should prompt the clinician to reconsider the diagnosis of sJIA. Unlike drug rashes or many viral exanthems, a characteristic feature is that it is sometimes only seen with fever episodes, and it fades or vanishes when the fever abates. The eruption typically localizes to the trunk, neck, and proximal extremities, but it can be more widespread. Macules tend to be less than 5 mm in diameter, although larger macules can be present with central fading. Typically migratory and nonpruritic, the degree of erythema can be variable in the same patient.[16] Mild pressure on the skin (such

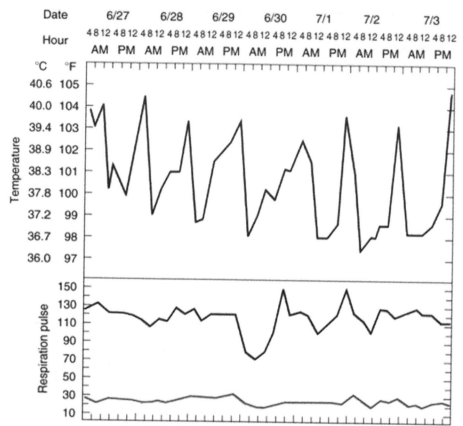

Fig. 1. Typical fever pattern in sJIA, showing a daily (quotidian) pattern. Note that in this patient the body temperature spikes at night and then falls to normal or below normal during the day. (*From* De Bendetti F, Schneider R. Chapter 16: systemic juvenile idiopathic arthritis. In: Petty RE, Laxer RM, Lindsley CB, et al, editors. Pediatric rheumatology. 7th edition. Philadelphia: Elsevier; 2016. p. 206; with permission.)

as stroking the skin) can evoke the *Koebner phenomenon*, where linear maculopapular lesions appear (**Fig. 2**).[17]

Musculoskeletal manifestations

In order to meet the classification criteria, the presence of arthritis must be confirmed. Although arthralgias are typically present at onset, arthritis may not necessarily be evident at initial presentation and can develop weeks, months, or rarely, years later. The vast majority of children will develop arthritis within the first 3 months of disease onset.[4,14] Because systemic symptoms often overshadow the features of arthritis, a detailed musculoskeletal examination should be performed in all patients who present with unexplained fever and elevated inflammatory markers.

Joint involvement can also be quite variable, ranging from oligoarticular (4 or fewer joints with arthritis) to polyarticular patterns. The most commonly involved joints include the wrists, knees, and ankles.[4] However, any joint can be affected, including the temporomandibular joints,[18] cervical spine,[19] hips,[20] and small joints of the hands and feet. A concerning feature of the arthritis, particularly before the availability of current biologic agents, is its rapidly destructive nature, leading to joint space loss,

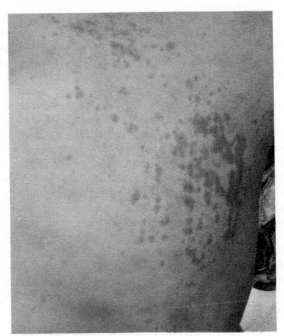

Fig. 2. sJIA patient with a maculopapular rash on the chest and abdomen. Note the linear streaks where the skin was scratched (Koebner phenomenon), which occurs in some children with sJIA.

erosions, and ankylosis.[4,21] Wrists and hips seem to be particularly vulnerable sites for joint destruction.[22] Other common musculoskeletal manifestations include myalgias and tenosynovitis.

Other organ involvement

Generalized lymphadenopathy, seen in more than 25% of patients at presentation, is nontender and can be quite prominent, raising the suspicion of a diagnosis of malignancy.[13] Hepatosplenomegaly occurs less frequently.[4] Chest pain, especially with an inability to lie supine, may suggest acute pericarditis, which occurs more commonly than pleuritis. Pericarditis can progress rapidly to cardiac tamponade that requires urgent systemic anti-inflammatory treatment and may require drainage of pericardial fluid. However, serositis is most frequently asymptomatic and may only be detectable on echocardiogram or chest radiograph. Sore throat is reported less commonly than in adult-onset Still disease, but is nevertheless a prominent symptom in some children and adolescents with active systemic disease. Less common clinical manifestations that have been reported in this population include aseptic meningitis,[23] nasal septal perforation,[24] pulmonary hypertension, interstitial lung disease, and pulmonary alveolar proteinosis.[25]

Macrophage Activation Syndrome

Macrophage activation syndrome (MAS), also known as secondary hemophagocytic lymphohistiocytosis (HLH), is a serious, potentially fatal, complication that is observed in sJIA patients, but rarely seen in other subtypes of JIA.[26] The reported prevalence of MAS in sJIA is approximately 10%,[27] although Behrens and colleagues[28] reported subtle clinical or laboratory features consistent with occult MAS in more than half of their sJIA cohort. The frequency of these features of MAS in sJIA suggests a shared pathogenetic pathway of these conditions. There are increasing reports that patients with sJIA-associated MAS have heterozygous sequence variations or mutations of unknown significance in genes commonly involved in autosomal recessive primary (genetic) HLH.[29,30] MAS can be seen at diagnosis, during a flare, and even when the disease is in remission.[3] This complication is not exclusively seen in sJIA patients and has been reported in patients with a variety of infections, malignancies, and other autoimmune conditions (see Stacey E. Tarvin and Kathleen M. O'Neil's article, "Systemic Lupus Erythematosus, Sjögren Syndrome, and MCTD in Children and Adolescents," in this issue and Ref.[31]). Furthermore, MAS can have numerous apparent triggers in sJIA patients, including infection, drugs, and inadequate control of underlying sJIA disease activity.[32]

MAS is an overwhelming inflammatory process associated with an overproduction of proinflammatory cytokines, also known as "cytokine storm." The overproduction of cytokines results in proliferation of T cells and well-differentiated macrophages, which can infiltrate and exhibit hemophagocytic activity in bone marrow and multiple organ systems. In the liver, for example, this infiltration and inflammation lead to impaired hepatic synthesis of proteins, such as albumin.[33] Clinical features in overt MAS are often dramatic. Children with MAS are often very unwell and can quickly progress to hemodynamic instability, requiring intensive care support. Clinical features include unremitting fever with hepatosplenomegaly, lymphadenopathy, encephalopathy, petechial rash, bruising, or frank bleeding (**Box 2**). The clinical features of MAS may be challenging to distinguish from sJIA flare or sepsis.

Box 2
Features that may suggest macrophage activation syndrome in systemic juvenile idiopathic arthritis

Clinical findings

- Sustained, nonremitting fever
- Worsening hepatosplenomegaly and lymphadenopathy
- New-onset encephalopathy
- Bruising, purpura, or mucosal bleeding
- Multiple organ failure

Laboratory findings

- Very high or increasing ferritin
- Decreasing ESR with persistently elevated or increasing CRP
- Low or decreasing platelet count, white blood cell count, neutrophil count, and hemoglobin
- Paradoxically normal platelet count in the setting of prominent inflammation
- Low or decreasing fibrinogen
- High or increasing transaminases and LDH
- High or increasing D-dimers, clotting times
- High or increasing triglycerides

Other

- Presence of hemophagocytosis on biopsy (such as in bone marrow, lymph node, liver, or spleen)

Abbreviations: LDH, lactate dehydrogenase; ESR, erythrocyte sedimentation rate; CRP, C-reactive protein.

Classic laboratory findings of MAS may include pancytopenia, elevated serum transaminases, hypertriglyceridemia, consumptive coagulopathy, and hyperferritinemia (see **Box 2**). However, it is very important to recognize that MAS can occur in the absence of profound cytopenias. Because substantial elevations of platelet, white blood cell, and neutrophil counts are typically seen in active sJIA, even unexpectedly normal counts, in the face of active systemic inflammation, should raise the suspicion of MAS. Moreover, the trends in sequential laboratory values may be more important than absolute values in making the diagnosis. The pathologic hallmark feature is the presence of numerous well-differentiated macrophages actively phagocytosing hematopoietic cells, but these abnormalities are only seen on examination of the bone marrow in 30% to 60% of patients and often do not correlate reliably with clinical features.[26,32,34]

Ravelli and colleagues[35] recently developed classification criteria for sJIA-associated MAS in patients with sJIA or suspected sJIA, to differentiate MAS from confounding conditions, particularly active sJIA or an infection (**Box 3**). Although these criteria will no doubt help to advance the study of MAS in sJIA, they are neither intended to be diagnostic criteria nor have they been validated as such. A key laboratory finding is elevation of serum ferritin; however, high ferritin can accompany active systemic inflammation in sJIA in the absence of overt MAS. Extreme hyperferritinemia, with serum levels greater than 10,000 µg/L (ng/mL), strongly suggests full-blown or at least rapidly evolving MAS. Because the level of serum ferritin alone is insufficient to make a diagnosis of MAS, careful monitoring of the clinical status of the patient and diligently following the laboratory features associated with MAS are critically important in making an early diagnosis. The authors recommend that suspected MAS in a patient with sJIA be evaluated immediately by, and managed in consultation with, a pediatric rheumatologist because patients with MAS can quickly develop multiorgan system involvement and failure. Consultation with a pediatric hematologist may also be needed.

Without appropriate treatment, MAS can rapidly worsen and become fatal. In a recent study by Minoia and colleagues[36] evaluating 362 patients with sJIA and MAS, one-third of patients required an admission to the intensive care unit, and the overall mortality was 8%. This potentially life-threatening condition requires vigilance, prompt recognition, and treatment.

DIFFERENTIAL DIAGNOSIS OR MIMICS OF SYSTEMIC JUVENILE IDIOPATHIC ARTHRITIS

The diagnosis of suspected sJIA may be challenging because of overlapping features with other conditions. Physicians need to carefully consider infections, malignancies,

---

Box 3
2016 Classification criteria of macrophage activation syndrome in systemic juvenile idiopathic arthritis patients

A febrile patient with known or suspected sJIA is classified as having MAS if the following are met:

Ferritin greater than 684 ng/mL and any 2 of the following:
1. Platelet count $\leq$181 × 10^9/L (181,000/µL)
2. AST greater than 48 units/L
3. Triglycerides greater than 156 mg/dL
4. Fibrinogen $\leq$360 mg/dL

Abbreviation: AST, aspartate aminotransferase.
   From Ravelli A, Minoia F, Davì S, et al. 2016 classification criteria for macrophage activation syndrome complicating systemic juvenile idiopathic arthritis: a European League Against Rheumatism/American College of Rheumatology/Paediatric Rheumatology International Trials Organisation collaborative initiative. Ann Rheum Dis 2016;75(3):481–9.

autoimmune, autoinflammatory, and other inflammatory diseases. A wide range of infectious diseases can mimic features of sJIA, so particular attention should be paid to excluding infectious endocarditis, osteomyelitis, viral infections, cat scratch disease, brucellosis, mycoplasma, and Lyme disease. Important differential diagnoses with features that may be helpful in differentiating these conditions from sJIA are listed in **Table 1**.

LABORATORY AND IMAGING STUDIES FOR DIAGNOSIS AND CARE

There is no pathognomonic laboratory feature that distinguishes sJIA from other conditions. The pattern of laboratory abnormalities may be supportive for the diagnosis of sJIA, but none is specific. **Box 4** summarizes the list of investigations and the typical findings that would be supportive of the diagnosis. See the MAS section above for more discussion of the pattern of laboratory findings in MAS.

Hematologic Abnormalities

Hematologic investigations typically reflect the inflammatory nature of sJIA, particularly with a reactive thrombocytosis. It is not uncommon to see moderate degrees of anemia and microcytosis due to the acute phase response initially, sometimes followed by deficiency in iron stores over time.[4,38] There may be a very marked leukemoid reaction with white blood cell counts exceeding 30,000/mm³ with predominant neutrophilia, making it imperative to exclude bacterial sepsis.

Inflammatory Markers

Inflammatory markers such as the erythrocyte sedimentation rate (ESR) and C-reactive protein (CRP) are usually elevated and can be helpful to monitor the response to treatment. Tracking the levels of leukocytosis, thrombocytosis, elevated ferritin and D-dimers, and other initial laboratory abnormalities is also important for monitoring response to treatment and potential adverse effects due to treatment. When there is a discrepancy between the ESR and CRP, with an elevated or increasing CRP but a normal or falling ESR, patients should be carefully evaluated for MAS, because the hypofibrinogenemia of MAS can result in the misleading decrease of the ESR. Because hyperferritinemia is a key laboratory feature of MAS, ferritin should be measured in any febrile patient with sJIA or suspected sJIA. Other markers reflecting the acute phase response include elevated complement levels, fibrinogen, and D-dimer levels. S100 proteins, particularly S100A12 and S100A8/A9, are significantly elevated in sJIA and, although not readily available in all locations currently, may be helpful in differentiating sJIA from infectious causes of fever in the future.[39]

Autoantibodies

Autoantibodies, such as antinuclear autoantibodies (ANA) and rheumatoid factor, are almost always negative and are not helpful in the diagnosis. Positive ANA is seen in approximately 4% to 6% of sJIA patients.[7,40]

Radiologic Examination

Soft tissue swelling and osteoporosis are the most common radiologic abnormalities, followed by subchondral irregularity, cartilage loss, and bone erosions, often seen within 2 years of the disease onset.[41] Routine surveillance using joint radiographs to monitor sJIA disease activity is not useful, but radiographs can be useful in demonstrating disease progression in persistently affected joints.

Table 1
Differential diagnosis and possible differentiating features from systemic juvenile idiopathic arthritis

Condition	Differentiating Features from sJIA
Infection and infection-related diseases	
Infection (viral, bacterial)	Positive cultures, sick contacts or exposures, continuous or less predictable fever patterns, persistent nonepisodic rash
Reactive arthritis (post–salmonella/ shigella/yersinia arthritis)	Positive cultures or antigen detection, preceding infectious symptoms, exposures, sick contacts
Acute rheumatic fever	Migratory asymmetric polyarthritis, endocarditis, evidence of a group A streptococcal infection (positive throat culture or high antistreptolysin O titers), dramatic response to NSAIDs
Malignancy	
Leukemla, lymphoma, neuroblastoma	Nonarticular bone pain, bone tenderness, history of night-time pain, severe constitutional symptoms including night sweats, petechiae, or purpura, abnormal peripheral blood smear, low or very high WBC, low-normal platelet count, and elevated LDH[37]
Genetic causes	
Primary HLH	Very early age at presentation (particularly <1 y), petechiae or purpura, continuous fevers, cytopenias, liver dysfunction
Systemic autoimmune or inflammatory diseases	
Serum sickness	Exposure to a responsible agent, continuous fevers, urticarial rash, hypocomplementemia
SLE	Characteristic dermatologic findings, including malar rash, discoid rash, photosensitivity, cutaneous vasculitis, oral or nasal ulcers, neuropsychiatric symptoms. Family history of SLE. Abnormal urinalysis, hypocomplementemia, positive ANA, and positive SLE-specific autoantibodies
Kawasaki disease	Sustained fever, mucocutaneous symptoms, swelling, erythema or peeling of hands and feet, coronary artery dilatation/aneurysms
Polyarteritis nodosa	Subcutaneous nodules, uveitis, peripheral neuropathy
IBD	Significant weight loss, oral ulcers, predominant gastrointestinal symptoms, family history of IBD, erythema nodosum
NOMID/CINCA	Neonatal onset, maculopapular rash, prominent neurologic features such as aseptic meningitis and papilledema, progression to sensorineural loss from infancy or childhood, characteristic bone deformity with enlargement of the ossified portions of the epiphyses. Pathogenic mutations in the NLRP3 gene (dominantly inherited or spontaneous)
Muckle-Wells syndrome	Conjunctivitis, arthralgia with less prominent arthritis, sensorineural hearing loss typically in adolescence, pathogenic mutations in the NLRP3 gene (dominantly inherited or spontaneous)
TRAPS	Regular periodicity of fever episodes, myalgias, erythema over muscles, periorbital edema, pathogenic mutation in TNFRSF1A gene (dominantly inherited)

Abbreviations: CINCA, chronic infantile neurologic cutaneous and articular syndrome; IBD, inflammatory bowel disease; NOMID, neonatal-onset multisystem inflammatory disease; SLE, systemic lupus erythematosus; TRAPS, TNF receptor-associated periodic syndrome; WBC, white blood cell count.

Box 4
Summary of typical laboratory findings in systemic juvenile idiopathic arthritis

Anemia (microcytic, hypochromic)

Neutrophilic leukocytosis

Thrombocytosis

High ESR, CRP

High ferritin

Low albumin

High IgG

Mildly elevated AST, alanine aminotransferase

High D-dimers

Negative autoantibodies

Bone Marrow Aspirate and Biopsy

Although a bone marrow aspirate or biopsy will not be helpful in diagnosing a patient with sJIA, it is often indicated to rule out hematologic malignancies. Musculoskeletal and systemic symptoms are common in children with acute lymphoblastic leukemia.[42] It is prudent for the clinician to exclude malignancy, particularly if systemic corticosteroid treatment is being considered. Studies have shown that preemptive steroid treatment in patients with malignancy can relieve symptoms but may ultimately lead to a delay in diagnosis and reduce subsequent response to chemotherapy.[43]

PATHOGENESIS

The cause of sJIA is not completely understood but has been attributed to a combination of environmental triggers and polygenic influences. One study investigated the role of infectious agents in triggering the disease by analyzing seasonal onset patterns of sJIA, but no consistent seasonal pattern or infectious pathogen was identified.[44]

Over the last decade, sJIA has increasingly been considered an autoinflammatory, rather than an autoimmune, disease,[45] distinguishing it from other subtypes of JIA. Autoimmune diseases are disorders of the adaptive immune system and are often characterized by the presence of autoantibodies, whereas autoinflammatory conditions are related to dysregulation of the innate immune system (described further in Kathleen E. Sullivan's article, "Pathogenesis of Pediatric Rheumatologic Diseases," in this issue). Elegant research has identified a key role of several proinflammatory cytokines of the innate immune system in mediating expression of the disease, particularly interleukin-1β (IL-1β) and IL-6.[46–48] Polymorphisms in the genes that encode or regulate these and other cytokines, such as tumor necrosis factor-alpha (TNF-α), appear to contribute to disease susceptibility.[45] The rapid response of symptoms of sJIA to antagonism of IL-1 or IL-6 lends further support to their pivotal roles. The notion of sJIA as a purely autoinflammatory condition, however, has been recently challenged by some researchers because of the strong association of some variants in the major histocompatibility class II locus with sJIA.[49] Readers can refer to Kathleen E. Sullivan's article, "Pathogenesis of Pediatric Rheumatologic Diseases," in this issue for more information about the pathogenesis of autoimmune and autoinflammatory diseases.

HOW SYSTEMIC JUVENILE IDIOPATHIC ARTHRITIS IS TREATED

The goal of treatment is to control active inflammation in order to alleviate symptoms and to prevent disease-related complications and comorbidities.[50] Because sJIA patients often need treatment with systemic corticosteroids and are at risk for developing MAS, the authors recommend all sJIA patients be treated in conjunction with a pediatric rheumatologist. Children with new-onset sJIA, who are stable, without severe systemic symptoms or MAS, typically receive a trial of nonsteroidal anti-inflammatory drugs (NSAIDs) as first-line therapy, whereas the initial diagnostic workup is being pursued. Most sJIA patients who receive NSAID monotherapy will have an incomplete response. Those who have not improved within 2 weeks of starting NSAIDs, or have more severe systemic symptoms, may need treatment with systemic corticosteroids and/or a biologic agent. The systemic manifestations of sJIA respond poorly to traditional disease-modifying antirheumatic drugs (DMARDs), such as methotrexate, and to TNF inhibitor biologic agents.[51] Their efficacy for joint disease is modest. Intra-articular corticosteroid injections may be used as adjunctive treatment of refractory arthritis, but the duration of response tends to be less than in other subtypes of JIA, particularly if there are active systemic symptoms.

Treatment with systemic corticosteroids has been commonly used for managing sJIA, but is associated with significant side effects. Intravenous pulses of methylprednisolone or oral corticosteroids may be used in accordance with the severity of the symptoms. In comparison to other subtypes, sJIA patients have the highest probability of starting systemic corticosteroids within the first 6 months of diagnosis.[52] More recently, alternative effective treatments with a lower frequency of serious side effects have been identified and may eventually replace use of corticosteroids for routine treatment of most patients.

Children with sJIA unresponsive to, or dependent on, systemic corticosteroid monotherapy, should be treated with a biologic agent.[50] Controlled clinical trials of anakinra (human recombinant IL-1 receptor antagonist),[53] canakinumab (monoclonal anti-IL-1β),[54] rilonacept (a fusion protein consisting of the IL-1-binding domains of human IL-1 receptor type 1 coupled to IL-1 receptor accessory protein and the Fc fragment of immunoglobulin G [IgG1]),[55] and tocilizumab (monoclonal anti-IL-6 receptor),[56,57] have shown impressive efficacy in sJIA. However, only 2 of these medications, canakinumab and tocilizumab, are currently approved by regulatory bodies in Canada and the United States for treatment of sJIA, so the others are much less likely to be covered by health care plans.

Ongoing research[12] is evaluating the use of an IL-1 or IL-6 inhibitor as first-line therapy.[50] Since there is a high likelihood of response to these agents, particularly of systemic symptoms, this approach has the potential to completely avoid using systemic corticosteroids for some patients. Failure to respond to an IL-1 or IL-6 inhibitor should prompt reconsideration of other diagnoses such as infection or malignancy.

Treatment of sJIA-associated MAS includes the prompt use of high-dose intravenous corticosteroid therapy. Intravenous immunoglobulin can be used before the administration of corticosteroid therapy if the child is stable and the diagnostic evaluation for MAS, particularly exclusion of malignancy, has not yet been completed.[58] Other medications that can be used if corticosteroids do not provide adequate control of MAS include cyclosporine A[59] and anakinra used off-label.[60] Anakinra may be effective in treating both MAS and active sJIA and may be helpful in achieving a more rapid reduction of systemic corticosteroid dose.[61] More severe episodes of MAS might require treatment with etoposide or antithymocyte globulin, typically in consultation with a hematologist. The level of supportive care required for hospitalized sJIA patients with severe MAS is best be provided in the intensive care unit of a pediatric tertiary care facility with a pediatric rheumatologist on staff.

Role of the Pediatric Primary Care Provider in the Management of a Child with Systemic Juvenile Idiopathic Arthritis

sJIA patients should be co-managed by a pediatric primary care provider and a pediatric rheumatologist for the most optimal and comprehensive care. The following are important aspects of care that require longitudinal monitoring and support.

Immunizations

Effective and safe vaccination is a key component in preventing infections. Inactivated vaccinations continue to remain safe in children with rheumatic disease who receive immunosuppressive agents. Providers should counsel patients to receive inactivated vaccines, particularly meningococcal, pneumococcal, and annual influenza vaccinations. Live virus vaccines are contraindicated in patients who are already on immunosuppressive therapy. See Gloria C. Higgins' article, "Complications of Treatments for Pediatric Rheumatic Diseases," in this issue for more information on vaccination and tuberculosis screening; tuberculosis screening should be done before initiating biologic therapy.

Growth

It is well recognized that chronic inflammation can lead to growth delay and poor weight gain, whereas cumulative doses and longer duration of oral corticosteroids can lead to growth delay and increased weight gain.[62] Despite recent advances in treatments that reduce corticosteroid requirements, Guzman and colleagues,[63] using a Canadian registry of newly diagnosed sJIA patients enrolled between 2005 and 2010, recently reported that the 3-year cumulative incidence for new-onset short stature and for obesity in sJIA patients was 9.3% and 34.4%, respectively, much higher than in other JIA subtypes. However, this outcome may be improved from the prebiologic era for sJIA treatment; in 2002, Simon and colleagues[64] documented that 30% of sJIA patients continued to experience impaired linear growth after prednisone discontinuation and disease remission.

There is promising evidence to suggest that biologic agents may have a beneficial impact on growth velocity. Tocilizumab and canakinumab were approved by US and Canadian regulatory agencies during time period 2011 to 2014. In 2015, De Benedetti and colleagues[65] reported that sJIA patients in a phase 3 clinical trial of tocilizumab infusions and lower doses of corticosteroids achieved normal growth velocities and catch-up growth on treatment. Improved growth may have been a result of better control of inflammation, and lower cumulative doses of corticosteroids, as well as the potential effects of tocilizumab itself on the growth hormone/insulin growth factor-1 axis and on bone metabolism. It will likely take many more years before the full impact of IL-1 and IL-6 inhibitors on growth of sJIA patients can be determined.

Providers are encouraged to regularly monitor anthropometric measurements, calculate growth velocity and body mass index and assess pubertal development. In children treated with systemic corticosteroids, primary care providers can play an important role in educating and counseling patients on healthy active living strategies, such as engaging in physical activity, reducing sedentary behaviors, and improving nutritional intake. Consultation with a pediatric endocrinologist may be helpful in patients with pubertal delay, significantly reduced growth velocity, or reduced height in comparison to predicted final height.[62] See Sharon Bout-Tabaku's article, "General Nutrition and Fitness for the Child with Rheumatic Disease," in this issue for more discussion of growth issues and treatment.

Medication side effects

Gloria C. Higgins' article, "Complications of Treatments for Pediatric Rheumatic Diseases," in this issue describes the common and important toxicities of the medications used frequently in sJIA. Children treated with chronic systemic corticosteroids should be monitored for hypertension (using the appropriate blood pressure cuff size) and steroid-induced diabetes and evaluated for optimal calcium and vitamin D intake for bone health. Bone mineral density measurements should be performed on an annual basis if patients continue to be on long-term corticosteroid therapy. Eye examinations should be done on an annual basis to screen for glaucoma and cataracts. It is important to address the psychological effects of systemic corticosteroids, especially in children with excessive weight gain, acne, striae, and mood changes.

All children who are immunosuppressed with corticosteroids or biologics require a contingency plan to deal with episodes of fever or infection. sJIA patients who develop fever on immunosuppressive treatment should seek medical attention, ideally within 24 hours of fever onset or immediately if they appear to have a more severe illness. In addition to evaluating for sJIA flare and MAS, providers should carefully check for possible infection. Simple bacterial infections, such as an acute otitis media, should be treated promptly with antibiotics. Oral corticosteroids are not discontinued when a patient is treated for an infection, and in some cases, additional stress dosing may be required in patients who are unwell due to concerns of adrenal insufficiency. The authors recommend close communication with the rheumatologist to determine whether biologics should be withheld during an infectious illness, because this decision may depend on the nature of the infection, the specific biologic agent being used, and disease activity. Infections can trigger a disease flare and MAS, both of which may be exacerbated by withdrawal of treatment.

Uveitis screening

The American Academy of Pediatrics recommends annual ophthalmologic examinations for patients with sJIA.[66] Uveitis is more commonly associated with other types of JIA (see Courtney B. Crayne and Timothy Beukelman's article, "Juvenile Idiopathic Arthritis: Oligoarthritis and Polyarthritis," in this issue), but has been reported in less than 2% of sJIA patients.[66] If applicable, eye examinations are also helpful to evaluate for corticosteroid-induced glaucoma or cataracts as previously mentioned and may need to be performed more frequently if such side effects develop.

Psychosocial aspects and burden of chronic disease

Providers need to be cognizant of the burden and challenge of living with a chronic illness on the child and the family. Frustration and anxiety may arise not only with the chronic daily physical symptoms and functional limitations related to the arthritis but also with the uncertainty of flares and prognosis. Numerous studies have reported lower and suboptimal health-related quality-of-life scores in JIA patients compared with their healthy peers, with a greater difference in scores in regards to pain, anxiety, and depression.[67–69] Primary care providers are well positioned to provide support and counseling for both the physical and the emotional challenges, because patients and families adjust to living with arthritis. Helping families communicate with the child's school may facilitate the necessary accommodations, because children may often miss school because of medical appointments, flares, or medication infusions. Connecting families with local or national arthritis organizations may help provide families with additional resources and support (**Box 5**).

WHAT IS THE PROGNOSIS FOR SYSTEMIC JUVENILE IDIOPATHIC ARTHRITIS?

Before the "biologic era," based on numerous longitudinal follow-up studies, there appeared to be 3 patterns of disease course seen in sJIA patients, leading to

---

Box 5
Helpful organizations and resources for families

About Kids Health (http://www.aboutkidshealth.ca/En/ResourceCentres/JuvenileIdiopathicArthritis/)

Arthritis Foundation (https://www.arthritis.org/)

Arthritis Society (https://www.arthritis.ca/)

Childhood Arthritis and Rheumatology Research Alliance (https://carragroup.org/)

Kids Get Arthritis Too (http://www.kidsgetarthritistoo.org/)

---

significantly different long-term outcomes. About half the sJIA patients followed a persistent course of disease activity, characterized by ongoing active systemic features and arthritis.[70,71] In many cases of persistent disease, the systemic symptoms eventually resolved, but the arthritis remained active[72] with the potential for functional disability. Singh-Grewal and colleagues[71] identified that polyarticular arthritis at presentation and evidence of ongoing disease activity at 3 months after diagnosis were independent risk factors for a persistent disease course. On the other hand, approximately 30% to 40% of sJIA patients had a monophasic disease course.[71] These patients had a single episode of systemic symptoms and arthritis, typically lasting less than 24 months, followed by complete remission off medication with no recurrence. These patients did very well and their likelihood for disability was low. Finally, a small proportion (<20%) had a polycyclic course with multiple recurrences of active disease alternating with periods (months or years) of remission off medication.

Other early studies generally indicated a disproportionately high burden of morbidity and mortality in sJIA compared with other JIA subtypes. Bowyer and colleagues[73] evaluated outcomes of sJIA patients from the 1990s and found that nearly two-thirds of patients had radiographic evidence of joint space narrowing within 2 years. Studies by Foster and colleagues[74] and Packham and Hall[21] described higher proportions of sJIA patients with severe functional impairment and a large proportion of patients (up to 75%) who had undergone joint replacement.

Presently, there is great interest in determining how much long-term outcomes have changed since many sJIA patients are treated with effective biologics such as IL-1 and IL-6 blockers. Some experts believe there is a "window of opportunity" whereby cytokine inhibition early in the disease course may positively alter the disease trajectory and prognosis.[75]

At this time, there is no reliable way of predicting, at disease onset, which disease course trajectory a child with sJIA will follow and who is at highest risk of poor functional outcome. Older predictors of poor outcomes (often defined as poor function or high level of articular burden) from various studies include persistent systemic symptoms, reliance on corticosteroid therapy 6 months from disease onset, thrombocytosis (>600 × 10^9/L or 600,000/μL) at 6 months, young age at onset (younger than 18 months), fever duration of more than 3 months, polyarticular arthritis in the first 3 months, early joint damage, and early hip involvement.[20,76,77]

Hashkes and colleagues[78] reported a standardized mortality ratio of 1.8 when evaluating newly diagnosed sJIA patients from 1992 to 2001. Previous studies have reported higher mortalities with sJIA deaths accounting for a disproportionate number of deaths in JIA.[79–81] A major cause of death is MAS,[36] as described previously. The other important cause of mortality is infection, typically exacerbated by the use of chronic immunosuppression. Treatment-related complications account for 10% of deaths of all pediatric rheumatic diseases.[78] Other serious disease-related complications that can result in increased mortalities in sJIA patients include interstitial lung disease, pulmonary alveolar proteinosis, pulmonary hypertension, myocarditis, arrhythmias, and cardiac tamponade. Amyloidosis was an important cause of death in earlier series but the incidence of amyloidosis in sJIA has declined significantly,[82,83] perhaps at least partly because of more aggressive treatment and better disease control.

REFERENCES

1. Harrold LR, Salman C, Shoor S, et al. Incidence and prevalence of juvenile idiopathic arthritis among children in a managed care population, 1996-2009. J Rheumatol 2013;40(7):1218–25.
2. Prakken B, Albani S, Martini A. Juvenile idiopathic arthritis. Lancet 2011; 377(9783):2138–49.
3. Ramanan AV, Grom AA. Does systemic-onset juvenile idiopathic arthritis belong under juvenile idiopathic arthritis? Rheumatology (Oxford) 2005;44(11):1350–3.
4. Behrens EM, Beukelman T, Gallo L, et al. Evaluation of the presentation of systemic onset juvenile rheumatoid arthritis: data from the Pennsylvania systemic onset juvenile arthritis registry (PASOJAR). J Rheumatol 2008;35(2):343–8.
5. Petty RE, Southwood TR, Manners P, et al. International League of Associations for Rheumatology classification of juvenile idiopathic arthritis: second revision, Edmonton, 2001. J Rheumatol 2004;31(2):390–2.
6. Fujikawa S, Okuni M. Clinical analysis of 570 cases with juvenile rheumatoid arthritis: results of a nationwide retrospective survey in Japan. Acta Paediatr Jpn 1997;39(2):245–9.
7. Seth V, Kabra SK, Semwal OP, et al. Clinico-immunological profile in juvenile rheumatoid arthritis–an Indian experience. Indian J Pediatr 1996;63(3):293–300.
8. Bywaters EG. Still's disease in the adult. Ann Rheum Dis 1971;30(2):121–33.
9. Yamaguchi M, Ohta A, Tsunematsu T, et al. Preliminary criteria for classification of adult Still's disease. J Rheumatol 1992;19(3):424–30.
10. Fautrel B, Zing E, Golmard JL, et al, CARRA Legacy Registry Investigators. Proposal for a new set of classification criteria for adult-onset still disease. Medicine (Baltimore) 2002;81(3):194–200.
11. Janow G, Schanberg LE, Setoguchi S, et al. The systemic juvenile idiopathic arthritis cohort of the childhood arthritis and rheumatology research alliance registry: 2010-2013. J Rheumatol 2016;43(9):1755–62.
12. DeWitt EM, Kimura Y, Beukelman T, et al, Juvenile idiopathic arthritis disease-specific research committee of childhood arthritis rheumatology and research alliance. Consensus treatment plans for new-onset systemic juvenile idiopathic arthritis. Arthritis Care Res (Hoboken) 2012;64(7):1001–10.
13. Calabro JJ, Holgerson WB, Sonpal GM, et al. Juvenile rheumatoid arthritis: a general review and report of 100 patients observed for 15 years. Semin Arthritis Rheum 1976;5(3):257–98.
14. Schneider R, Laxer RM. Chapter 3: systemic juvenile idiopathic arthritis. In: Cimaz R, Lehman T, editors. Handbook of systemic autoimmune diseases, vol. 6. Elsevier BV; 2007. p. 35–274.
15. Gurion R, Lehman TJ, Moorthy LN. Systemic arthritis in children: a review of clinical presentation and treatment. Int J Inflam 2012;2012:271569.
16. Calabro JJ, Marchesano JM. Rash associated with juvenile rheumatoid arthritis. J Pediatr 1968;72(5):611–9.
17. Bywaters EG, Isdale IC. The rash of rheumatoid arthritis and Still's disease. Q J Med 1956;25(99):377–87.

18. Ringold S, Cron RQ. The temporomandibular joint in juvenile idiopathic arthritis: frequently used and frequently arthritic. Pediatr Rheumatol Online J 2009;7(1):11.
19. Ornilla E, Ansell BM, Swannell AJ. Cervical spine involvement in patients with chronic arthritis undergoing orthopaedic surgery. Ann Rheum Dis 1972;31:364–8.
20. Modesto C, Woo P, García-Consuegra J, et al. Systemic onset juvenile chronic arthritis, polyarticular pattern and hip involvement as markers for a bad prognosis. Clin Exp Rheumatol 2001;19(2):211–7.
21. Packham JC, Hall MA. Long-term follow-up of 246 adults with juvenile idiopathic arthritis: functional outcome. Rheumatology 2002;41(12):1428–35.
22. Oen K. Long-term outcomes and predictors of outcomes for patients with juvenile idiopathic arthritis. Best Pract Res Clin Rheumatol 2002;16(3):347–60.
23. Blockmans DE, Knockaert DC, Bobbaers HJ. Still's disease can cause neutrophilic meningitis. Neurology 2000;54(5):1203.
24. Avcin T, Silverman ED, Forte V, et al. Nasal septal perforation: a novel clinical manifestation of systemic juvenile idiopathic arthritis/adult onset Still's disease. J Rheumatol 2005;32(12):2429–31.
25. Kimura Y, Weiss JE, Haroldson KL, et al. Pulmonary hypertension and other potentially fatal pulmonary complications in systemic juvenile idiopathic arthritis. Arthritis Care Res (Hoboken) 2013;65(5):745–52.
26. Grom AA. Macrophage activation syndrome and reactive hemophagocytic lymphohistiocytosis: the same entities? Curr Opin Rheumatol 2003;15(5):587–90.
27. Sawhney S, Woo P, Murray KJ. Macrophage activation syndrome: a potentially fatal complication of rheumatic disorders. Arch Dis Child 2001;85(5):421–6.
28. Behrens EM, Beukelman T, Paessler M, et al. Occult macrophage activation syndrome in patients with systemic juvenile idiopathic arthritis. J Rheumatol 2007; 34(5):1133–8.
29. Vastert SJ, van Wijk R, D'Urbano LE, et al. Mutations in the perforin gene can be linked to macrophage activation syndrome in patients with systemic onset juvenile idiopathic arthritis. Rheumatology 2010;49(3):441–9.
30. Hazen MM, Woodward AL, Hofmann I, et al. Mutations of the hemophagocytic lymphohistiocytosis-associated gene UNC13D in a patient with systemic juvenile idiopathic arthritis. Arthritis Rheum 2008;58(2):567–70.
31. Schulert GS, Grom AA. Macrophage activation syndrome and cytokine directed therapies. Best Pract Res Clin Rheumatol 2014;28(2):277–92.
32. Ravelli A, Grom AA, Behrens EM, et al. Macrophage activation syndrome as part of systemic juvenile idiopathic arthritis: diagnosis, genetics, pathophysiology and treatment. Genes Immun 2012;13(4):289–98.
33. Schulert GS, Grom AA. Pathogenesis of macrophage activation syndrome and potential for cytokine-directed therapies. Annu Rev Med 2015;66:145–59.
34. Ho C, Yao X, Tian L, et al. Marrow assessment for hemophagocytic lymphohistiocytosis demonstrates poor correlation with disease probability. Am J Clin Pathol 2014;141(1):62–71.
35. Ravelli A, Minoia F, Davì S, et al. 2016 classification criteria for macrophage activation syndrome complicating systemic juvenile idiopathic arthritis: a European League Against Rheumatism/American College of Rheumatology/Paediatric Rheumatology International Trials Organisation collaborative initiative. Ann Rheum Dis 2016;75(3):481–9.
36. Minoia F, Davì S, Horne A, et al. Clinical features, treatment, and outcome of macrophage activation syndrome complicating systemic juvenile idiopathic arthritis: a multinational, multicenter study of 362 patients. Arthritis Rheumatol 2014;66(11):3160–9.

37. Cabral DA, Tucker LB. Malignancies in children who initially present with rheumatic complaints. J Pediatr 1999;134(1):53–7.
38. Harvey AR, Pippard MJ, Ansell BM. Microcytic anaemia in juvenile chronic arthritis. Scand J Rheumatol 1987;16(1):53–9.
39. Wittkowski H, Frosch M, Wulffraat N, et al. S100A12 is a novel molecular marker differentiating systemic-onset juvenile idiopathic arthritis from other causes of fever of unknown origin. Arthritis Rheum 2008;58(12):3924–31.
40. Ozdogan H, Kasapçopur O, Dede H, et al. Juvenile chronic arthritis in a Turkish population. Clin Exp Rheumatol 1991;9(4):431–5.
41. Lang BA, Schneider R, Reilly BJ, et al. Radiologic features of systemic onset juvenile rheumatoid arthritis. J Rheumatol 1995;22(1):168–73.
42. Tamashiro MS, Aikawa NE, Campos LM, et al. Discrimination of acute lymphoblastic leukemia from systemic-onset juvenile idiopathic arthritis at disease onset. Clinics (Sao Paulo) 2011;66(10):1665–9.
43. Revesz T, Kardos G, Kajtár P, et al. The adverse effect of prolonged prednisolone pretreatment in children with acute lymphoblastic leukemia. Cancer 1985;55(8):1637–40.
44. Feldman BM, Birdi N, Boone JE, et al. Seasonal onset of systemic-onset juvenile rheumatoid arthritis. J Pediatr 1996;129(4):513–8.
45. Mellins ED, Macaubas C, Grom AA. Pathogenesis of systemic juvenile idiopathic arthritis: some answers, more questions. Nat Rev Rheumatol 2011;7(7):416–26.
46. Pascual V, Allantaz F, Arce E, et al. Role of interleukin-1 (IL-1) in the pathogenesis of systemic onset juvenile idiopathic arthritis and clinical response to IL-1 blockade. J Exp Med 2005;201(9):1479–86.
47. Yokota S, Miyamae T, Imagawa T, et al. Therapeutic efficacy of humanized recombinant anti-interleukin-6 receptor antibody in children with systemic-onset juvenile idiopathic arthritis. Arthritis Rheum 2005;52(3):818–25.
48. Gattorno M, Piccini A, Lasigliè D, et al. The pattern of response to anti-interleukin-1 treatment distinguishes two subsets of patients with systemic-onset juvenile idiopathic arthritis. Arthritis Rheum 2008;58(5):1505–15.
49. Ombrello MJ, Remmers EF, Tachmazidou I, et al. HLA-DRB1*11 and variants of the MHC class II locus are strong risk factors for systemic juvenile idiopathic arthritis. Proc Natl Acad Sci U S A 2015;112(52):15970–5.
50. Ringold S, Weiss PF, Beukelman T, et al. 2013 update of the 2011 American College of Rheumatology recommendations for the treatment of juvenile idiopathic arthritis: recommendations for the medical therapy of children with systemic juvenile idiopathic arthritis and tuberculosis screening among children receiving biologic medications. Arthritis Rheum 2013;65(10):2499–512.
51. Horneff G, Schulz AC, Klotsche J, et al. Experience with etanercept, tocilizumab, and interleukin-1 inhibitors in systemic onset juvenile idiopathic arthritis patients from the BIKER registry. Arthritis Res Ther 2017;19:256.
52. Guzman J, Oen K, Tucker LB, et al. The outcomes of juvenile idiopathic arthritis in children managed with contemporary treatments: results from the ReACCh-Out cohort. Ann Rheum Dis 2015;74(10):1854–60.
53. Quartier P, Allantaz F, Cimaz R, et al. A multicentre, randomised, double-blind, placebo-controlled trial with the interleukin-1 receptor antagonist anakinra in patients with systemic-onset juvenile idiopathic arthritis (ANAJIS trial). Ann Rheum Dis 2011;70(5):747–54.
54. Ruperto N, Brunner HI, Quartier P, et al. Two randomized trials of canakinumab in systemic juvenile idiopathic arthritis. N Engl J Med 2012;367(25):2396–406.

55. Ilowite NT, Prather K, Lokhnygina Y, et al. Randomized, double-blind, placebo-controlled trial of the efficacy and safety of rilonacept in the treatment of systemic juvenile idiopathic arthritis. Arthritis Rheumatol 2014;66(9):2570–9.

56. Yokota S, Imagawa T, Mori M, et al. Efficacy and safety of tocilizumab in patients with systemic-onset juvenile idiopathic arthritis: a randomised, double-blind, placebo-controlled, withdrawal phase III trial. Lancet 2008;371(9617): 998–1006.

57. De Benedetti F, Brunner HI, Ruperto N, et al. Randomized trial of tocilizumab in systemic juvenile idiopathic arthritis. N Engl J Med 2012;367(25):2385–95.

58. Emmenegger U, Frey U, Reimers A, et al. Hyperferritinemia as indicator for intravenous immunoglobulin treatment in reactive macrophage activation syndromes. Am J Hematol 2001;68(1):4–10.

59. Mouy R, Stephan JL, Pillet P, et al. Efficacy of cyclosporine A in the treatment of macrophage activation syndrome in juvenile arthritis: report of five cases. J Pediatr 1996;129(5):750–4.

60. Shakoory B, Carcillo JA, Chatham WW, et al. Interleukin-1 receptor blockade is associated with reduced mortality in sepsis patients with features of the macrophage activation syndrome: re-analysis of a prior phase III trial. Crit Care Med 2016;44(2):275–81.

61. Grom A, Horne A, De Benedetti F, et al. Macrophage activation syndrome in the era of biologic therapy. Nat Rev Rheumatol 2016;12:259–68.

62. Erguven M, Guven S, Okumus O. Growth in Juvenile idiopathic arthritis. In: Preedy VR, editor. Handbook of growth and growth monitoring in health and disease. New York: Springer New York; 2012. p. 1959–75.

63. Guzman J, Kerr T, Ward LM, et al. Growth and weight gain in children with juvenile idiopathic arthritis: results from the ReACCh-Out cohort. Pediatr Rheumatol Online J 2017;15(1):68.

64. Simon D, Fernando C, Czernichow P, et al. Linear growth and final height in patients with systemic juvenile idiopathic arthritis treated with long-term glucocorticoids. J Rheumatol 2002;29(6):1296–300.

65. De Benedetti F, Brunner H, Ruperto N, et al. Catch-up growth during tocilizumab therapy for systemic juvenile idiopathic arthritis: results from a phase III trial. Arthritis Rheumatol 2015;67(3):840–8.

66. American Academy of Pediatrics Section on Rheumatology and Section on Ophthalmology: guidelines for ophthalmologic examinations in children with juvenile rheumatoid arthritis. Pediatrics 1993;92(2):295.

67. Shaw KL, Southwood TR, Duffy CM, et al. Health-related quality of life in adolescents with juvenile idiopathic arthritis. Arthritis Rheum 2006;55(2):199–207.

68. Barth S, Haas JP, Schlichtiger J, et al. Long-term health-related quality of life in German patients with juvenile idiopathic arthritis in comparison to German general population. PLoS One 2016;11(4):e0153267.

69. Gutierrez-Suarez R, Pistorio A, Cespedes Cruz A, et al. Health-related quality of life of patients with juvenile idiopathic arthritis coming from 3 different geographic areas. The PRINTO multinational quality of life cohort study. Rheumatology (Oxford) 2007;46(2):314–20.

70. Lomater C, Gerloni V, Gattinara M, et al. Systemic onset juvenile idiopathic arthritis: a retrospective study of 80 consecutive patients followed for 10 years. J Rheumatol 2000;27(2):491–6.

71. Singh-Grewal D, Schneider R, Bayer N, et al. Predictors of disease course and remission in systemic juvenile idiopathic arthritis: significance of early clinical and laboratory features. Arthritis Rheum 2006;54(5):1595–601.

72. Martini A. It is time to rethink juvenile idiopathic arthritis classification and nomenclature. Ann Rheum Dis 2012;71(9):1437–9.
73. Bowyer SL, Roettcher PA, Higgins GC, et al. Health status of patients with juvenile rheumatoid arthritis at 1 and 5 years after diagnosis. J Rheumatol 2003;30(2):394.
74. Foster HE, Marshall N, Myers A, et al. Outcome in adults with juvenile idiopathic arthritis: a quality of life study. Arthritis Rheum 2003;48(3):767–75.
75. Nigrovic PA. Review: is there a window of opportunity for treatment of systemic juvenile idiopathic arthritis? Arthritis Rheumatol 2014;66(6):1405–13.
76. Spiegel LR, Schneider R, Lang BA, et al. Early predictors of poor functional outcome in systemic-onset juvenile rheumatoid arthritis: a multicenter cohort study. Arthritis Rheum 2000;43(11):2402–9.
77. Russo RA, Katsicas MM. Patients with very early-onset systemic juvenile idiopathic arthritis exhibit more inflammatory features and a worse outcome. J Rheumatol 2013;40(3):329–34.
78. Hashkes PJ, Wright BM, Lauer MS, et al. Mortality outcomes in pediatric rheumatology in the US. Arthritis Rheum 2010;62(2):599–608.
79. Stoeber E. Prognosis in juvenile chronic arthritis. Follow-up of 433 chronic rheumatic children. Eur J Pediatr 1981;135(3):225–8.
80. French AR, Mason T, Nelson AM, et al. Increased mortality in adults with a history of juvenile rheumatoid arthritis: a population-based study. Arthritis Rheum 2001;44(3):523–7.
81. Wallace CA, Levinson JE. Juvenile rheumatoid arthritis: outcome and treatment for the 1990s. Rheum Dis Clin North Am 1991;17(4):891–905.
82. Youngstein T-B, Lane T, Gilbertson J, et al. THU0076 disease-modifying treatment regimens have been insufficient to reduce the incidence of systemic aa amyloidosis associated with rheumatoid arthritis in contrast to a significant reduction in those with juvenile idiopathic arthritis. Ann Rheum Dis 2017;76(Suppl 2):227.
83. Immonen K, Savolainen HA, Hakala M. Why can we no longer find juvenile idiopathic arthritis-associated amyloidosis in childhood or in adolescence in Finland? Scand J Rheumatol 2007;36(5):402–3.

Systemic Lupus Erythematosus, Sjögren Syndrome, and Mixed Connective Tissue Disease in Children and Adolescents

Stacey E. Tarvin, MD, MS, Kathleen M. O'Neil, MD*

KEYWORDS

- Juvenile systemic lupus erythematosus • Juvenile mixed connective tissue disease
- Juvenile Sjögren syndrome • Autoantibodies • Lupus nephritis
- Antinuclear antibodies

KEY POINTS

- Juvenile systemic lupus erythematosus (jSLE) is a multisystem inflammatory disease with autoantibodies to nuclear antigens and complement consumption. It causes rapidly progressive damage if not recognized and treated promptly.
- Juvenile mixed connective tissue disease (jMCTD) presents with features similar to jSLE, with higher likelihood of prominent Raynaud phenomenon and high antibodies to ribonucleoprotein. Many children develop systemic scleroderma features over time.
- Juvenile Sjögren syndrome (jSS) usually presents with recurrent sialadenitis and causes dry eyes and mouth, arthralgia, arthritis, and systemic symptoms. Rarely it predisposes to lymphoma.
- Outcomes for jSLE, jMCTD, and jSS depend on early recognition and referral to rheumatology and other specialists depending on the organ system affected. Treatments involve control of inflammation and autoimmunity to minimize the risk for morbidity and mortality.

INTRODUCTION

Systemic lupus erythematous (SLE), mixed connective tissue disease (MCTD), and Sjögren syndrome (SS) are lifelong autoimmune diseases that present special challenges in the pediatric population because they are rare (<1 in 2000 children), and often associated with severe morbidity including mortality. These diseases are characterized by immune dysregulation and chronic multisystem inflammation

Disclosure: The authors have no relevant disclosures.
Division of Rheumatology, Department of Pediatrics, University of Indiana School of Medicine, Riley Hospital for Children at Indiana University Health, 699 Riley Hospital Drive, Riley Research 307, Indianapolis, IN 46202, USA
* Corresponding author.
E-mail address: kmoneil@iu.edu

Pediatr Clin N Am 65 (2018) 711–737
https://doi.org/10.1016/j.pcl.2018.04.001
0031-3955/18/© 2018 Elsevier Inc. All rights reserved.

pediatric.theclinics.com

leading to a myriad of clinical features of varying severity. Optimal care requires ongoing evaluation and management by a pediatric rheumatologist. This article discusses common disease characteristics, provides an overview of diagnosis and principles of treatment, outlines common mechanisms in pathogenesis, and highlights distinctions between juvenile SLE (jSLE), juvenile MCTD (jMCTD), and juvenile SS (jSS).

INCIDENCE AND PREVALENCE OF JUVENILE SYSTEMIC LUPUS ERYTHEMATOUS, JUVENILE MIXED CONNECTIVE TISSUE DISEASE, AND JUVENILE SJÖGREN SYNDROME

Children account for 20% of all cases of SLE.[1]

- SLE yearly incidence: 2.22 per 100,000 children in the United States.[2]
- SLE prevalence: 9.73 per 100,000 children ages 3 to 18 years.[2]
- jMCTD and jSS incidence and prevalence are not known. Based on small case series, MCTD is approximately 5-fold to 10-fold less common than jSLE, and jSS is less common still.[3,4]

DEMOGRAPHICS
Age

- jSLE mean age of diagnosis is 13 years.[5]
- jMCTD mean age of diagnosis is 13 years[3]
- jSS: median age at diagnosis is 10 years.[4]

Gender

- jSLE female/male ratio is 4:3 before age 10 years, increasing to 9:1 at puberty.[2]
- jMCTD and jSS: female predominance, similar to jSLE

Race and Ethnicity

- jSLE higher incidence rate in children of African, Asian, or Native American descent; these genetic groups also have high severity.[6]
- jMCTD and jSS: not known.

MAJOR DIFFERENCES FROM ADULT DISEASE

Compared with adults with SLE, children generally have more aggressive disease and worse outcomes.[7] Onset in childhood carries a higher risk of nephritis, malar rash, anti–double-stranded DNA (anti-dsDNA) antibodies, and hemolytic anemia compared with adults with SLE.[8] Pulmonary hypertension, a common cause of morbidity and death in adults with MCTD, is rarer and less severe in children with jMCTD.[9] Children with jSS present with recurrent parotitis and less commonly with sicca symptoms, although adults are more likely to have sicca symptoms.[4,10]

DELAYS IN DIAGNOSIS ARE COMMON FOR JUVENILE MIXED CONNECTIVE TISSUE DISEASE AND JUVENILE SJÖGREN SYNDROME

jMCTD can confuse diagnosticians because symptoms change during the development of the disease.[9] However, data on time to diagnosis are not known. The diagnosis of jSS is often delayed (mean, 3 years). The swelling of cheeks and lymph nodes in jSS are often attributed to obstructive sialadenitis or infection until recurrences happen. The autoantibodies associated with jSS, anti–Sjögren syndrome A (anti-SSA) (Ro) and anti–Sjögren syndrome B (anti-SSB) (La), are often detectable before overt glandular dysfunction is detected.[11,12]

WHEN TO CONSIDER JUVENILE SYSTEMIC LUPUS ERYTHEMATOUS, JUVENILE MIXED CONNECTIVE TISSUE DISEASE, OR JUVENILE SJÖGREN SYNDROME

These diseases should be considered in adolescent girls with complaints in several organ systems, as outlined in **Table 1**. Fatigue and malaise are common to all 3 diseases, with other symptoms shared to varying degrees. Adolescents with jSLE often have a malar rash (**Fig. 1**), oral ulcers (**Fig. 2**), joint swelling and tenderness, muscle pain with proximal weakness, fatigue, and sometimes fever and weight loss.

Patients with jMCTD, more than jSLE or jSS, present with cool and dusky extremities, with digits that may blanch and turn purple with cold exposure, then turn red and tingle on rewarming (Raynaud phenomenon). Adolescents with jMCTD may also have arthralgia or arthritis, diffusely puffy hands (**Fig. 3**), vasculitic rashes, proximal muscle pain, and weakness.[3,13] Over time, sclerodermalike manifestations often become prominent in jMCTD.

Children with jSS may have persistent lymphadenopathy with dry eyes and mouth, and visible parotid gland enlargement (**Fig. 4**); these symptoms and findings are also seen in children with jSLE.

Table 1
Features of Juvenile systemic lupus erythematosus, mixed connective tissue disease, and Sjögren syndrome

Features of the Diseases	jSLE	jMCTD	jSS
Fatigue, malaise	+++	+++	+++
Rash	++++	+++	+/−
Lymphadenopathy	++	+/−	+++
Raynaud phenomenon	+++	++++	+
Arthralgia/arthritis	+++	++++	++
Oral ulcers	+++	+	+/−
Myalgia/myositis	++	++++	+
Cytopenias	+++	++	+/−
Neurologic disease	+++	+	+++
Glomerulonephritis	+++	+/−	+/−
Pulmonary disease	+	+++	+/−
Autoantibodies (High vs Low Titers)			
ANA	++++	++++	++
Anti-dsDNA	+++	+/−	−
Anti-RNP	+/− early	++++	−
Anti-Sm	+++	−	−
Anti-SSA/SSB	++	+/−	+++
Major morbidity and complications	Kidney disease, central nervous system damage, rash, arthritis, oral ulcers, antiphospholipid syndrome, infection, early atherosclerosis	33% in remission at 16 y, most still need medication. 5% mortality (from infection, lung disease, pulmonary hypertension)[71]	Lymphoma is a rare complication in childhood; corneal abrasions; dental caries

Abbreviations: ANA, antinuclear antibody; dsDNA, double-stranded DNA; RNP, ribonucleoprotein; SSA, Sjögren syndrome A; SSB, Sjögren syndrome B.

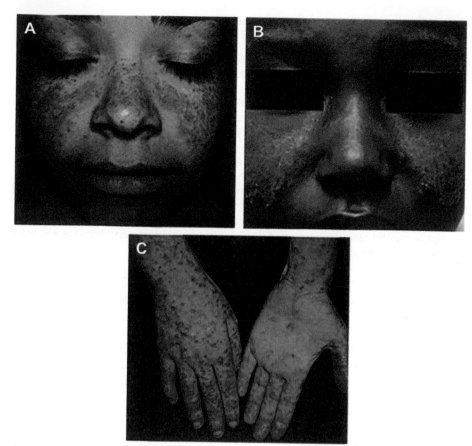

Fig. 1. Common rashes in juvenile systemic lupus erythematosus. (*A*) Malar rash, common in jSLE, is fixed erythema in a butterfly distribution across the malar eminences sparing naso-labial folds. It is often brought on by sun exposure. (*B*) Discoid rash has deeper dermal inflammation. It can cause follicular plugging, dyspigmentation, and scarring. (*C*) Maculo-papular rash with palmar erythema. Note the palmar thinning, wrinkling, and punctate areas of atrophy. (*Data from* Kristal L, Prose N. Weinberg's color atlas of pediatric derma-tology, 5e. New York: McGraw-Hill Education; 2016; with permission.)

Clinical Presentations

There are no validated diagnostic criteria for jSLE, jMCTD, and jSS. Classification criteria for research purposes exist and have been validated in adults.[14]

SLE classification criteria are summarized in **Table 2** and help clinicians understand the disease spectrum. The certainty of the diagnosis of SLE increases with the number of classification criteria identified, but experienced clinicians diagnose and initiate treatment of SLE before some patients fulfill these criteria. For example, some children have no other criteria for diagnosis than lupus nephritis, but begin standard lupus nephritis treatment.[14,15] For pediatric practitioners, a practical approach in consid-ering referral for possible jSLE is to identify 2 or more symptoms or manifestations from the 3 major subgroups of features in either classification scheme, then look for supporting laboratory features. These major subgroups are (1) mucocutaneous find-ings, (2) inflammatory conditions of organs and tissues (so-called organitis), and (3) laboratory abnormalities (see **Table 2**). Clues from the history and physical

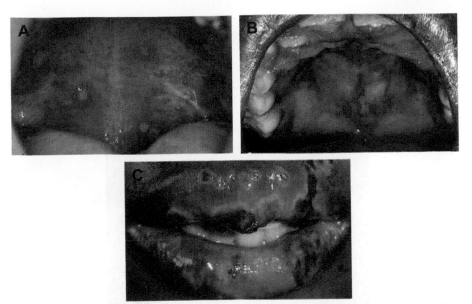

Fig. 2. Oral ulceration in juvenile systemic lupus erythematosus. (*A*) Aphthae that often involve the palate with superficial erosion. (*B*) Deeper, more chronic palatal ulceration of the hard palate in a child with jSLE. The ischemic ulceration typical of a patient with jSLE with antiphospholipid antibodies may be painless; the denuded areas of mucosa tend to be very painful. (*C*) Ulceration of the lips and buccal mucosa in a child with lupus. This extensive mucosal ulceration can make oral alimentation impossible. (*Reproduced from* Rodsaward P, Prueksrisakul T, Deekajorndech T, et al. Oral ulcers in juvenile-onset systemic lupus erythematosus: A review of the literature. Am J Clin Dermatol 2017;18:758.)

examination are essential to an appropriate laboratory investigation and timely referral to a pediatric rheumatologist.

Malar rash and arthritis are seen in more than 60% of children with jSLE at diagnosis. The typical butterfly rash is nonpruritic, nonscarring, fixed erythema that crosses the

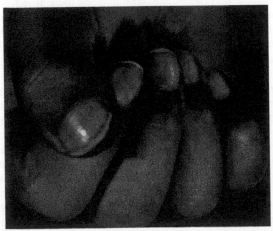

Fig. 3. Diffuse finger and hand swelling of jMCTD. This child cannot make a fist, as shown. Diffuse nonpitting edema of soft tissues and tendon sheaths with or without synovitis is characteristic of jMCTD. (*From* Deepak S, Warrier KC. Mixed connective disease in children – a case series. Rheumatol Orthop Med 2017;2(2):4; with permission.)

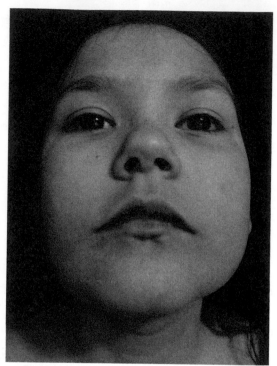

Fig. 4. Recurrent sialadenitis in jSS. This 8-year-old girl has lymphadenopathy and the recurrent parotitis and painful swelling of submandibular salivary glands seen in jSS. Antibody to SSA and sometimes SSB nuclear antigen (Ro and La) is a frequent finding in jSS.

nasal bridge and spares the nasolabial folds (see **Fig. 1**A). Discoid rash scars and is less common (see **Fig. 1**B). Photosensitivity is common. Nonscarring alopecia occurs occasionally. If jSLE is suspected, special attention should also be given to the musculoskeletal, cardiac, pulmonary, and neurologic examinations (**Box 1**).

Joint pain is one of the most common complaints in adults and children with lupus. Warmth, effusions, limited motion, and pain with motion help confirm arthritis, rather than arthralgia. Malar rash, antiribonucleoprotein (anti-RNP) antibodies, anemia, and thrombocytopenia are all findings associated with arthritis in jSLE.[16] Rheumatoid factor–positive erosive arthritis occurs in 12% of patients with jSLE.[17]

Renal disease may bring a child to medical attention, with oliguria; fluid overload; hypertensive headache; or red, foamy, or tea-colored urine. Seventy percent of patients with jSLE develop lupus nephritis.[18] If not detected early, renal damage can lead to dialysis or death within days to weeks.

Serositis is the most common cardiopulmonary presentation of jSLE: 30% of patients with jSLE have pleuritis or pericarditis.[19] Findings of tachycardia, tachypnea, pericardial friction rub, diminished basal breath sounds, and dullness to percussion may be clues. Any portion of the heart or lungs may be affected by lupus. Screening pulmonary function tests help assess for interstitial lung disease, and echocardiography tests for structural cardiac changes or signs of pulmonary hypertension. Up to one-third of patients with jSLE display rhythm or conduction abnormalities on electrocardiography.[19]

The spectrum of neurologic findings in jSLE spans from headache to cognitive changes to seizures and stroke. Some neurologic manifestation is seen at diagnosis in 11% of jSLE, and another 16% develop neurologic symptoms within the first

Table 2
American College of Rheumatology and Systemic Lupus International Collaborating Clinics classification criteria for systemic lupus erythematosus

ACR Criteria (4 of 11 Needed)	Description	SLICC Criteria (4 of 17 Needed Including ≥1 Clinical and ≥1 Immunologic)	Description
Mucocutaneous Features (4 Criteria)			
Malar rash	Fixed erythema over malar eminences tending to spare nasolabial folds	Acute cutaneous lupus	Lupus malar rash (do not count if discoid rash in malar distribution); bullous lupus; toxic epidermal necrolysis of SLE; maculopapular lupus rash; photosensitive lupus rash[a]
Photosensitivity	Persistent rash caused by sun exposure		
Discoid rash	Erythematous raised patches, scaling and follicular plugging, atrophic scarring, and dyspigmentation may occur	Chronic cutaneous lupus	Discoid rash; localized (head & neck); generalized (above and below neck); hypertrophic (verrucous) lupus; lupus panniculitis (profundus); mucosal lupus; lupus erythematosus tumidus; chilblain lupus; or discoid lupus/lichen planus overlap
		Non-scarring alopecia	Diffuse thinning or visible broken hairs[a]
Oral ulcers	Oral or nasopharyngeal ulcers, usually painless, observed by a clinician	Oral ulcers[a]	Ulcers of palate, tongue, buccal mucosa, or nasal ulcers[a]
Inflammatory Disorders of Organs or Tissues (4 Criteria)			
Serositis	Pleuritis or pericarditis	Serositis	Pleurisy for >1 d, pleural effusion, or pleural rub Pericardial pain for >1 d, pericardial rub or effusion, or pericarditis by EKG[a]
Arthritis (joint inflammation)	Nonerosive arthritis with tenderness, swelling, or effusion in ≥2 peripheral joints	Joint disease	Synovitis of ≥2 joints with swelling or joint effusion OR Tenderness of ≥2 joints and ≥30 min of morning stiffness

(continued on next page)

Table 2
(continued)

ACR Criteria (4 of 11 Needed)	Description	SLICC Criteria (4 of 17 Needed Including ≥1 Clinical and ≥1 Immunologic)	Description
Renal disorder (nephritis)	Persistent proteinuria >500 mg/24 h or >3+ OR Cellular casts: red blood cells, hemoglobin, granular, tubular, or mixed	Renal disease	Urine protein to creatinine ratio >0.2, or 24-h urine protein ≥500 mg/24 h OR Red blood cell casts
Neurologic disorder[a]	Seizures OR Psychosis[a]	Neurologic disease[a]	Seizures, psychosis, mononeuritis multiplex, myelitis, peripheral or cranial neuropathy OR Acute confusional state[a]
Hematologic disorder			
Hemolytic anemia OR	With reticulocytosis	Hemolytic anemia	Hemolytic anemia
Leukopenia OR	<4000/mm³ on ≥2 occasions	Leukopenia OR	Leukopenia: WBC<4000/mm³ OR
Lymphopenia OR	<1000/mm³	Lymphopenia[a]	Lymphopenia (<1000/mm³) ≥once[a]
Immune thrombocytopenia	<100,000/mm³	Thrombocytopenia[a]	Thrombocytopenia (<100,000/mm³) ≥ once[a]
Immunologic Abnormality[a] (any of)		*Immunologic Criteria*	
dsDNA antibody OR	Antibody to native DNA in abnormal titer	Anti-dsDNA	Anti-dsDNA antibody above reference range (or >2-fold the laboratory reference range if performed by ELISA)
Sm antibody OR	Antibody to Sm nuclear antigen	Anti-Sm antibody	Presence of antibody to Sm nuclear antigen
Antiphospholipid antibody	Positive test for lupus anticoagulant OR False-positive test for RPR OR Anticardiolipin or anti–beta-2 glycoprotein I antibody (IgA, IgG, or	Antiphospholipid antibody	Antiphospholipid antibody determined by any of the following: • Positive lupus anticoagulant • False-positive RPR • Medium- or high-titer anticardiolipin antibody (IgA, IgG, or IgM)

(continued on next page)

Table 2
(continued)

ACR Criteria (4 of 11 Needed)	Description	SLICC Criteria (4 of 17 Needed Including ≥1 Clinical and ≥1 Immunologic)	Description
	IgM) of medium or high titer		• Anti–beta-2 glycoprotein I (IgA, IgG, or IgM)
		Low complement	Low C3 low C4 low CH50
ANA	ANA titer > normal range for laboratory by immuno-fluorescence or equivalent assay	ANA	ANA above laboratory reference range
		Direct Coombs test	Direct Coombs test in the absence of hemolytic anemia

Abbreviations: ACR, American College of Rheumatology; C3, complement component 3; C4, complement component 4; CH50, 50% hemolytic complement activity; EKG, electrocardiogram; ELISA, enzyme-linked immunosorbent assay; IgA, immunoglobulin A; IgG, immunoglobulin G; IgM, immunoglobulin M; RPR, rapid plasma reagin; SLE, systemic lupus erythematosus; SLICC, Systemic Lupus International Collaborating Clinics; WBC, white blood cell count.

ᵃ In the absence of other causes.
Data from Refs.[14,15,76]

Box 1
The physical examination in suspected juvenile systemic lupus erythematosus, juvenile mixed connective tissue disease, and juvenile Sjögren syndrome

- Blood pressure: in jSLE, hypertension may signal glomerulonephritis

- Growth parameters: weight loss and stalled linear growth are common in all 3 diseases; sudden weight gain may be fluid retention in jSLE nephritis

- Skin and membrane examination: Rashes – in jSLE, malar, discoid, or other fixed rash especially in sun-exposed areas; alopecia or vitiligo; oral ulcers. In jSLE and jMCTD poor perfusion – Raynaud phenomenon, digital ischemia, ulcers or scarring, delayed capillary refill; tortuous or thrombosed periungual capillaries

- Salivary and lacrimal gland enlargement, dry mucous membranes: seen in jSS>jSLE, jMCTD

- Lymphatic examination: generalized adenopathy seen in any of the diseases

- Heart and lungs: In all of these diseases, tachypnea, tachycardia, heart murmurs, pleural or pericardial rubs may signal pleuritis, pericarditis, valvulitis, heart failure, interstitial pneumonitis, or pulmonary hypertension

- Abdomen: hyperactive bowel sounds (enterocolitis), hepatomegaly, splenomegaly, tenderness (jSLE, jMCTD>jSS)

- Genitourinary: delayed puberty in jSLE, jSS, jMCTD; enlarged kidneys in lupus nephritis

- Extremities: in all diseases, joint swelling, effusion, tenderness, limited range of motion (arthritis); impaired digital perfusion, muscle wasting, muscle tenderness, peripheral edema if renal disease; diffuse non-pitting hand swelling in jSS

- Neurologic: altered mental status; signs of slow processing or dyscalculia; sensory examination for stroke (jSLE) or peripheral neuropathy (jSS>jSLE and jMCTD); muscle power for proximal weakness (jMCTD>jSLE); rapid alternating movements (jSLE)

year.[20] If lupus is suspected, a full neurologic examination should be performed with attention to higher cortical function: memory, complex problem solving, serial 7 recall, and coordination. Patients with neuropsychiatric symptoms often have dyscalculia, dysdiadochokinesis, and past-pointing. It is important to ask about changes in academic performance, hallucinations, and personality change. If a neurologic deficit is identified, evaluation may require imaging, electroencephalogram, and/or neurocognitive evaluation.

Other key presentations that should prompt astute primary care providers to consider lupus as a diagnosis are outlined in **Box 2**. jSLE may present as recurrent pancreatitis,[21] chronic/recurrent immune cytopenias such as immune thrombocytopenic purpura,[22] autoimmune hemolytic anemia, or Evans syndrome.[23–25]

Juvenile mixed connective tissue disease

jMCTD is a distinct disease rather than an undifferentiated rheumatic condition.[26] Classification criteria in adults,[27] although not rigorously validated in children, are used for jMCTD.[28,29] The criteria require either Raynaud phenomenon or swollen hands or fingers, plus high-titer anti-U1 RNP antibody and at least 1 sign from at least 2 of the following diseases: SLE, systemic sclerosis, or polymyositis.[27] Early manifestations include polyarthritis, Raynaud phenomenon, diffuse hand swelling (see **Fig. 3**), muscle inflammation, swallowing difficulty, and systemic symptoms (fever, fatigue, and malaise).[13] Sclerodactyly often follows diffuse finger swelling.[3] Over time, the disease may involve pulmonary, renal, cardiac, gastrointestinal, and neurologic manifestations. See **Box 1** for physical examination clues for jMCTD.

Juvenile Sjögren syndrome

SS is seen occasionally in children with SLE, but it also is a distinct autoimmune disease. The classification criteria for adult SS are a points-based system requiring at

---

Box 2
Key presentations that suggest juvenile systemic lupus erythematosus

- Chronic idiopathic immune thrombocytopenia, autoimmune hemolytic anemia
- Evans syndrome (autoimmune destruction of white blood cells, red blood cells, platelets)
- Pancreatitis, especially if recurrent
- Unexplained fever with high total protein but low albumin levels
- Insidious weight loss + generalized lymphadenopathy
- Proximal, symmetric muscle weakness and mildly increased muscle enzyme levels (aspartate transaminase, creatine kinase, lactate dehydrogenase)
- Arthritis of hands with prominent effusions

Disorders that could suggest SLE but are likely benign if in isolation; other possible causes in parentheses.

- Raynaud phenomenon (thin teens, stimulant medications, others)
- Hair thinning without patches of alopecia (nutritional problems, hypothyroidism, hair treatments)
- Arthralgia without joint swelling (chondromalacia patellae, hypermobility syndrome, pes planus)
- Antinuclear antibody without multisystem inflammation (normal child, family history of rheumatic disease, recent viral infection, Epstein-Barr virus)

least 4 points. Three points each are given for anti-SSA antibody and focal lympho-cytic sialadenitis, and 1 point each for low salivary flow, low tear secretion, or corneal lesions from dry eye.[30] More study is needed to evaluate criteria for these children, because only 8% of children with jSS present with traditional sicca symptoms; instead most (62%) present with parotitis.[4,10] Other common problems include arthralgia (23%), renal disease (12%), neurologic symptoms (12%), and rash (4%). In long-standing jSS, the most common clinical features were sicca symptoms (47%) and arthralgia or arthritis (36%), followed by fevers (18%). Lymphadenopathy, fatigue, rash, renal disease, neurologic complaints, Raynaud symptoms, myalgia, increased hepatic enzyme levels, or complete blood count (CBC) abnormalities were uncommon (see **Table 1**). Sicca syndrome can lead to recurrent dental caries, dysphagia, cheek swelling, and corneal abrasions. See **Box 1** for physical examination clues for jSS; the disease can be subtle so clinicians must maintain a high index of suspicion for jSS.

UNCOMMON BUT IMPORTANT JUVENILE SYSTEMIC LUPUS ERYTHEMATOUS MANIFESTATIONS
Antiphospholipid Antibody Syndrome

Autoantibodies directed against phospholipids (antiphospholipid antibodies [APL]) can trigger intravascular thrombosis and severe ischemic manifestations of jSLE. In jSLE, symptoms can range from poor skin perfusion causing livedo reticularis (**Fig. 5**) to limb or organ necrosis, to major vessel thrombosis and stroke. In jSLE, anti-phospholipid antibodies are associated with a 3-fold risk of irreversible organ damage.[31] Vascular events are more likely to happen in the face of infection or severe systemic inflammation, and treatment requires control of the inflammation and long-term anticoagulation. It is critical that antiphospholipid antibody syndrome (APS) be recognized rapidly, to preserve organ function and prevent mortality.

Macrophage Activation Syndrome

Macrophage activation syndrome (MAS) occurs in patients with very active jSLE.[31,32] MAS is discussed in detail in Jennifer J.Y. Lee and Rayfel Schneider's article, "Systemic Juvenile

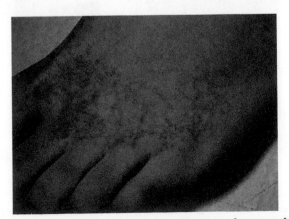

Fig. 5. Livedo reticularis. The characteristic lacy cyanotic areas of poor perfusion can be seen in jSLE and related autoimmune inflammatory disease, and when present should prompt testing for antiphospholipid antibodies. There is a risk of major arterial or venous throm-bosis in these children. (*Reprinted from* Avcin T, O'Neil KM. Antiphospholipid syndrome. In: Cassidy JT, Petty RE, Laxer RM, et al, editors. Textbook of pediatric rheumatology. 7th edition. Philadelphia: Elsevier; 2011. p. 344–60; with permission.)

Idiopathic Arthritis (JIA)," in this issue. Compared with MAS in systemic juvenile idiopathic arthritis, central nervous system (CNS) complications and hyponatremia were seen more commonly in jSLE-related MAS.[32] In children with active SLE, unexplained fever, cytopenia, and hyperferritinemia should prompt further investigation into MAS.[33] As in systemic juvenile idiopathic arthritis, it can be rapidly progressive and carries a high mortality.

Neonatal Lupus Erythematosus

Rarely, a lupus rash (**Fig. 6**) in a newborn, neonatal thrombocytopenia, or congenital heart block may indicate previously unsuspected maternal autoimmune disease. Antibodies to SSA, or Ro60, cause the rash and variable injury to cardiac intraventricular Purkinje fibers. This condition can cause intrauterine heart failure (hydrops fetalis) and sometimes fetal demise. Complete conduction block from NLE is irreversible by the time it is detected, and a permanent pacemaker is required. Mothers may be asymptomatic, may have overt SLE, or may have sicca symptoms of SS. Autoantibodies to platelets can cause profound neonatal thrombocytopenia.[34] Increased serum aminotransferase levels in an infant represent an autoimmune hepatitis.[35] The rash usually begins shortly after birth and can take several months to resolve. As maternal autoantibody is cleared from the infant's body, most manifestations resolve, except heart block. Neonatal lupus erythematosus (NLE) can recur in subsequent pregnancies.[36] A recent review summarizes the important progress in understanding the pathophysiology of this rare disease.[37]

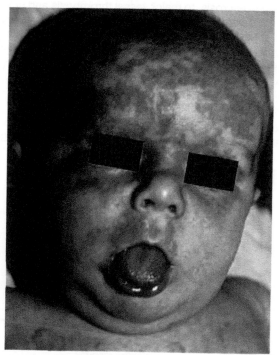

Fig. 6. Neonatal lupus. Infants born to women with high-titer SSA antibody (most of whom have SLE or SS) may develop the neonatal lupus syndrome. Photosensitive annular rash is a common manifestation; heart block may be severe because of antibody to Ro60 (SSA) reacting to fetal conducting system cells. Thrombocytopenia, liver disease, and other systemic manifestations are less frequent features of the neonatal lupus syndrome. (*Reprinted from* Buyon JP, Lindsley CB, Silverman ED. Antiphospholipid syndrome. In: Cassidy JT, Petty RE, Laxer RM, et al, editors. Textbook of pediatric rheumatology. 7th edition. Philadelphia: Elsevier; 2011; with permission.)

DIFFERENTIAL DIAGNOSIS AND MIMICS

The most common misleading situation that makes clinicians consider jSLE is an adolescent with pain near many joints but localizing to muscles. The child may have disordered sleep, may have recovered from infectious mononucleosis, or may spend hours bent over an electronic device in an inefficient posture. Depression and/or anxiety are often present and disguised as a pain syndrome. This condition may be the prodrome of fibromyalgia. The root issues of stress, depression, physical inactivity, and sleep disorder must be addressed for a return to health (see Jennifer E. Weiss and Jennifer N. Stinson's article, "Pediatric Pain Syndromes and Noninflammayory Musculoskeletal Pain," in this issue.). Particularly following infection with Epstein-Barr virus, antinuclear antibodies (ANAs) may be present, but complement proteins are normal in serum and other markers of inflammation are absent.

The differential diagnosis of jSLE includes jMCTD, and patients with jSLE may also have SS with sialadenitis and sicca symptoms. Serology and phenotype help distinguish among these 3 autoimmune diseases (see **Table 1**). jMCTD has overlapping features with juvenile idiopathic arthritis, dermatomyositis, and, over time, systemic scleroderma, so distinguishing it from other rheumatic conditions depends on laboratory findings.[3]

Other diseases in the differential for jSLE, jMCTD, and jSS include sarcoidosis and malignancy. Sarcoidosis can present with arthritis, adenopathy, and sialadenitis, but pulmonary nodules or granulomatous interstitial lung disease and high serum angiotensin converting enzyme levels distinguish this diagnosis. Childhood leukemias and lymphomas can have very similar presentation to these autoimmune diseases, and a bone marrow examination may be needed.

Many other diseases are in the differential for jSLE, with an extensive differential list included in the 2012 *Pediatric Clinics of North America* jSLE review.[18] In patients with evidence of nephritis, another glomerulonephritic condition may be the cause. Given the huge variety of symptoms that may be associated with lupus, other autoimmune disorders and immunodeficiency should be considered. Inappropriate vascular thrombosis without other evidence of jSLE may represent the primary antiphospholipid syndrome. Thrombocytopenia in jSLE resembles idiopathic thrombocytopenic purpura, consumptive coagulopathy (eg, thrombotic thrombocytopenic purpura), primary antiphospholipid syndrome, or malignancy. Primary immunodeficiency diseases may share features of jSLE, although nephritis is not typically seen. Recurrent, severe, or unusual infections and abnormal quantitative immunoglobulins help make that diagnosis.

PATHOGENESIS OF JUVENILE SYSTEMIC LUPUS ERYTHEMATOUS, JUVENILE MIXED CONNECTIVE TISSUE DISEASE, JUVENILE SJÖGREN SYNDROME

jSLE, jMCTD, and jSS are considered autoimmune diseases because of prominent autoantibody formation and altered lymphocyte populations and activation states, and their association with genes in the major histocompatibility complex on chromosome 6 that regulate immune responses (see Kathleen E. Sullivan's article, "Pathogenesis of Pediatric Rheumatologic Diseases," in this issue.). Different human leukocyte antigen genotypes are associated with MCTD than with SLE.[38] The concordance rate of identical twins for jSLE is approximately 30%, supporting the role of genetics in lupus. First-degree relatives have a 5% risk of developing the disease.[39] In these diseases, inappropriate activation of humoral, cell-mediated, and complement pathways cause chronic inflammation and organ damage.[40] Patients have circulating autoantibodies to nuclear constituents, including small nuclear RNA-binding proteins (SSA, SSB, anti-Sm, RNP) in jSLE, RNP in jMCTD, and SSA/SSB in jSS.[41] A constant barrage of autoantibodies reacting with autoantigens produces immune complexes, complement activation, dysregulation of type I interferon (interferon alpha), inflammatory cytokine production, disruption of cellular life cycle, altered differentiation and immune cell development, and abnormal tumor suppression.[42,43]

Increasingly, scientists are recognizing the importance of the innate immune system (neutrophils, receptors for danger signals like Toll-like receptors that trigger inflammation following activation by lipopolysaccharides, nucleic acids and glycans, the complement, coagulation, and kinin cascades, and type I interferons) in mediating the inflammation and autoantibody formation seen in these diseases (**Fig. 7**). It now seems that abnormalities in innate immunity are at least as important to the pathogenesis of jSLE and related conditions as are abnormalities of lymphocyte function.

LABORATORY AND IMAGING STUDIES FOR DIAGNOSIS AND CARE

There is no single laboratory test that identifies jSLE, jMCTD, or jSS, but laboratory abnormalities are common. More than 50% of patients with jSLE present with hematologic abnormalities, especially thrombocytopenia, lymphopenia, or Coombs-positive hemolytic anemia; 37% of patients with jSLE present with evidence of glomerulonephritis.[5,44,45] The initial laboratory evaluation (**Box 3**) should include a CBC with differential and platelets evaluating for cytopenias; lymphopenia (<1000/mm^3) is common,

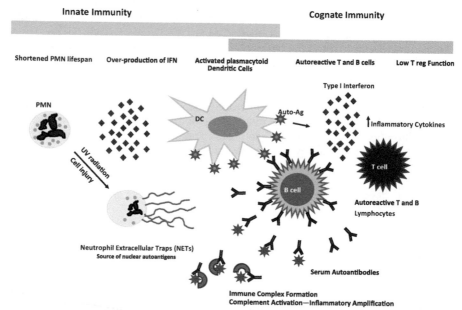

Fig. 7. Pathogenesis of the autoimmune and inflammatory diseases jSLE, jMCTD, and jSS. This cartoon represents some of the complex interactions between mechanisms involved in inflammation and the autoimmunity that is seen in these diseases. The primary defects in these diseases are not yet certain. However, complex interactions between the innate immune system (intrinsic host defense based on pattern recognition, not specific antigens) initiate inflammation and trigger the antigen-specific or cognate immune responses (represented by T cells, B cells, and antibodies), making these diseases a complex blend of autoimmune and autoinflammatory disorders. Auto-Ag, autoantigen; DC, dendritic cell; PMN, polymorphonuclear neutrophil; T reg, T regulatory cell; UV, ultraviolet.

Box 3
Screening laboratory tests for juvenile systemic lupus erythematosus

Complete blood count with differential and platelets
Comprehensive metabolic profile
Urinalysis with spot first morning urine protein to creatinine ratio
Screening complement studies (C3 and C4)
Antinuclear antibody titer
Anti-dsDNA antibody titer

---

particularly in jSLE. A comprehensive metabolic profile and urinalysis with microscopic examination may identify proteinuria, blood, or casts indicating lupus nephritis, but these may be seen in jMCTD as well. The chemistry profile can show high total protein level with low albumin level, implying high globulin levels from immune overactivation and inflammation, and the serum creatinine level may increase very rapidly in patients with jSLE with renal disease. A spot first morning urine protein to creatinine ratio helps differentiate pathologic from orthostatic proteinuria. Increasing protein level or a ratio greater than 0.2 suggests a renal biopsy may be needed.

Specific screening tests for jSLE include complement C3 and C4 and selected serologies; high-yield assessment includes an ANA titer and anti–double-stranded DNA (dsDNA). Extensive autoantibody panels should only be done after establishing a positive ANA and other features of rheumatic disease.[46] In jSLE, a high ANA titer is nearly universal.[47] ANA in low titers (1:40, 1:80 and higher) may be present in up to 30% of healthy children and some with nonimmune conditions (infection, neoplasms). A titer of 1:160 or higher in the setting of other suspicious symptoms warrants further evaluation.[48] High titers of anti-dsDNA antibody and very low serum C3 and C4 or albumin levels should prompt careful assessment for lupus nephritis.

Patients with jMCTD with extensive synovitis may have a positive rheumatoid factor, and autoantibodies to U1-RNP seem to be pathogenic in pulmonary arterial hypertension.[49] Although complement activation occurs in skin lesions of MCTD, complement depletion is not seen as it is in SLE.[50,51] In jSS, patients often have a positive autoantibody, whether an ANA, anti-SSA, or anti-SSB, with 76% having only a positive anti-SSA.[4]

Additional evaluation should be based on symptoms. If coagulopathy or vasculopathy is suspected, a prolonged activated partial thromboplastin time and antiphospholipid antibody titers can support the diagnosis. **Box 3** provides a list of suggested screening studies if a practitioner suspects jSLE or related disorders. If serositis is suspected, chest radiograph and echocardiogram can confirm effusion and carditis. Echocardiography is indicated with hypertension or suspected valve disease; rarely Libman-Sacks endocarditis occurs in jSLE; myocarditis occurs rarely in any of these diseases. Pulmonary function testing to screen for pulmonary fibrosis should be considered if cough or dyspnea are present, and as a baseline in jMCTD.

Decisions on invasive testing should be deferred to a pediatric subspecialist (usually rheumatologist or nephrologist). In the setting of proteinuria with or without hematuria, renal biopsy assesses the nature of the glomerulonephritis and confirms the diagnosis. These biopsy findings affect treatment choice and prognosis. For jSS, minor salivary gland biopsies from the lip are often done for diagnosis, with 97% found to have lymphocytic salivary nests.[4] Eye examinations are also helpful, with evidence of retinal vasculitis, episcleritis, and scleritis found in jSLE. In jSS, keratoconjunctivitis sicca can be found, and specific tests to diagnose decreased tear production, such as the Schirmer test, can be done by ophthalmologists.

Following diagnosis, laboratory monitoring is important to identify new disease manifestations, monitor established problems, and ensure medication tolerance. Serial testing is often more important than a single value in an individual patient. Patients with jSLE must be examined at every medical encounter for possible new glomerulonephritis, because renal disease can appear at any time in the disease course. In jSLE, CBC, serum creatinine, anti-dsDNA titer, C3 and C4, and urinalyses are important to predict clinical flares before tissue injury is apparent, and to guide intensity of treatment.

Because of the high risk of early-onset atherosclerosis in inflammatory disease, particularly in SLE, lipid profiles should be monitored periodically. Serum vitamin D concentrations may indicate need for supplementation, particularly for patients taking corticosteroids. DEXA (dual-energy x-ray absorptiometry) scans are very important to monitor bone health, and should be performed on children who require long-term steroid therapy and those with renal impairment. Periodic pulmonary function tests and echocardiograms help monitor cardiopulmonary complications of jSLE, jMCTD, and jSS, if present. Pregnancy testing in sexually mature girls taking mycophenolate, cyclophosphamide, methotrexate, or angiotensin-converting enzyme inhibitors is an important part of monitoring. Esophagrams and swallowing studies are important for children with features of esophageal dysmotility or proximal muscle weakness in jMCTD.

HOW ARE JUVENILE SYSTEMIC LUPUS ERYTHEMATOUS, JUVENILE MIXED CONNECTIVE TISSUE DISEASE, AND JUVENILE SJÖGREN SYNDROME TREATED?

These 3 diseases are complex and require the coordination of a full spectrum of pediatric subspecialists for optimal outcomes. Rheumatologists are the central managers of subspecialty care for these diseases, and referral should be made as soon as the primary care provider has strong suspicion that the diagnosis is one of these conditions. Even a short delay can make the difference between irreversible organ damage and treatable disease, particularly in jSLE. The primary care provider remains a very important part of care for these children. Important roles for the primary care provider include patient and family education, evaluation for changed symptoms and possible infections, routine laboratory monitoring, and optimizing communication among subspecialists.

Juvenile Systemic Lupus Erythematous Therapy

When a patient presents with a pattern of organ dysfunction and features of inflammation, the primary care provider should refer rapidly to a pediatric rheumatologist for further assessment. New-onset lupus is considered a relative medical emergency in pediatric rheumatology and patients should be evaluated and treated quickly to prevent organ damage. Management is predicated on the specific manifestations. Medication options for jSLE are derived from studies in adult lupus; most drugs used to treat jSLE are prescribed off-label. Only aspirin and prednisone are approved for use in jSLE in the United States.

The cornerstones of management are immunosuppression and inflammation control. More than 90% of patients with jSLE receive glucocorticoids.[52,53] Compared with adults, children with SLE accrue more steroid-associated damage, including growth disturbance, cataracts, and avascular necrosis, so steroid-sparing immunosuppressants are routinely used.[53] Antimalarial agents such as hydroxychloroquine (HCQ), are a mainstay of therapy. HCQ decreases flare rates, reduces organ damage, and limits the thrombotic effects of antiphospholipid antibodies.[54]

Treatment of active APS requires anticoagulation and control of underlying inflammation. Hydroxychloroquine is recommended for prophylaxis in patients with jSLE with high-titer antiphospholipid antibody[55]; low-dose aspirin at 3 to 5 mg/kg/d may be considered in addition. Thrombotic events require heparin for both thrombolysis and complement inhibition. Long-term APS treatment may require change to oral anticoagulants. Patients taking long-term HCQ should have regular eye examinations for retinal changes.

Nonsteroidal antiinflammatory medications (NSAIDs) are used for mild arthritis or serositis, but close monitoring is needed in children at risk for nephritis, hypertension, and thrombocytopenia. Arthritis and serositis in jSLE may be treated with methotrexate, although it is used less frequently than in adult lupus.[53] Azathioprine is the gold standard therapy for patients with lupus during pregnancy and is effective for arthritis, cytopenias, and serositis.

Renal and CNS involvement are severe manifestations often treated with mycophenolate mofetil or cyclophosphamide. Pediatric consensus treatment plans (CTPs) have been developed to help standardize therapy. The lupus nephritis CTPs support use of either cyclophosphamide or mycophenolate mofetil.[56] Hypertension is common in patients with lupus nephritis and should be tightly controlled with a target blood pressure of the 50th percentile for age. Proteinuria can further impair renal tubular function, and efforts to decrease intraglomerular pressure with angiotensin-converting enzyme inhibitors or receptor blockers is a mainstay of management.

B cell–targeting therapies have been used off-label in jSLE. Rituximab is used for severe, refractory renal and neuropsychiatric disease. Small pediatric cohorts have shown that rituximab is steroid sparing and has reasonable safety.[57] Belimumab, a monoclonal antibody against B cell–activating factor, has been used in a small cohort of pediatric patients and was effective for arthritis, rash, and worsening serologies.[57] This drug has been approved for adults but not yet for jSLE. Treatment of MAS in jSLE varies but high-dose glucocorticoid therapy is a mainstay. Interleukin-1 antagonists, cyclosporine, mycophenolate mofetil, and cyclophosphamide are adjunctive therapies.[32]

Photoprotection is extremely important in everyone with jSLE and jMCTD. Broad-spectrum sunblock of at least sun protection factor 30 should be worn every day, with more aggressive photoprotection for more intense sun exposure. Several factors combine to promote osteopenia in jSLE, jMCTD, and jSS. Sun avoidance leads to vitamin D deficiency, chronic glucocorticoid use promotes calcium resorption from bone and loss in urine, and chronic inflammation leads to calcium mobilization from bone. Renal impairment further compromises bone integrity by impairing renal hydroxylation of vitamin D. Vitamin D supplements combat hypovitaminosis D and help ensure adequate calcium absorption for bone accrual. Calcium supplementation is important for patients taking glucocorticoids. Low-estrogen or no-estrogen contraception is important in young women of child-bearing age.

Juvenile Mixed Connective Tissue Disease Therapy

Similar to jSLE, treatment of jMCTD is guided by disease manifestations. Low-dose glucocorticoids, hydroxychloroquine, methotrexate, and NSAIDs are used. Vasodilators such as calcium channel blockers help manage Raynaud phenomenon. Severe myositis or lung or renal disease may require potent immunosuppression, including cyclophosophamide.[58] Pulmonary hypertension necessitates aggressive treatment with prostacyclin analogs[58] or endothelin receptor antagonists and systemic immunosuppression.[59] B cell–depletion therapies, including rituximab, have not been studied in jMCTD.[60]

Juvenile Sjögren Syndrome Treatment

Coordinated care among pediatric subspecialists including dentistry, ophthalmology, otorhinolaryngology, and rheumatology is needed for children with jSS. Adults with SS develop B-cell lymphomas, but this is uncommon in children. Treatment of xerophthalmia includes eliminating medications that slow lacrimation, and the use of lubricants, topical cyclosporine, and systemic antiinflammatory treatment.[61] Xerostomia responds to topical agents to promote saliva, and fluoride to prevent caries. Hydroxychloroquine reduces malaise and fatigue in many patients, and may help with musculoskeletal pain. Methotrexate and NSAIDs help control arthritis. Often, low-dose glucocorticoids are used for short periods. Biologic agents (abatacept, rituximab and belimumab, and anticytokine antibodies) are used anecdotally in adult SS.[62] Safety and efficacy of these medications have not been tested in jSS, either as a discrete rheumatic disease or as a manifestation of SLE.

ROLE OF PRIMARY PEDIATRIC CLINICIANS IN MANAGEMENT OF CHILDREN WITH SYSTEMIC LUPUS ERYTHEMATOUS

Once the diagnosis is made, pediatric practitioners remain the medical home for patients, and play a very important role in the children's health. **Box 4** contains several care suggestions that can be implemented in the primary care setting and that benefit patients with jSLE and related disorders. Remind any child with jSLE or jMCTD to avoid sun exposure and use daily sunscreen year-round. Ultraviolet light can increase disease activity in skin and prompt systemic flares. To screen for lupus nephritis, primary care providers should check the children's weight and blood pressure, comparing these results with age-related norms at each visit. Abrupt increases in either can indicate renal disease. A urine dipstick test for proteinuria and blood is a useful tool for early detection of nephritis. Children with jSLE and related chronic inflammatory disease are at risk for atherosclerosis, so testing for lipid abnormalities should be performed, and abnormalities treated. Lifestyle modifications such as diet change, regular aerobic exercise, and tobacco avoidance should be encouraged to minimize this risk.

Box 4
Care suggestions for the medical home in jSLE

- Use of sunscreen *every day* is imperative to help reduce the risk of lupus flare
- Live vaccines (live attenuated influenza, varicella, measles, mumps and rubella) should be avoided; all other usual vaccines are recommended, especially meningococcal and pneumococcal vaccines. Vaccination schedules may require modification to optimize response.
- Blood pressure at every visit to target 50th to 75th percentiles for age
- Screening yearly (at minimum) eye examinations should be done to evaluate for disease-associated pathology and side effects from medications
- Urinalysis at every visit and urine pregnancy test if appropriate
- Avoid sulfa-containing medications because of the risk of hemolytic anemia and disease flare
- Screen for sexual activity and provide appropriate low-estrogen or no-estrogen contraception
- Consider iatrogenic adrenal insufficiency and provide stress-dose steroids if appropriate
- Contact pediatric rheumatology with any questions or concerns

---

Assess the Severity of Infections and Treat

Children with these systemic inflammatory conditions develop typical childhood infections, but they might also have unusual infections. Two important concepts to keep in mind in children who seems to have an intercurrent infection are that (1) the immunosuppressive medications used to control rheumatic disease can obscure symptoms and signs of infection, and (2) the inflammation caused by infection may cause underlying disease flares. When fever occurs, clinicians must seek a source and treat appropriately. Stopping immune suppression, except for glucocorticoids, may be necessary until fever abates but should always be discussed with the patient's rheumatologist. Any child with SLE with substantial fever while on immunosuppressive medication should be admitted to the hospital for observation and receive empiric antimicrobial treatment, unless a source of the fever is identified allowing targeted treatment.

Long-term immunosuppressive medications increase the risk for opportunistic infection. Importantly, with prolonged corticosteroid use, iatrogenic adrenal insufficiency may require short-term stress-dose steroid coverage. A call to the subspecialty consultant should help assess how to manage stress coverage.

Give Immunizations

Because children with jSLE consume C3 and C4 in immune complexes, they are at risk for bacteremia caused by encapsulated organisms such as *Streptococcus pneumoniae*, *Haemophilus*, and *Neisseria* species. Immunization with 23-valent pneumococcal and the meningococcal vaccines helps ensure that immunoglobulin (Ig) G antibody, the other major opsonin, is protective. Nearly all children with jSLE and related diseases should receive the annual killed influenza vaccine. Live attenuated vaccines including live influenza, varicella and measles, mumps and rubella should be avoided in immune-suppressed children. When patients are very ill or taking high doses of immune suppressive medication it may be best to delay immunizations until the child is better able to respond to them. See Gloria C. Higgins' article, "Complications of Treatments for Pediatric Rheumatic Diseases," in this issue for additional discussion of immunizations. An excellent preventive measure against infection is good hand-washing and avoidance of ill contacts. At primary care visits, reminding the patient and family of these measures is crucial to protecting health.

Other General Pediatric Care

Many medications that treat these diseases are teratogenic. When a patient is sexually active, the primary care provider should help provide appropriate low-estrogen or no-estrogen contraception or referral for those services. Screening urine pregnancy tests are recommended. Pregnancy should be planned carefully in women with jSLE, jMCTD, and jSS, ideally when disease is well controlled, and medication is minimal, to limit fetal toxicity. Lupus pregnancies should be managed by high-risk obstetricians.

Some medications deserve special consideration in jSLE, jMCTD, and jSS. Sulfa-containing medications are relatively contraindicated in jSLE because of possible association with flares and risk of hemolytic anemia. Prophylactic doses of trimethoprim-sulfamethoxazole are recommended by some for children at risk for Pneumocystis jiroveci pneumonia; alternative prophyactic regimens can be used. Other medications, including some antiepileptics and antihypertensives, can cause drug-induced lupus. Minocycline causes a variety of rheumatic syndromes, including arthritis and drug-induced lupus. Minocycline should be stopped in anyone who has new rheumatic complaints, thrombocytopenia, and/or new autoantibodies.

Supporting Transition

Transition is a difficult time for adolescent and young adult patients with jSLE and related diseases. On average, patients with jSLE transition at age 19 years. More than half have transition difficulties, with loss of insurance and emotional adjustment issues leaving pediatric providers.[63] The lag between the last pediatric visit and establishing adult care averages 9 months with three-quarters of patients having at least 1 gap in care.[64] Anxiety and depression are prevalent at this time, increasing from 10% to 26% of patients in one study.[64] Pediatric care providers should consider staggering the transition process from their own care and the pediatric specialists' care to help prevent major lapses of health care in youth. Additional information on transition is given in Stacy P. Ardoin's article, "Transitions in Rheumatic Disease: Pediatric to Adult Care," in this issue.

Helping to Manage Stress

The stress of chronic disease is increasingly recognized as detrimental to patients with rheumatic disease. Depression and anxiety are prevalent in jSLE.[65] Children may develop jSLE-related psychosis and cognitive dysfunction requiring increased immunosuppression with prolonged lag times to remission.[66] Fatigue, pain, anxiety, and depression contribute to poor health-related quality of life.[67] The financial burden of disease is apparent but not well described in jSLE, jMCTD, or jSS. A study from 2006 estimated the direct cost of jSLE per quality-adjusted life year was $30,908,[68] compared with adult estimates of annual direct medical cost in the United States ranging from $13,735 to $20,926, including medications, hospitalization, and outpatient care. This estimate does not account for the indirect costs of parental sick-leave, absence from school, and strain on the entire family. Close collaboration among subspecialists and primary care providers is essential for patients with jSLE, jMCTD, and jSS.

WHAT IS THE PROGNOSIS FOR JUVENILE SYSTEMIC LUPUS ERYTHEMATOUS, JUVENILE MIXED CONNECTIVE TISSUE DISEASE, AND JUVENILE SJÖGREN SYNDROME?

These diseases remain idiopathic, and although treatments are available, cures are not. Some information about survival has been published, but therapies are rapidly changing, and any published statistics are out-of-date. The outcomes of each disease are tied to rapid diagnosis and treatment, close monitoring, and adherence to prescribed treatments. Important life-threatening complications include glomerulonephritis and MAS (jSLE), CNS disease and pulmonary involvement (jSLE and jMCTD), and, in all, premature atherosclerosis and infection. Medication toxicities, especially severe infection, can be life limiting as well, with much morbidity and mortality related to chronic high-dose glucocorticoid use. Children with jSLE, jMCTD, and jSS are at risk for avascular necrosis of bone, with further risk associated with glucocorticoid treatment. **Table 3** identifies the severe and more common complications seen in jSLE and related conditions.

Damage is common in jSLE; one-third of patients have some damage after a mean follow-up of 3.5 years.[5] Damage was more common in patients with jSLE who had renal (5.6%) and/or CNS disease (25%), with CNS damage attributed as cerebral vascular accident, cognitive impairment, persistent seizures, or transverse myelitis.[5] Compared with an adult cohort, children with SLE had more severe renal and neuropsychiatric damage.[7] Mortality in jSLE occurred in 2.3%.[5] jMCTD outcome relates to pulmonary hypertension and interstitial lung disease, which are less common in jMCTD than in adult MCTD.[3] In adults, one-third had a predominantly vascular course with pulmonary hypertension, Raynaud phenomenon, livedo reticularis, and vascular thrombosis; a third had interstitial lung disease, esophageal dysmotility, and myositis;

Table 3
Severe and common complications of juvenile systemic lupus erythematosus and related conditions

Complications	jSLE	jMCTD	jSS
Neurologic	Severe: seizures, stroke, cerebral hemorrhage, psychosis, transverse myelitis, peripheral neuropathy Common: depression, dyscalculia, memory problems, lupus "brain fog"	Severe: jSLE-like neurologic features Common: depression, "brain fog", and fatigue	Severe: peripheral neuropathy Common: fatigue, "brain fog"
Renal	Severe: hypertension, acute or chronic renal insufficiency, glomerulonephritis Common: glomerulonephritis, hypertension	Severe: glomerulonephritis is less common and usually less severe than in jSLE	Rarely an issue
Musculoskeletal	Severe: effusive polyarthritis, Jaccoud arthropathy, joint deformities or erosions, avascular necrosis of bone, osteoporosis Common: arthralgia, nondeforming arthritis. osteopenia, hypovitaminosis D	Severe: proximal inflammatory myositis, increased muscle enzyme levels, osteoporosis Common: arthritis, myalgia and arthralgia, osteopenia	Severe: severe arthritis or inflammatory myositis, osteoporosis Common: arthralgia and myalgia, osteopenia
Gastrointestinal	Severe: GI vasculitis with perforation More common: pancreatitis, sterile peritonitis, enteritis with malabsorption (including medications), chronic diarrhea, and nutrient malabsorption	Severe: dysphagia from sclerodermatous esophageal changes, thickening of any bowel wall segments with malabsorption, GI motility problems, small bowel bacterial overgrowth Common: milder dysmotility of the GI tract	Severe: dental caries Common: dry mouth can interfere with swallowing
Cardiovascular	Severe: pericarditis, sterile endocarditis, chordae tendinae rupture, premature atherosclerosis, renovascular hypertension, thromboembolic disease (antiphospholipid syndrome) Common: hyperlipidemia, Raynaud phenomenon (may be severe)	Severe: most SLE-related complications may occur in jMCTD; pulmonary hypertension from sclerodermatous involvement of major vessels and lung tissue	Severe: advanced atherosclerosis risk is anticipated because of chronic inflammatory disease; not yet well documented in jSS

(continued on next page)

Table 3
(continued)

Complications	jSLE	jMCTD	jSS
Pulmonary	Severe: lupus pneumonitis, chronic interstitial lung disease, pulmonary hypertension, interstitial pulmonary fibrosis, pulmonary infarctions or emboli with antiphospholipid syndrome Common: pleuritis, pleuritic chest pain	Severe: scleroderma lung disease with lymphocytic pneumonitis, fibrosis; sudden pulmonary vasospasm precipitating pulmonary hypertension and right heart failure Common: minor respiratory infections	Severe: interstitial pneumonitis, pulmonary hypertension, mediastinal lymphoma
Mucosal lesions	Severe: oral ulcerations if extensive, can be life-threatening. Common: epistaxis, oral aphthae	Severe: fibrosis of gut wall, watermelon stomach Common: dyspepsia, constipation	Severe: corneal abrasions from dry eyes Common: dry mouth, dry eyes, dental caries, swallowing difficulty
Infections (caused by disease and medications)	Severe: septicemia with gram-positive encapsulated organisms, *Haemophilus* and *Neisseria* spp because of complement depletion; protracted, severe, or opportunistic infection related to immunosuppressive medication and leukopenia Common: protracted respiratory infections, sinusitis	Severe: bacteremia as in jSLE, depending on degree of immune suppression; may have opportunistic infections also Common: protracted respiratory infections, sinusitis	Severe: opportunistic infection from severe immune suppression Common: protracted respiratory infections, sinusitis
Others	Severe: MAS, infertility related to cyclophosphamide or other immunosuppressive medication, diabetes	Severe: systemic scleroderma complications: calcinosis, digit ischemia, and autoamputation. Infertility rarely, depending on medications	Severe: lymphoma (few reports in children)

Abbreviation: GI, gastrointestinal

and about 25% had erosive arthritis with anticyclic citrullinated peptide antibodies and osteoporosis.[69] Long-term follow-up data in jMCTD are sparse, but, in the available literature, the acute inflammatory myositis and arthritis features tend to wane over time, and scleroderma features persist.[70] In one study, 33% attained remission by 16 years after diagnosis, but there was a 5% mortality (from infection, lung disease, and pulmonary hypertension).[71]

Outcome of jSS is variable and depends on rapidity of diagnosis, the level of inflammation and glandular damage, and the development of lymphoma. Markers of high lymphoma risk are low serum C3 and C4 levels, germinal centers in minor salivary gland biopsies, chronic parotid enlargement, purpura, mixed cryoglobulinemia, and high-titer rheumatoid factor.[72] Mortality was low, at approximately 5% at 16 years from diagnosis in one study.[10]

Adults with chronic inflammatory disease have high mortalities from atherosclerotic disease and from lipid derangement related to steroid medication.[73] Early atherosclerosis in jSLE has been documented as well as a significant risk of cardiovascular disease (CVD), including increased risk of myocardial infarction with earlier onset (first myocardial infarction at mean age of 32 years), and in early adulthood, a 100-fold to 300-fold increased risk of death from CVD compared with age-matched controls.[74,75]

SUMMARY

Childhood-onset SLE, MCTD, and SS are a group of related but distinct inflammatory diseases with significant autoimmunity and specific autoantibodies that help define the different disorders. They all have broad-reaching effects on the health of children with these diseases and have the potential to limit life expectancy and quality of life. Early detection is crucial in controlling the diseases before the occurrence of permanent damage. Collaboration and communication among all care providers is necessary for optimal outcomes for these children.

REFERENCES

1. Klein-Gitelman M, Reiff A, Silverman ED. Systemic lupus erythematosus in childhood. Rheum Dis Clin North Am 2002;28(3):561–77, vi-vii.
2. Mina R, Brunner HI. Update on differences between childhood-onset and adult-onset systemic lupus erythematosus. Arthritis Res Ther 2013;15(4):218.
3. Berard RA, Laxer RM. Pediatric mixed connective tissue disease. Curr Rheumatol Rep 2016;18(5):28.
4. Mehta J, Lieberman SN. A comparison of clinical and serologic profiles of children with Sjogren syndrome based on the presence or absence of parotitis. American College of Rheumatology Annual Scientific Meeting. Boston, MA, November 14–19, 2014.
5. Hiraki LT, Benseler SM, Tyrrell PN, et al. Clinical and laboratory characteristics and long-term outcome of pediatric systemic lupus erythematosus: a longitudinal study. J Pediatr 2008;152(4):550–6.
6. Barsalou J, Levy DM, Silverman ED. An update on childhood-onset systemic lupus erythematosus. Curr Opin Rheumatol 2013;25(5):616–22.
7. Tucker LB, Uribe AG, Fernandez M, et al. Adolescent onset of lupus results in more aggressive disease and worse outcomes: results of a nested matched case-control study within LUMINA, a multiethnic US cohort (LUMINA LVII). Lupus 2008;17(4):314–22.

8. Webb R, Kelly JA, Somers EC, et al. Early disease onset is predicted by a higher genetic risk for lupus and is associated with a more severe phenotype in lupus patients. Ann Rheum Dis 2011;70(1):151–6.

9. Tsai YY, Yang YH, Yu HH, et al. Fifteen-year experience of pediatric-onset mixed connective tissue disease. Clin Rheumatol 2010;29(1):53–8.

10. Yokogawa N, Lieberman SM, Sherry DD, et al. Features of childhood Sjogren's syndrome in comparison to adult Sjogren's syndrome: considerations in establishing child-specific diagnostic criteria. Clin Exp Rheumatol 2016;34(2):343–51.

11. Jonsson R, Theander E, Sjostrom B, et al. Autoantibodies present before symptom onset in primary Sjogren syndrome. JAMA 2013;310(17):1854–5.

12. Theander E, Jonsson R, Sjostrom B, et al. Prediction of Sjogren's syndrome years before diagnosis and identification of patients with early onset and severe disease course by autoantibody profiling. Arthritis Rheumatol 2015;67(9):2427–36.

13. Ortega-Hernandez OD, Shoenfeld Y. Mixed connective tissue disease: an overview of clinical manifestations, diagnosis and treatment. Best Pract Res Clin Rheumatol 2012;26(1):61–72.

14. Tan EM, Cohen AS, Fries JF, et al. The 1982 revised criteria for the classification of systemic lupus erythematosus. Arthritis Rheum 1982;25(11):1271–7.

15. Petri M, Orbai AM, Alarcon GS, et al. Derivation and validation of the Systemic Lupus International Collaborating Clinics classification criteria for systemic lupus erythematosus. Arthritis Rheum 2012;64(8):2677–86.

16. Sule SD, Moodalbail DG, Burnham J, et al. Predictors of arthritis in pediatric patients with lupus. Pediatr Rheumatol Online J 2015;13:30.

17. Gormezano NW, Silva CA, Aikawa NE, et al. Chronic arthritis in systemic lupus erythematosus: distinct features in 336 paediatric and 1830 adult patients. Clin Rheumatol 2016;35(1):227–31.

18. Levy DM, Kamphuis S. Systemic lupus erythematosus in children and adolescents. Pediatr Clin North Am 2012;59(2):345–64.

19. Yeh TT, Yang YH, Lin YT, et al. Cardiopulmonary involvement in pediatric systemic lupus erythematosus: a twenty-year retrospective analysis. J Microbiol Immunol Infect 2007;40(6):525–31.

20. Muscal E, Brey RL. Neurologic manifestations of systemic lupus erythematosus in children and adults. Neurol Clin 2010;28(1):61–73.

21. Limwattana S, Dissaneewate P, Kritsaneepaiboon S, et al. Systemic lupus erythematosus-related pancreatitis in children. Clin Rheumatol 2013;32(6):913–8.

22. Sipurzynski J, Fahrner B, Kerbl R, et al. Management of chronic immune thrombocytopenia in children and adolescents: lessons from an Austrian national cross-sectional study of 81 patients. Semin Hematol 2016;53(Suppl 1):S43–7.

23. Gormezano NW, Kern D, Pereira OL, et al. Autoimmune hemolytic anemia in systemic lupus erythematosus at diagnosis: differences between pediatric and adult patients. Lupus 2017;26(4):426–30.

24. Lube GE, Ferriani MP, Campos LM, et al. Evans syndrome at childhood-onset systemic lupus erythematosus diagnosis: a large multicenter study. Pediatr Blood Cancer 2016;63(7):1238–43.

25. Velo-Garcia A, Castro SG, Isenberg DA. The diagnosis and management of the haematologic manifestations of lupus. J Autoimmun 2016;74:139–60.

26. Cappelli S, Bellando Randone S, Martinovic D, et al. "To be or not to be," ten years after: evidence for mixed connective tissue disease as a distinct entity. Semin Arthritis Rheum 2012;41(4):589–98.

27. Kasukawa R. Mixed connective tissue disease. Intern Med 1999;38(5):386–93.

28. Kotajima L, Aotsuka S, Sumiya M, et al. Clinical features of patients with juvenile onset mixed connective tissue disease: analysis of data collected in a nationwide collaborative study in Japan. J Rheumatol 1996;23(6):1088–94.

29. Sedej K, Toplak N, Praprotnik M, et al. Autoimmune hepatitis as a presenting manifestation of mixed connective tissue disease in a child. Case report and review of the literature. Pediatr Rheumatol Online J 2015;13(1):47.

30. Shiboski CH, Shiboski SC, Seror R, et al. 2016 American College of Rheumatology/European League against Rheumatism classification criteria for primary Sjogren's syndrome: a consensus and data-driven methodology involving three international patient cohorts. Arthritis Rheumatol 2017;69(1):35–45.

31. Descloux E, Durieu I, Cochat P, et al. Paediatric systemic lupus erythematosus: prognostic impact of antiphospholipid antibodies. Rheumatology (Oxford) 2008;47(2):183–7.

32. Bennett TD, Fluchel M, Hersh AO, et al. Macrophage activation syndrome in children with systemic lupus erythematosus and children with juvenile idiopathic arthritis. Arthritis Rheum 2012;64(12):4135–42.

33. Parodi A, Davi S, Pringe AB, et al. Macrophage activation syndrome in juvenile systemic lupus erythematosus: a multinational multicenter study of thirty-eight patients. Arthritis Rheum 2009;60(11):3388–99.

34. Zuppa AA, Riccardi R, Frezza S, et al. Neonatal lupus: follow-up in infants with anti-SSA/Ro antibodies and review of the literature. Autoimmun Rev 2017;16(4):427–32.

35. Lee LA, Sokol RJ, Buyon JP. Hepatobiliary disease in neonatal lupus: prevalence and clinical characteristics in cases enrolled in a national registry. Pediatrics 2002;109(1):E11.

36. Brucato A, Cimaz R, Caporali R, et al. Pregnancy outcomes in patients with autoimmune diseases and anti-Ro/SSA antibodies. Clin Rev Allergy Immunol 2011; 40(1):27–41.

37. Brito-Zeron P, Izmirly PM, Ramos-Casals M, et al. The clinical spectrum of autoimmune congenital heart block. Nat Rev Rheumatol 2015;11(5):301–12.

38. Flam ST, Gunnarsson R, Garen T, et al. The HLA profiles of mixed connective tissue disease differ distinctly from the profiles of clinically related connective tissue diseases. Rheumatology (Oxford) 2015;54(3):528–35.

39. Sestak A, O'Neil KM. Familial lupus and antiphospholipid syndrome. Lupus 2007; 16(8):556–63.

40. Tsokos GC, Lo MS, Costa Reis P, et al. New insights into the immunopathogenesis of systemic lupus erythematosus. Nat Rev Rheumatol 2016;12(12):716–30.

41. Ghodke-Puranik Y, Niewold TB. Immunogenetics of systemic lupus erythematosus: a comprehensive review. J Autoimmun 2015;64:125–36.

42. Jensen MA, Niewold TB. Interferon regulatory factors: critical mediators of human lupus. Transl Res 2015;165(2):283–95.

43. Zhao GN, Jiang DS, Li H. Interferon regulatory factors: at the crossroads of immunity, metabolism, and disease. Biochim Biophys Acta 2015;1852(2):365–78.

44. Livingston B, Bonner A, Pope J. Differences in clinical manifestations between childhood-onset lupus and adult-onset lupus: a meta-analysis. Lupus 2011; 20(13):1345–55.

45. Malattia C, Martini A. Paediatric-onset systemic lupus erythematosus. Best Pract Res Clin Rheumatol 2013;27(3):351–62.

46. Man A, Shojania K, Phoon C, et al. An evaluation of autoimmune antibody testing patterns in a Canadian health region and an evaluation of a laboratory algorithm aimed at reducing unnecessary testing. Clin Rheumatol 2013;32(5):601–8.

47. Wichainun R, Kasitanon N, Wangkaew S, et al. Sensitivity and specificity of ANA and anti-dsDNA in the diagnosis of systemic lupus erythematosus: a comparison using control sera obtained from healthy individuals and patients with multiple medical problems. Asian Pac J Allergy Immunol 2013;31(4):292–8.

48. Breda L, Nozzi M, De Sanctis S, et al. Laboratory tests in the diagnosis and follow-up of pediatric rheumatic diseases: an update. Semin Arthritis Rheum 2010;40(1):53–72.

49. Bodolay E, Csipo I, Gal I, et al. Anti-endothelial cell antibodies in mixed connective tissue disease: frequency and association with clinical symptoms. Clin Exp Rheumatol 2004;22(4):409–15.

50. Magro CM, Crowson AN, Regauer S. Mixed connective tissue disease. A clinical, histologic, and immunofluorescence study of eight cases. Am J Dermatopathol 1997;19(3):206–13.

51. Hameenkorpi R, Ruuska P, Forsberg S, et al. More evidence of distinctive features of mixed connective tissue disease. Scand J Rheumatol 1993; 22(2):63–8.

52. Brunner HI, Klein-Gitelman MS, Ying J, et al. Corticosteroid use in childhood-onset systemic lupus erythematosus-practice patterns at four pediatric rheumatology centers. Clin Exp Rheumatol 2009;27(1):155–62.

53. Brunner HI, Gladman DD, Ibanez D, et al. Difference in disease features between childhood-onset and adult-onset systemic lupus erythematosus. Arthritis Rheum 2008;58(2):556–62.

54. Ponticelli C, Moroni G. Hydroxychloroquine in systemic lupus erythematosus (SLE). Expert Opin Drug Saf 2017;16(3):411–9.

55. Avcin T, O'Neil KM. Antiphospholipid syndrome. In: Cassidy JT, Petty RE, Laxer RM, et al, editors. Textbook of pediatric rheumatology. 7th edition. Philadelphia: Elsevier; 2011. p. 344–60.

56. Mina R, von Scheven E, Ardoin SP, et al. Consensus treatment plans for induction therapy of newly diagnosed proliferative lupus nephritis in juvenile systemic lupus erythematosus. Arthritis Care Res (Hoboken) 2012;64(3):375–83.

57. Hui-Yuen JS, Nguyen SC, Askanase AD. Targeted B cell therapies in the treatment of adult and pediatric systemic lupus erythematosus. Lupus 2016;25(10): 1086–96.

58. Jais X, Launay D, Yaici A, et al. Immunosuppressive therapy in lupus- and mixed connective tissue disease-associated pulmonary arterial hypertension: a retrospective analysis of twenty-three cases. Arthritis Rheum 2008;58(2): 521–31.

59. Denton CP, Humbert M, Rubin L, et al. Bosentan treatment for pulmonary arterial hypertension related to connective tissue disease: a subgroup analysis of the pivotal clinical trials and their open-label extensions. Ann Rheum Dis 2006; 65(10):1336–40.

60. Jovancevic B, Lindholm C, Pullerits R. Anti B-cell therapy against refractory thrombocytopenia in SLE and MCTD patients: long-term follow-up and review of the literature. Lupus 2013;22(7):664–74.

61. Foulks GN, Forstot SL, Donshik PC, et al. Clinical guidelines for management of dry eye associated with Sjogren disease. Ocul Surf 2015;13(2):118–32.

62. Carsons SE, Vivino FB, Parke A, et al. Treatment guidelines for rheumatologic manifestations of Sjogren's syndrome: use of biologic agents, management of fatigue, and inflammatory musculoskeletal pain. Arthritis Care Res (Hoboken) 2017; 69(4):517–27.

63. Felsenstein S, Reiff AO, Ramanathan A. Transition of care and health-related outcomes in pediatric-onset systemic lupus erythematosus. Arthritis Care Res (Hoboken) 2015;67(11):1521–8.
64. Son MB, Sergeyenko Y, Guan H, et al. Disease activity and transition outcomes in a childhood-onset systemic lupus erythematosus cohort. Lupus 2016;25(13): 1431–9.
65. Knight A, Weiss P, Morales K, et al. Depression and anxiety and their association with healthcare utilization in pediatric lupus and mixed connective tissue disease patients: a cross-sectional study. Pediatr Rheumatol Online J 2014;12:42.
66. Lim LS, Lefebvre A, Benseler S, et al. Longterm outcomes and damage accrual in patients with childhood systemic lupus erythematosus with psychosis and severe cognitive dysfunction. J Rheumatol 2013;40(4):513–9.
67. Jones JT, Cunningham N, Kashikar-Zuck S, et al. Pain, fatigue, and psychological impact on health-related quality of life in childhood-onset lupus. Arthritis Care Res (Hoboken) 2016;68(1):73–80.
68. Brunner HI, Sherrard TM, Klein-Gitelman MS. Cost of treatment of childhood-onset systemic lupus erythematosus. Arthritis Rheum 2006;55(2):184–8.
69. Szodoray P, Hajas A, Kardos L, et al. Distinct phenotypes in mixed connective tissue disease: subgroups and survival. Lupus 2012;21(13):1412–22.
70. Mier RJ, Shishov M, Higgins GC, et al. Pediatric-onset mixed connective tissue disease. Rheum Dis Clin North Am 2005;31(3):483–96, vii.
71. Hetlevik SO, Flato B, Rygg M, et al. Long-term outcome in juvenile-onset mixed connective tissue disease: a nationwide Norwegian study. Ann Rheum Dis 2017;76(1):159–65.
72. Papageorgiou A, Voulgarelis M, Tzioufas AG. Clinical picture, outcome and predictive factors of lymphoma in Sjögren syndrome. Autoimmun Rev 2015;14(7): 641–9.
73. Ku IA, Imboden JB, Hsue PY, et al. Rheumatoid arthritis: model of systemic inflammation driving atherosclerosis. Circ J 2009;73(6):977–85.
74. Ardoin SP, Schanberg LE, Sandborg CI, et al. Secondary analysis of APPLE study suggests atorvastatin may reduce atherosclerosis progression in pubertal lupus patients with higher C reactive protein. Ann Rheum Dis 2014;73(3):557–66.
75. Barsalou J, Bradley TJ, Silverman ED. Cardiovascular risk in pediatric-onset rheumatological diseases. Arthritis Res Ther 2013;5(3):212.
76. Hochberg MC. Updating the American College of Rheumatology revised criteria for the classification of systemic lupus erythematosus. Arthritis Rheum 1997; 40(9):1725.

Juvenile Idiopathic Inflammatory Myopathies

Adam M. Huber, MSc, MD

KEYWORDS

- Juvenile idiopathic inflammatory myopathy • Juvenile dermatomyositis
- Juvenile polymyositis

KEY POINTS

- The juvenile idiopathic inflammatory myopathies (JIIM) are several acquired, autoimmune disorders that affect muscle and, to a lesser extent, skin.
- JIIM should be considered in children presenting with either signs of muscle weakness or typical rash.
- The diagnosis of juvenile polymyositis should be made cautiously, with careful consideration and evaluation of other differentials.
- Consultation and referral to a provider with expertise in diagnosis and management of JIIM should occur before initiation of treatment.

INTRODUCTION

Juvenile dermatomyositis (JDM) is a rare disease but is the most common and recognizable of the systemic inflammatory myopathies. The term juvenile idiopathic inflammatory myopathy (JIIM) is used to emphasize that there are several acquired autoimmune disorders that affect muscle and, to a lesser extent, skin. In addition to JDM, this group includes juvenile polymyositis (JPM), immune-mediated necrotizing myositis (a disorder recently distinguished from JPM and characterized by severe weakness marked increase in muscle enzyme levels, poor response to therapy, and specific autoantibody associations[1]), and myositis associated with another connective tissue disease. A more complete listing of other disorders can be found in **Box 1**.[2]

All forms of JIIM have muscle involvement as a common feature, which presents as weakness, poor endurance, and reductions in physical function. Skin manifestations are important in some forms, particularly JDM, and children may have several pathognomonic and typical skin lesions. Involvement of organ systems outside the muscle and skin is possible and may have a major impact on both morbidity and mortality.

Historically, the JIIMs were severe, chronic illnesses with mortality in excess of 30%.[3] However, with current therapy, mortality is uncommon but morbidity remains a concern.

Disclosure: The author has no relevant financial disclosures.
Division of Pediatric Rheumatology, IWK Health Centre, Dalhousie University, 5850 University Avenue, Halifax, Nova Scotia B3K 6R8, Canada
E-mail address: adam.Huber@iwk.nshealth.ca

Pediatr Clin N Am 65 (2018) 739–756
https://doi.org/10.1016/j.pcl.2018.04.006
0031-3955/18/© 2018 Elsevier Inc. All rights reserved.

> **Box 1**
> **Forms of juvenile idiopathic inflammatory myopathy**
>
> JDM
>
> JPM
>
> Immune-mediated necrotizing myositis
>
> Focal/nodular myositis
>
> Orbital/ocular myositis
>
> Granulomatous myositis
>
> Eosinophilic myositis
>
> Macrophagic myofasciitis
>
> Myositis associated with another rheumatic illness[a]
>
> [a] Myositis when seen with another rheumatic illness, such as lupus, is considered to be a form of JIIM by some clinicians, whereas others view this as a potential mimic of JIIM.
> *Data from* Rider LG, Nistala K. The juvenile idiopathic inflammatory myopathies: pathogenesis, clinical and autoantibody phenotypes, and outcomes. J Intern Med 2016;280(1):24–38.

New diagnostic approaches hold promise to identify patients at higher risk of poor outcomes, leading to more tailored therapy. Given the rarity and complexity of these disorders, early referral to providers with expertise in the management of the JIIMs is necessary.

INCIDENCE OF JUVENILE IDIOPATHIC INFLAMMATORY MYOPATHIES

All of the JIIMs are rare. The most common is JDM, with an incidence of approximately 2.5 per million per year[4] and prevalence of approximately 2.5 per 100,000.[5] Data are more limited for other forms of JIIM, although JPM is estimated to be about one-tenth as common as JDM, with the other forms rarer still.[4]

DEMOGRAPHICS OF JUVENILE IDIOPATHIC INFLAMMATORY MYOPATHIES
Age

For JDM[6–10]
- Median age at onset 5.7 to 6.9 years
- Median age at diagnosis 7.4 to 7.7 years
For JPM[9]
- Median age at onset 11 years
- Median age at diagnosis 12.1 years

Race and Ethnicity

The impact of race or ethnicity has not been adequately studied, but patients from all races and ethnicities have been reported. However, a study conducted in the United States suggests a similar incidence of JDM for white, non-Hispanic and African American, non-Hispanic children, and possibly slightly lower incidences for Hispanic children.[10]

DELAYS IN DIAGNOSIS ARE COMMON

Most studies report delays in diagnosis, averaging approximately 6 months from disease onset to diagnosis.[6,11] However, much longer delays are common. It is important to make the diagnosis of JIIM in a timely fashion, because delays in diagnosis are associated with important negative outcomes, including increased risks of calcinosis[12] and mortality.[11]

MAJOR DIFFERENCES FROM ADULT IDIOPATHIC INFLAMMATORY MYOPATHIES

Although the idiopathic inflammatory myopathies share several features in adults and children, including proximal muscle weakness and similar rashes, there are important differences.

- Children with JIIM are more likely to develop calcinosis: approximately 40% (10%–70%)[13] versus 10% to 20%.[14]
- Common myositis-specific autoantibodies (MSAs) are different in children and adults. In children, the most common are anti–transcriptional intermediary factor (TIF1)-gamma, anti–nuclear matrix protein (NXP)-2 (previously anti-MJ), and anti–melanoma differentiation-associated protein 5 (anti-MDA5).[2] In contrast, the most common MSA in adults are anti–transfer RNA (tRNA) synthetase autoantibodies (most frequently anti-Jo-1) and anti-Mi-2 autoantibodies.[15]
- Interstitial lung disease is less frequent in children, although it is associated with similar MSA (anti-tRNA synthetase and anti-MDA5).[9]
- Mortality is lower in children with JIIM than in adults: 0.7% to 4.2%[6,7,11,16] versus 9% in the first year after diagnosis and up to 30% overall in adults.[17]
- Malignancy is not associated with JIIM in children, whereas this association is well established in adults.[18] For this reason, routine screening for malignancy is not indicated in JIIM.[19]

WHEN TO CONSIDER A JUVENILE IDIOPATHIC INFLAMMATORY MYOPATHY

Children with a JIIM most commonly present with both typical rashes and signs of muscle dysfunction (weakness and/or loss of muscular endurance). However, JIIM should be considered in any child presenting with either of these complaints or findings. On occasion, children are found to have unexpected increases in muscle enzyme levels on routine blood work, which should lead to consideration of the possibility of JIIM.

Muscle enzymes include creatine phosphokinase (creatine kinase [CPK or CK]), alanine transaminase (ALT), aspartate transaminase (AST), lactate dehydrogenase (LDH), and aldolase. Some of these enzymes may be derived from multiple sources besides skeletal muscle, such as liver or cardiac muscle, and so interpretation may be challenging. In addition, many routine blood work panels include only AST and/or ALT, which may lead to errors if a muscle source is not considered.

HOW CHILDREN WITH JUVENILE IDIOPATHIC INFLAMMATORY MYOPATHY PRESENT

Historically, criteria for JIIM were described by Bohan and Peter.[20] They proposed the following criteria for inflammatory myopathy in both children and adults:

- Proximal muscle weakness
- Characteristic muscle biopsy changes
- Increased serum muscle enzyme levels
- Electromyography abnormalities: (1) polyphasic, short, small motor-unit potentials; (2) fibrillation, positive sharp waves, insertional irritability; and (3) bizarre, high-frequency repetitive discharges
- Characteristic skin rash

Children with JDM were considered to have typical rash with other features indicating muscle disease. Children with JPM lacked rash but had the same features of muscle disease. These criteria have not been validated in JIIM, although they are refer-enced in most of the JIIM literature. In addition, many children with JIIM no longer un-dergo electromyography or muscle biopsy, making their application challenging. More recently, new classification criteria for adult and JIIM have been developed.[21] These criteria assign a score to several characteristics, such as presence of rashes, biopsy findings, and distribution of weakness. Patients are said to have idiopathic inflamma-tory myopathy if they reach certain thresholds. It is currently unknown whether these criteria can be successfully applied in the clinical setting.

Skin Disease in Juvenile Idiopathic Inflammatory Myopathy

Skin manifestations are a key feature of JDM but are usually absent in other forms of JIIM.

In JDM, the presence of either of 2 pathognomonic rashes should strongly suggest the diagnosis. Gottron papules (**Fig. 1**) are erythematous, raised, and scaly lesions, classically located over the metacarpophalangeal joints, the proximal and distal inter-phalangeal joints of the fingers, and less frequently the toes. They may also be seen over the elbows, knees, and medial malleoli. The appearance may be suggestive of psoriasis, and it is common for this to be the initial diagnosis. The classic distribution is an indicator of the correct diagnosis. Sometimes, only erythema is seen in the same distribution, in which case the lesions are called Gottron sign.

The second pathognomonic rash is the heliotrope rash (**Fig. 2**). It is a red or purple discoloration of the upper eyelid, often with diffuse swelling. It may be subtle and

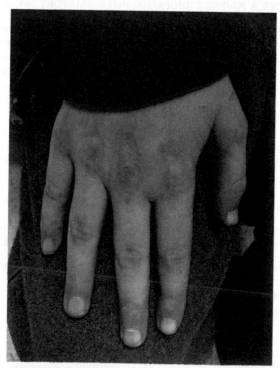

Fig. 1. Gottron papules distributed over metacarpophalangeal and proximal and distal interphalangeal joints of a child with JDM.

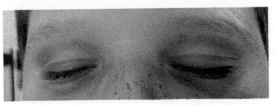

Fig. 2. Heliotrope rash of JDM, demonstrating red/purple discoloration of the eyelids with mild swelling.

therefore easily missed. It may also be accompanied by an accentuation of the vasculature along the lash line, called the eyeliner sign.

A large number of other skin and mucous membrane lesions may also be seen in JDM. Some are similar to those seen in other systemic rheumatic illnesses, particularly systemic lupus erythematosus, and include malar rash, photosensitive erythema, oral ulcers (typically on the hard palate; see Figure 2 for examples in Stacey E. Tarvin and Kathleen M. O'Neil's article, "Systemic Lupus Erythematosus, Sjögren Syndrome, and MCTD in Children and Adolescents," in this issue), alopecia, and Raynaud phenomenon. Sometimes it can be difficult to distinguish JDM and lupus on initial evaluation. Other erythematous, scaly rashes can also be seen, particularly on the extremities, but can appear anywhere, including on both sun-exposed and sun-unexposed skin. Cutaneous ulcerations can be seen in children with JIIM. These ulcerations may be shallow and painless but may also be full thickness and painful. They occur in up to 20% of children.[9] The presence of skin ulcers is particularly important because they can be associated with ulceration of the gastrointestinal tract, which may lead to bleeding, sometimes massive, or perforation. Periungual (nailfold) capillary abnormalities (**Fig. 3**) and cuticular hypertrophy are often present. A more complete list of skin and mucous membrane lesions may be found in **Box 2**, and the reader is directed to Refs.[22,23] for a more complete discussion. Validated tools for the assessment of skin disease in JDM are available, including the Cutaneous Dermatomyositis Disease Area and Severity Index[24] and the Cutaneous Assessment Tool.[25]

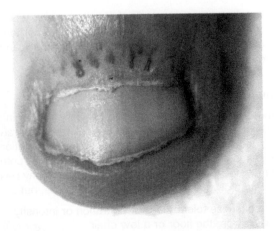

Fig. 3. Severe nailfold capillary loop changes in a child with JDM, including dilatation of capillary loops, areas of capillary dropout, and increased tortuosity. Many patients with JDM have less prominent changes.

Box 2
Skin lesions seen in juvenile dermatomyositis (not exhaustive)

Considered to indicate active disease[a]
  Gottron papules/sign
  Heliotrope rash
  Malar/facial erythema
  Linear extensor erythema
  V-sign rash
  Shawl-sign rash
  Non–sun-exposed erythema
  Erythroderma
  Livedo reticularis
  Skin ulcers
  Mucous membrane lesions (including oral ulcers)
  Periungual capillary loop changes
  Mechanic's hands
  Cuticular overgrowth
  Subcutaneous edema
  Panniculitis
  Alopecia

Considered to indicate chronic disease/damage[a]
  Calcinosis
  Lipoatrophy
  Depressed scar
  Poikiloderma vasculare atrophicans

[a] Some skin lesions may reflect activity or damage, depending on circumstances. For other lesions, there is some controversy about whether they reflect activity or damage (eg, calcinosis).

Calcinosis, deposits of calcium in the skin and subcutaneous tissues, is a particular problem in JIIM. It is usually a later complication but may be present at diagnosis. It may present in several ways.[13] Many patients have a mixture of forms.[13] For some patients, this is the most important and lasting aspect of their illness.

- Calcinosis circumscripta: superficial nodules or plaques; the most common form (**Fig. 4**)
- Tumoral calcinosis: larger masses of calcium that may extend into deeper tissues
- Collections of calcium along fascial planes, ligaments, or tendons
- Exoskeletal calcinosis: extensive plates of calcium that can result in joint contractures and dysfunction

Muscle Disease in Juvenile Idiopathic Inflammatory Myopathy

Involvement of muscle in JIIM, including JDM, typically results in weakness, loss of endurance, and alterations in physical function. Weakness may range from profound, with patients being bed-bound, to virtually imperceptible. Presentation of muscle disease may vary with age. Although older children and adolescents may complain of weakness, younger children may not. Observations of family or school may be much more important. Possible indicators of weakness are potentially endless, but could include:

- Reductions in exercise tolerance, both duration or intensity
- Difficulties rising from the floor or a low chair
- Difficulty/inability to squat while playing
- Difficulty climbing stairs or failing to alternate feet on stairs when the child has done so previously

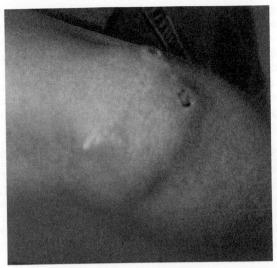

Fig. 4. Elbow with several calcinosis lesions caused by JDM, some with superficial skin breakdown and mild redness.

- Reductions in performance in sports activities
- Difficulty in activities that require raising arms above head, including brushing or curling hair, or putting an object on a high shelf
- Changes in ability to perform self-care, such as dressing, bathing, or toileting

Weakness is typically symmetric and greater proximally (hip and shoulder girdles) than distally. It is important to keep in mind that axial muscles (including those required to perform a sit-up and support the head and neck) are proximal and are commonly involved. Deviations from the typical pattern should stimulate consideration of alternative diagnoses. In the office, observation of simple maneuvers, such as getting the child to stand up from a seated position on the floor or raise the arms directly above the head, can be very helpful. Validated measures of strength and physical function in JIIM include the Childhood Myositis Assessment Scale,[26] the Childhood Health Assessment Questionnaire,[27] and Manual Muscle Testing.[28] Formal assessment of muscle strength often requires considerable experience, because expected strength varies with age, size of the patient, and the differential in strength between the patient and the examiner. Presentation of weakness may also vary with baseline levels of strength and physical fitness. Assessment of change from usual abilities should be considered as well as assessment of absolute strength.

Muscle weakness may be severe, demanding urgent evaluation and intervention. Concerning characteristics include difficulty swallowing or controlling secretions, difficulty breathing, falling, or an inability to rise safely from the floor.

Involvement Outside the Skin and Muscle in Juvenile Idiopathic Inflammatory Myopathy

Children with JIIM may present with other symptoms and signs.[8] Evidence of systemic disease is common (80% in one series[7]), and may include fever, fatigue, malaise, and weight loss. Pulmonary disease, particularly interstitial lung disease, is usually a later finding but presents early in some of the more severe phenotypes.[9,29] Any suggestion of lung involvement should be investigated urgently, as this is associated with poor outcomes and mortality.[11] Gastrointestinal involvement, including pain, constipation, or nausea, can also be an early feature. If severe, abdominal pain can be a sign of bowel vasculitis, which may be associated with severe complications such as gastrointestinal bleeding or perforation. Any indication of bleeding, such as hematemesis or melena, should be taken very seriously and investigated quickly, because it may become massive and life threatening. Arthritis is common, affecting up to 40% of children, and, if extensive, may make assessment of weakness challenging.[30] Involvement of other organ systems, such as cardiac or neurologic systems, is described, although fortunately very rare.

Atypical Presentations of Juvenile Idiopathic Inflammatory Myopathy

Some children with JDM may have no appreciable muscle involvement, even with detailed clinical and imaging assessments. These children have typical rashes of JDM and approximately 25% are at risk of developing clinical weakness.[31] In the literature, these patients may be called amyopathic JDM, clinically amyopathic JDM, hypomyopathic JDM, and more recently skin predominant JDM.[32] In adults, this phenotype may be associated with malignancy,[33] but this is not the case in children.

DIFFERENTIAL DIAGNOSIS AND MIMICS
Rheumatologic

As noted earlier, there is overlap between JDM and other systemic rheumatic diseases. Lupus, scleroderma, and mixed connective tissue disease may all have cutaneous features that suggest JDM and may include myositis as one of their manifestations. A positive antinuclear autoantibody (ANA) test does not distinguish among these conditions. In children presenting with apparently acquired muscle weakness without rash, considerable care must be taken. Although the diagnosis may be JPM, this condition is much rarer and more likely to be misdiagnosed because of difficulties in distinguishing from other disorders.

Myopathic and Dystrophic

There are many myopathies and muscular dystrophies that may present with isolated muscle weakness. The pattern of weakness may be a hint to some of these diagnoses (such as distal weakness or asymmetry). In circumstances such as these, muscle biopsy and the involvement of a clinician skilled in neuromuscular disease are recommended.

Infectious

Several infections may be associated with muscle inflammation and symptoms. The most common of these is postinfluenza myositis, which follows an influenza illness and is typically associated with calf pain and marked increase in muscle enzyme levels. This condition is self-limited and requires only symptomatic treatment. Several other viral illnesses may also cause myositis, including Coxsackie group B and human immunodeficiency virus. In addition, some parasitic infections may be associated with chronic muscle disease, such as toxoplasma and trichinae, and should be considered in appropriate clinical circumstances.

Endocrinologic or Metabolic

Endocrine disorders, including adrenal and thyroid disease, may be associated with muscle weakness, although other symptoms associated with these problems are likely to suggest the correct diagnosis. Metabolic diseases, such as glycogen storage diseases or lipid storage diseases, may also be associated with muscle weakness.

Other Rashes

Many of the rashes of JDM are erythematous and scaly. They can be mistaken for psoriasis lesions, although the distribution may suggest the correct diagnosis. Consideration of other erythematous rashes is also needed, including eczema and fungal infections.

A summary of differential diagnoses and mimics of JIIM can be found in **Box 3**.[34,35]

PATHOGENESIS

The JIIMs are autoimmune disorders, as suggested by their association with autoantibodies and frequent family history of other autoimmune illnesses. It is recognized that there are both genetic factors and environmental factors involved. In particular, infections seem to be important triggers.[2,12,36–38] Associations with season[12] and ultraviolet exposure[37] have also been documented.

At its heart, JIIM seem to be associated with a vasculopathy of small capillaries, related to swelling of the capillary cells and subsequent limitation of blood flow. At least part of the disorder seems to be related to microscopic areas of ischemia. At the same time, inflammation occurs, which seems to be related to involvement of interferons and interferon-related gene products.[2,39] Perpetuation of the inflammatory process is thought to be related to a complex interplay of the interferon system and ischemic damage, although it remains incompletely understood.

The vasculopathic process is present throughout the body. It can be directly visualized by examination of the digital nailfold capillaries.[40] Visualization is often improved by application of a thin coat of lubricant to the nailfold. Using an ophthalmoscope as a magnifier in the clinic, the findings of capillary dropout, dilatation, hemorrhage, and tortuosity can be seen (see **Fig. 3**, see also Figure 8 for examples in Suzanne C. Li's article, "Scleroderma in Children and Adolescents: Localized Scleroderma and Systemic Sclerosis," in this issue). Vasculopathy is thought to contribute to the manifestations in skin and muscle, and possibly other end organs.

Lung disease in JIIM, in the form of progressive fibrosis, is now recognized as an important problem.[11,29,41] Pathogenesis is not well understood but is associated with, and may be pathogenically related to, certain autoantibodies (in particular anti-tRNA synthetase and anti-MDA5 autoantibodies).

LABORATORY AND IMAGING STUDIES FOR DIAGNOSIS AND CARE
At Diagnosis

Evaluation of muscle enzyme levels is a key part of initial evaluation. As noted previously, they include CK, ALT, AST, LDH, and aldolase. There is no consensus on which muscle enzyme is the most sensitive or most useful. Most children with JIIM have increases in the levels of 1 or more of these enzymes. It is important to measure several to minimize the possibility of missing the diagnosis. However, in any given child, some may be normal, and, in 10% to 15% of children, all are normal.[42] Normal muscle enzyme levels do not rule out JIIM. Very high values (CK>100,000 units/L) are possible but less likely, and should prompt additional consideration of alternative diagnoses, such as Duchenne or Becker muscular dystrophy.

Evaluation of MSA has become recognized as an important aspect of diagnosis of JIIM.[43] They assist with identifying JIIM phenotypes and are associated with both important complications (such as interstitial lung disease) and prognosis. At this time, the biggest challenge with obtaining MSA is that only a handful of laboratories in the world are considered accurate, and both false-positive and

Box 3
Differential diagnoses and mimics to consider for juvenile idiopathic inflammatory myopathies

Without typical skin lesions
  Neuromuscular diseases
    Dystrophies
      Duchenne muscular dystrophy
      Becker muscular dystrophy
      Dysferlin deficiency (limb-girdle muscular dystrophy type 2B)
      Other limb-girdle muscular dystrophy
      Merosin deficiency (infantile polymyositis)
      Congenital muscular dystrophy
      Emery-Dreifuss muscular dystrophy
      Facioscapulohumeral muscular dystrophy
      Myotonic muscular dystrophy
      Oculopharyngeal muscular dystrophy
    Myopathies
      Nemaline rod myopathy
      Multicore/minicore myopathy
      Centronuclear/myotubular myopathy
      Mitochondrial myopathies
  Disorders of metabolism
    Glycogen storage diseases
    Lipid storage diseases
    Vitamin D deficiency
    Disorders of sodium, potassium, calcium, magnesium, or phosphorus metabolism
  Endocrine myopathies
    Hypothyroidism/hyperthyroidism
    Hypoparathyroidism/hyperparathyroidism
    Adrenal disorders (excess or deficient glucocorticoid, hyperaldosteronism)
    Excess growth hormone (acromegaly)
  Myopathy/myositis associated with infection[a]
    Viral
      Influenza, influenza, coxsackievirus B, human immunodeficiency virus, others
    Parasitic
      Toxoplasma, Trypanosoma, Trichinae, cysticerci
    Other
      Borrelia burgdorferi, Legionella pneumophila
  Drug-related/toxin-related myopathies
    Lipid-level-lowering agents (fibrates, statins, niacin)
    Corticosteroids
    Chronic alcohol exposure
    Other (D-penicillamine, procainamide, cimetidine, phenytoin, propylthiouracil, amiodarone, chloroquine, hydroxychloroquine, colchicine, zidovudine)

With typical skin lesions[b]
  Other rheumatic illnesses
    Systemic lupus erythematosus
    Scleroderma
    Mixed connective tissue disease
    Overlap syndromes
  Other erythematous rashes with scaling
    Psoriasis
    Eczema
    Fungal infections
    Secondary syphilis

[a] Rash associated with the relevant infection may be present, and may mimic typical dermatomyositis rashes.
[b] Skin lesions may be absent or atypical.
Data from Chawla J. Stepwise approach to myopathy in systemic disease. Front Neurol 2011;2:49; and Hoffman EP, Rao D, Pachman LM. Clarifying the boundaries between the inflammatory and dystrophic myopathies: insights from molecular diagnostics and microarrays. Rheum Dis Clin North Am 2002;28(4):743–57.

false-negative results are common with most techniques. Consultation with an expert in the diagnosis of JIIM is recommended before having this testing performed.

The original Bohan and Peter[20] criteria included muscle biopsy and electromyography (EMG). Muscle biopsy has become much less used over time, because of its invasiveness and concerns about missing an affected area because of the patchiness of muscle disease.[8] However, recent literature has described several additional evaluations that can be done on tissue specimens to assist in diagnosis.[44] In addition, biopsy results have recently been shown to correlate with disease prognosis, resulting in recommendations to increase the role of muscle biopsy in diagnosis.[45] Typical features in JDM include mononuclear infiltrates in the perivascular region and perifascicular atrophy under light microscopy. The exact role of muscle biopsy at the present time is not entirely clear. However, when the diagnosis is uncertain (suspected polymyositis, atypical distribution of weakness, or other unusual features), biopsy is recommended, and it should be performed by a surgeon experienced in the collection and handling of muscle for this purpose. Muscle biopsies should be interpreted by a pathologist with experience in differentiating between different muscle diseases and assessing their severity.

The role of EMG has diminished considerably.[8] It is invasive and requires cooperation sometimes from very young children. In JIIM, it is often not necessary. However, it remains a potential tool in identifying those children with an alternative diagnosis. In this case, consultation with a neuromuscular expert is recommended.

The diminished use of biopsy and EMG is largely related to marked increase in the use of MRI.[8] This modality has several advantages, including being relatively noninvasive, offering the ability to assess many muscles simultaneously, and sensitivity to low levels of inflammation. Most commonly the short-tau inversion recovery (STIR) sequence is used to image the hip girdle and/or shoulder girdle, looking for inflammatory changes within the proximal muscles[46,47] (Fig. 5). Total-body MRI has also been advocated.[48] MRI is expensive, requires sedation in young children, and is not available to all patients. Expertise in assessment of muscle MRI in children is not available in all centers. However, most children with JIIM in recent studies have received MRI as part of their diagnostic evaluation.

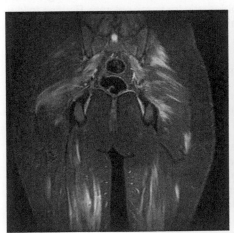
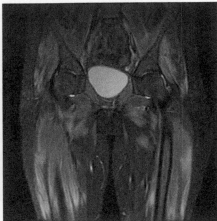

Fig. 5. STIR MRI, without contrast, of a child with JDM showing extensive but patchy increased signal through muscles of the pelvis and thighs, consistent with inflammation.

At the time of diagnosis, most children have had routine hematology and chemistry evaluation, including muscle enzyme levels. Except for 1 or more muscle enzymes, most of these results are normal, including minimal if any changes in inflammatory markers. Blood work to assist in ruling out other diagnoses is also recommended, including routine ANA testing, which is helpful to rule out lupus if negative but does not necessarily identify a specific rheumatic disease if positive. If the ANA is positive, the rheumatologist to whom the patient is referred will investigate the possibility of lupus and other rheumatic disorders by checking antibodies against double-stranded DNA and extractable nuclear antigens, levels of complement C3 and C4, and coagulation parameters. Infectious disease serologies should be checked as suggested by signs, symptoms, and history consistent with possible exposure. For primary care providers, these evaluations probably constitute an appropriate work-up. Given issues around access and interpretation, imaging (including MRI), MSA, other specific autoantibodies, and muscle biopsy should be deferred until specialist consultation.

Baseline chest radiographs are probably appropriate, looking for either evidence of ground-glass changes or signs of fibrosis/scarring, given the potential for interstitial lung disease in a subset of patients with JIIM. Baseline cardiac evaluation may also be appropriate to assess for signs of myocardial or valvular dysfunction, although formal recommendations are not available.

At Follow-up

In follow-up, clinical examination remains key. However, laboratory testing may be helpful. It is important to recognize that the correlation between muscle enzyme levels and disease activity is limited once treatment has begun.[49] Monitoring of muscle enzyme levels should still be done on a regular basis, because they may point to a flare. However, they should not be relied on, because a flare may occur without a significant change. Monitoring of blood counts and transaminase levels is also important to detect possible medication toxicity but is complicated by the overlap of muscle and liver enzymes and the requirement for interpretation.

There is some suggestion that repeat assessment of MSA can be used as a marker of disease response.[50] However, it is not routine at this time, and, given the difficulty and costs of obtaining these tests, is not recommended.

Follow-up MRI may be helpful in assessing disease response or identifying disease flare; however, cost and access remain problematic for some patients. Routine follow-up EMG or biopsy is not recommended, although either may have a role in selected patients.

HOW JUVENILE IDIOPATHIC INFLAMMATORY MYOPATHIES ARE TREATED

In general, it is recommended that treatment in JIIM be initiated by or in direct consultation with specialists with expertise in the management of these rare disorders.[46] The primary goals of treatment are to:

1. Normalize muscle strength and physical function.
2. Control other extramuscular disease features, in particular skin disease.
3. Minimize toxicity related to long-term steroids. Given the predictable toxicity of prolonged courses of corticosteroids (see Gloria C. Higgins's article, "Complications of Treatment for Pediatric Rheumatic Disease," in this issue), use of steroid-sparing therapies is critical.

It should be noted that many experts consider persistent skin disease to be a manifestation of ongoing systemic disease.[51]

Several nonpharmacologic approaches are important. Given the potential role of sun exposure in disease flares,[52,53] appropriate sun protection measures are recommended for all patients with JIIM.[53] These measures include avoidance of the sun during peak hours, use of sunscreen, and appropriate clothing. Calcium and vitamin D supplementation are usually given to reduce steroid effects on bone metabolism.[46] Involvement of both physiotherapy and occupational therapy, where available, is also helpful to minimize contractures, promote strength recovery, and support normal physical functioning.[46,54] More recently, the use of graduated strengthening programs as an so-called exercise prescription has been advocated, although specific recommendations are not available.[46]

Few clinical trials exist on which to base treatment recommendations in JIIM. However, there has been consensus work that has led to general agreement on treatment approaches.

A recent effort in Europe resulted in general recommendations for the evaluation and treatment of children with JIIM.[46] This group agreed that, for most patients, the combination of corticosteroids and methotrexate was appropriate. They also recommended weaning of steroids as clinically indicated. They did not make recommendations about dosage.

These recommendations are consistent with the findings of the Pediatric Rheumatology International Trials Organization, which conducted a randomized, open-label trial comparing prednisone alone, prednisone plus methotrexate, and prednisone plus cyclosporin.[55] They found that the 2 combination groups had better outcomes and that the prednisone plus methotrexate group experienced less toxicity. Prednisone was started at 2 mg/kg/d and tapered over 24 months, whereas the methotrexate dose was 15 to 20 mg/m^2 weekly either subcutaneously or intramuscularly.

The Childhood Arthritis and Rheumatology Research Alliance (CARRA) has developed several consensus clinical treatment plans (CTP) for children with JDM.[32,56–58] These plans are not intended to be treatment recommendations but reflect typical treatment approaches of North American pediatric rheumatologists. In the CTPs for children with moderate JDM, all 3 approaches included both prednisone and methotrexate. Prednisone was started at 2 mg/kg/d (maximum 60 mg) and the methotrexate dose was the lesser of 15 mg/m^2 or 1 mg/kg weekly. A consensus tapering schedule for prednisone extended over approximately 1 year, although, as the investigators point out, there was considerable controversy, with opinion ranging from 4 to 24 months.[57] Some experts advocate the use intravenous methylprednisolone in initial treatment, because of concerns of possible inadequate absorption of oral medication.[59] Although treatment with corticosteroids is tapered to discontinuation over approximately 1 year, other therapies (eg, methotrexate) are usually continued for at least a year after corticosteroids are stopped.

For children who are severely ill, for example with severe weakness, breathing or swallowing difficulties, bowel vasculitis, rapidly progressive lung disease, or other serious organ involvement, initial treatment with daily pulse intravenous steroids is usually given (typically 30 mg/kg/d methylprednisolone, up to 1000 mg). For such patients, and for those who are unresponsive to initial therapy, several other agents have been used. Intravenous immunoglobulin is often helpful, with relatively few side effects.[60] Reports have also documented the successful use of cyclophosphamide with acceptable toxicity.[61] Other possible agents include cyclosporin[55] or mycophenolate.[62] The Rituximab in Myositis (RIM) trial did not meet its primary end point, but results did suggest that rituximab may be a useful agent in children with JDM, particularly those with MSA.[63,64]

Side effects and appropriate monitoring for these medications used to treat JIIM can be found in Gloria C. Higgins's article, "Complications of Treatment for Pediatric Rheumatic Disease," in this issue.

WHAT IS THE PROGNOSIS FOR JUVENILE IDIOPATHIC INFLAMMATORY MYOPATHIES?

In general, the prognosis for JIIM is good, with many patients making complete recoveries and returning to normal function. However, over the last few years, it has become clear that there are more patients with long-term morbidities than was previously recognized. About 25% of patients experience a monocyclic course, recovering and successfully discontinuing medications within approximately 2 years.[9] Another 25% of patients have a polyphasic course, with clear periods of complete remission and recurrence, sometimes with prolonged periods off therapy.[9] The remaining 50% have a chronic course, meaning that they continue to require therapy (and often continue to have disease manifestations) for more than 2 years.[9] For some patients, their illness can stretch over much longer than 2 years.

Several reports have documented that approximately 40% of patients with JDM experience long persistence of their disease.[65–67] This persistence may be reflected as persistent skin rash or persistent impairments in physical function, including weakness, reduced muscular endurance, or contractures. In one study, approximately one-third of patients were still on immunosuppressive or immunomodulatory medications at a median of 7.2 years of follow-up. More research is needed in this area.

Calcinosis is a particular problem in JIIM, primarily JDM. Up to 40% of patients develop calcinosis to some degree over the course of their illness.[13,65] In one study, about one-quarter continued to have calcinosis after a median 7.2 years of follow-up.[65] Although some calcinosis is very mild, and other cases resolve completely, an unknown proportion continue to have pain, disfigurement, impairments in physical function, and overall impact on quality of life for many years.

Mortality in JIIM is generally low. Reliable statistics are lacking, but it is accepted that mortality is no greater than 2% and may be less.[11] Factors associated with an increased risk of death include having a non-JDM form of JIIM, pulmonary disease, and anti-tRNA synthetase autoantibodies.[11] The recently described anti-MDA5 autoantibody is probably also a risk for mortality, given the association with severe and rapidly progressive pulmonary disease.[29,41]

SUMMARY

The JIIMs are a group of rare, chronic, autoimmune, and complex disorders affecting muscles. They are associated with several signs and symptoms in other organ systems, particularly the skin. Diagnosis may be straightforward when patients present with typical features but is frequently challenging. Early involvement of specialists with expertise in diagnosis and management of these disorders is strongly recommended.

REFERENCES

1. Ernste FC, Reed AM. Idiopathic inflammatory myopathies: current trends in pathogenesis, clinical features, and up-to-date treatment recommendations. Mayo Clin Proc 2013;88(1):83–105.
2. Rider LG, Nistala K. The juvenile idiopathic inflammatory myopathies: pathogenesis, clinical and autoantibody phenotypes, and outcomes. J Intern Med 2016; 280(1):24–38.
3. Bitnum S, Daeschner CW Jr, Travis LB, et al. Dermatomyositis. J Pediatr 1964;64: 101–31.
4. Meyer A, Meyer N, Schaeffer M, et al. Incidence and prevalence of inflammatory myopathies: a systematic review. Rheumatology (Oxford) 2015;54(1):50–63.

5. Darin N, Tulinius M. Neuromuscular disorders in childhood: a descriptive epidemiological study from western Sweden. Neuromuscul Disord 2000;10(1):1–9.

6. Guseinova D, Consolaro A, Trail L, et al. Comparison of clinical features and drug therapies among European and Latin American patients with juvenile dermatomyositis. Clin Exp Rheumatol 2011;29(1):117–24.

7. McCann LJ, Juggins AD, Maillard SM, et al. The Juvenile Dermatomyositis National Registry and Repository (UK and Ireland)–clinical characteristics of children recruited within the first 5 yr. Rheumatology (Oxford) 2006;45(10):1255–60.

8. Robinson AB, Hoeltzel MF, Wahezi DM, et al. Clinical characteristics of children with juvenile dermatomyositis: the childhood arthritis and rheumatology research alliance registry. Arthritis Care Res (Hoboken) 2014;66(3):404–10.

9. Shah M, Mamyrova G, Targoff IN, et al. The clinical phenotypes of the juvenile idiopathic inflammatory myopathies. Medicine (Baltimore) 2013;92(1):25–41.

10. Mendez EP, Lipton R, Ramsey-Goldman R, et al. US incidence of juvenile dermatomyositis, 1995-1998: results from the National Institute of Arthritis and Musculoskeletal and Skin Diseases Registry. Arthritis Rheum 2003;49(3):300–5.

11. Huber AM, Mamyrova G, Lachenbruch PA, et al. Early illness features associated with mortality in the juvenile idiopathic inflammatory myopathies. Arthritis Care Res (Hoboken) 2014;66(5):732–40.

12. Pachman LM, Hayford JR, Chung A, et al. Juvenile dermatomyositis at diagnosis: clinical characteristics of 79 children. J Rheumatol 1998;25(6):1198–204.

13. Hoeltzel MF, Oberle EJ, Robinson AB, et al. The presentation, assessment, pathogenesis, and treatment of calcinosis in juvenile dermatomyositis. Curr Rheumatol Rep 2014;16(12):467.

14. Valenzuela A, Chung L, Casciola-Rosen L, et al. Identification of clinical features and autoantibodies associated with calcinosis in dermatomyositis. JAMA Dermatol 2014;150(7):724–9.

15. Satoh M, Tanaka S, Ceribelli A, et al. A comprehensive overview on myositis-specific antibodies: new and old biomarkers in idiopathic inflammatory myopathy. Clin Rev Allergy Immunol 2017;52(1):1–19.

16. Hashkes PJ, Wright BM, Lauer MS, et al. Mortality outcomes in pediatric rheumatology in the US. Arthritis Rheum 2010;62(2):599–608.

17. Dobloug GC, Svensson J, Lundberg IE, et al. Mortality in idiopathic inflammatory myopathy: results from a Swedish nationwide population-based cohort study. Ann Rheum Dis 2018;77(1):40–7.

18. Qiang JK, Kim WB, Baibergenova A, et al. Risk of malignancy in dermatomyositis and polymyositis. J Cutan Med Surg 2017;21(2):131–6.

19. Tansley SL, McHugh NJ, Wedderburn LR. Adult and juvenile dermatomyositis: are the distinct clinical features explained by our current understanding of serological subgroups and pathogenic mechanisms? Arthritis Res Ther 2013;15(2):211.

20. Bohan A, Peter JB. Polymyositis and dermatomyositis (second of two parts). N Engl J Med 1975;292(8):403–7.

21. Lundberg IE, Tjarnlund A, Bottai M, et al. 2017 European League Against Rheumatism/American College of Rheumatology classification criteria for adult and juvenile idiopathic inflammatory myopathies and their major subgroups. Arthritis Rheumatol 2017;69(12):2271–82.

22. Dugan EM, Huber AM, Miller FW, et al. Review of the classification and assessment of the cutaneous manifestations of the idiopathic inflammatory myopathies. Dermatol Online J 2009;15(2):2.

23. Dugan EM, Huber AM, Miller FW, et al. Photoessay of the cutaneous manifestations of the idiopathic inflammatory myopathies. Dermatol Online J 2009; 15(2):1.

24. Tiao J, Feng R, Berger EM, et al. Evaluation of the reliability of the cutaneous dermatomyositis disease area and severity index and the cutaneous assessment tool-binary method in juvenile dermatomyositis among paediatric dermatologists, rheumatologists and neurologists. Br J Dermatol 2017;177(4):1086–92.

25. Huber AM, Dugan EM, Lachenbruch PA, et al. Preliminary validation and clinical meaning of the cutaneous assessment tool in juvenile dermatomyositis. Arthritis Rheum 2008;59(2):214–21.

26. Huber AM, Feldman BM, Rennebohm RM, et al. Validation and clinical significance of the Childhood Myositis Assessment Scale for assessment of muscle function in the juvenile idiopathic inflammatory myopathies. Arthritis Rheum 2004;50(5):1595–603.

27. Huber AM, Hicks JE, Lachenbruch PA, et al. Validation of the Childhood Health Assessment Questionnaire in the juvenile idiopathic myopathies. Juvenile dermatomyositis disease activity collaborative study group. J Rheumatol 2001;28(5): 1106–11.

28. Rider LG, Koziol D, Giannini EH, et al. Validation of manual muscle testing and a subset of eight muscles for adult and juvenile idiopathic inflammatory myopathies. Arthritis Care Res (Hoboken) 2010;62(4):465–72.

29. Sato S, Uejima Y, Nanbu M, et al. Clinical analysis and outcome of interstitial lung disease complicated with juvenile dermatomyositis and juvenile polymyositis. Mod Rheumatol 2017;27(4):652–6.

30. Tse S, Lubelsky S, Gordon M, et al. The arthritis of inflammatory childhood myositis syndromes. J Rheumatol 2001;28(1):192–7.

31. Walling HW, Gerami P, Sontheimer RD. Juvenile-onset clinically amyopathic dermatomyositis: an overview of recent progress in diagnosis and management. Paediatr Drugs 2010;12(1):23–34.

32. Huber AM, Kim S, Reed AM, et al. Childhood arthritis and rheumatology research alliance consensus clinical treatment plans for juvenile dermatomyositis with persistent skin rash. J Rheumatol 2017;44(1):110–6.

33. Udkoff J, Cohen PR. Amyopathic dermatomyositis: a concise review of clinical manifestations and associated malignancies. Am J Clin Dermatol 2016;17(5): 509–18.

34. Chawla J. Stepwise approach to myopathy in systemic disease. Front Neurol 2011;2:49.

35. Hoffman EP, Rao D, Pachman LM. Clarifying the boundaries between the inflammatory and dystrophic myopathies: insights from molecular diagnostics and microarrays. Rheum Dis Clin North Am 2002;28(4):743–57.

36. Feldman BM, Rider LG, Reed AM, et al. Juvenile dermatomyositis and other idiopathic inflammatory myopathies of childhood. Lancet 2008;371(9631):2201–12.

37. Habers GE, Huber AM, Mamyrova G, et al. Brief report: association of myositis autoantibodies, clinical features, and environmental exposures at illness onset with disease course in juvenile myositis. Arthritis Rheumatol 2016;68(3):761–8.

38. Manlhiot C, Liang L, Tran D, et al. Assessment of an infectious disease history preceding juvenile dermatomyositis symptom onset. Rheumatology (Oxford) 2008;47(4):526–9.

39. Ernste FC, Reed AM. Recent advances in juvenile idiopathic inflammatory myopathies. Curr Opin Rheumatol 2014;26(6):671–8.

40. Barth Z, Witczak BN, Flato B, et al. Microvascular abnormalities assessed by nail-fold capillaroscopy in juvenile dermatomyositis after medium to long-term follow-up. Arthritis Care Res (Hoboken) 2018;70(5):768–76.
41. Kobayashi N, Takezaki S, Kobayashi I, et al. Clinical and laboratory features of fatal rapidly progressive interstitial lung disease associated with juvenile derma-tomyositis. Rheumatology (Oxford) 2015;54(5):784–91.
42. Stringer E, Singh-Grewal D, Feldman BM. Predicting the course of juvenile der-matomyositis: significance of early clinical and laboratory features. Arthritis Rheum 2008;58(11):3585–92.
43. Tansley SL, Simou S, Shaddick G, et al. Autoantibodies in juvenile-onset myositis: Their diagnostic value and associated clinical phenotype in a large UK cohort. J Autoimmun 2017;84:55–64.
44. Varsani H, Charman SC, Li CK, et al. Validation of a score tool for measurement of histological severity in juvenile dermatomyositis and association with clinical severity of disease. Ann Rheum Dis 2015;74(1):204–10.
45. Deakin CT, Yasin SA, Simou S, et al. Muscle biopsy findings in combination with myositis-specific autoantibodies aid prediction of outcomes in juvenile dermato-myositis. Arthritis Rheumatol 2016;68(11):2806–16.
46. Enders FB, Bader-Meunier B, Baildam E, et al. Consensus-based recommenda-tions for the management of juvenile dermatomyositis. Ann Rheum Dis 2017; 76(2):329–40.
47. Kimball AB, Summers RM, Turner M, et al. Magnetic resonance imaging detection of occult skin and subcutaneous abnormalities in juvenile dermato-myositis. Implications for diagnosis and therapy. Arthritis Rheum 2000;43(8): 1866–73.
48. Castro TC, Lederman H, Terreri MT, et al. Whole-body magnetic resonance imag-ing in the assessment of muscular involvement in juvenile dermatomyositis/poly-myositis patients. Scand J Rheumatol 2014;43(4):329–33.
49. Guzman J, Petty RE, Malleson PN. Monitoring disease activity in juvenile derma-tomyositis: the role of von Willebrand factor and muscle enzymes. J Rheumatol 1994;21(4):739–43.
50. Betteridge Z, McHugh N. Myositis-specific autoantibodies: an important tool to support diagnosis of myositis. J Intern Med 2016;280(1):8–23.
51. Christen-Zaech S, Seshadri R, Sundberg J, et al. Persistent association of nailfold capillaroscopy changes and skin involvement over thirty-six months with duration of untreated disease in patients with juvenile dermatomyositis. Arthritis Rheum 2008;58(2):571–6.
52. Mamyrova G, Rider LG, Ehrlich A, et al. Environmental factors associated with disease flare in juvenile and adult dermatomyositis. Rheumatology (Oxford) 2017;56(8):1342–7.
53. Shah M, Targoff IN, Rice MM, et al, Childhood Myositis Heterogeneity Collabora-tive Study Group. Brief report: ultraviolet radiation exposure is associated with clinical and autoantibody phenotypes in juvenile myositis. Arthritis Rheum 2013;65(7):1934–41.
54. Habers GE, Bos GJ, van Royen-Kerkhof A, et al. Muscles in motion: a random-ized controlled trial on the feasibility, safety and efficacy of an exercise training programme in children and adolescents with juvenile dermatomyositis. Rheuma-tology (Oxford) 2016;55(7):1251–62.
55. Ruperto N, Pistorio A, Oliveira S, et al. Prednisone versus prednisone plus ciclo-sporin versus prednisone plus methotrexate in new-onset juvenile dermatomyosi-tis: a randomised trial. Lancet 2016;387(10019):671–8.

56. Huber AM, Giannini EH, Bowyer SL, et al. Protocols for the initial treatment of moderately severe juvenile dermatomyositis: results of a Children's Arthritis and Rheumatology Research Alliance Consensus Conference. Arthritis Care Res (Hoboken) 2010;62(2):219–25.

57. Huber AM, Robinson AB, Reed AM, et al. Consensus treatments for moderate juvenile dermatomyositis: beyond the first two months. Results of the second Childhood Arthritis and Rheumatology Research Alliance consensus conference. Arthritis Care Res (Hoboken) 2012;64(4):546–53.

58. Kim S, Kahn P, Robinson AB, et al. Childhood Arthritis and Rheumatology Research Alliance consensus clinical treatment plans for juvenile dermatomyositis with skin predominant disease. Pediatr Rheumatol Online J 2017;15(1):1.

59. Rouster-Stevens KA, Gursahaney A, Ngai KL, et al. Pharmacokinetic study of oral prednisolone compared with intravenous methylprednisolone in patients with juvenile dermatomyositis. Arthritis Rheum 2008;59(2):222–6.

60. Lam CG, Manlhiot C, Pullenayegum EM, et al. Efficacy of intravenous Ig therapy in juvenile dermatomyositis. Ann Rheum Dis 2011;70(12):2089–94.

61. Riley P, Maillard SM, Wedderburn LR, et al. Intravenous cyclophosphamide pulse therapy in juvenile dermatomyositis. A review of efficacy and safety. Rheumatology (Oxford) 2004;43(4):491–6.

62. Rouster-Stevens KA, Morgan GA, Wang D, et al. Mycophenolate mofetil: a possible therapeutic agent for children with juvenile dermatomyositis. Arthritis Care Res (Hoboken) 2010;62(10):1446–51.

63. Aggarwal R, Bandos A, Reed AM, et al. Predictors of clinical improvement in rituximab-treated refractory adult and juvenile dermatomyositis and adult polymyositis. Arthritis Rheumatol 2014;66(3):740–9.

64. Oddis CV, Reed AM, Aggarwal R, et al. Rituximab in the treatment of refractory adult and juvenile dermatomyositis and adult polymyositis: a randomized, placebo-phase trial. Arthritis Rheum 2013;65(2):314–24.

65. Huber A, Feldman BM. Long-term outcomes in juvenile dermatomyositis: how did we get here and where are we going? Curr Rheumatol Rep 2005;7(6):441–6.

66. Mathiesen P, Hegaard H, Herlin T, et al. Long-term outcome in patients with juvenile dermatomyositis: a cross-sectional follow-up study. Scand J Rheumatol 2012; 41(1):50–8.

67. Sanner H, Kirkhus E, Merckoll E, et al. Long-term muscular outcome and predisposing and prognostic factors in juvenile dermatomyositis: a case-control study. Arthritis Care Res (Hoboken) 2010;62(8):1103–11.

Scleroderma in Children and Adolescents

Localized Scleroderma and Systemic Sclerosis

Suzanne C. Li, MD, PhD[a,b,*]

KEYWORDS

- Juvenile localized scleroderma • Juvenile systemic sclerosis • Pediatric scleroderma
- Morphea • Pediatric rheumatology • Extracutaneous involvement • Morbidity

KEY POINTS

- Scleroderma is a complex disease associated with inflammation, vasculopathy, and fibrosis. Extracutaneous involvement is common.
- There are 2 main forms: localized scleroderma and systemic sclerosis (SSc), each with several subtypes. Juvenile localized scleroderma (jLS) and juvenile systemic sclerosis (jSSc) represent different diseases with some shared pathophysiology.
- Both jLS and jSSc are associated with a high prevalence of major morbidity from skin and extracutaneous disease. jSSc also has a significant mortality risk, although much lower than adult SSc.
- No cure is available; treatment is directed at controlling inflammation to minimize damage severity, and managing specific skin and other organ problems.
- Assessment and management of jLS and jSSc are often difficult. Earlier diagnosis and initiation of appropriate treatment can greatly improve outcome.

INTRODUCTION

Scleroderma comes from the Greek word for "hard skin" and refers to diseases associated with excessive production of collagen resulting in fibrosis of skin and other affected organs. There are 2 main forms, localized scleroderma (LS) and systemic sclerosis (SSc), with LS about 6 to 10 times more common than SSc in children. Dermatologists often refer to LS as morphea. Although LS and SSc share some pathophysiologic pathways, they represent different diseases rather than a

Disclosure Statement: The author has received consulting fees from Bristol-Myers Squibb and funding from Childhood Arthritis and Rheumatology Research Alliance (CARRA), Arthritis Foundation, and Scleroderma Foundation.
[a] Department of Pediatrics, Hackensack Meridian School of Medicine at Seton Hall University, 30 Prospect Avenue, Hackensack, NJ 07601, USA; [b] Division of Pediatric Rheumatology, Joseph M. Sanzari Children's Hospital, Hackensack University Medical Center, 30 Prospect Avenue, Hackensack, NJ 07601, USA
* 30 Prospect Avenue, Hackensack, NJ 07601.
E-mail address: suzanne.li@hackensackmeridian.org

Pediatr Clin N Am 65 (2018) 757–781
https://doi.org/10.1016/j.pcl.2018.04.002
0031-3955/18/© 2018 Elsevier Inc. All rights reserved.

pediatric.theclinics.com

single disease continuum. Juvenile localized scleroderma (jLS) is not thought to evolve into juvenile systemic sclerosis (jSSc); rarely, some patients have both forms of scleroderma.[1] Both are chronic diseases that can present in different patterns (subtypes) and are usually associated with extracutaneous involvement. Overall morbidity and mortality are much worse for jSSc with patients at risk for life-threatening lung, heart, and other visceral organ fibrosis and vasculopathy. Mortality is extremely rare in jLS, but morbidity is common, with patients at risk for major disfigurement and functional impairment from extracutaneous involvement. This article reviews the different forms of jLS, and jSSc, common presenting features of both diseases, and provides an overview of management and prognosis. Early diagnosis and initiation of treatment for juvenile scleroderma can greatly improve outcome, and long-term shared management with a pediatric rheumatologist is strongly recommended.

INCIDENCE

Scleroderma is a rare condition. About one-third of LS cases begin in childhood,[2] whereas less than 10% of SSc begins in childhood.[3,4]

- jLS: incidence is 0.34 to 2.7 cases per 100,000 per year[2,5]
- jSSc: incidence in a recent UK study was 0.27 per million children per year[5]

DEMOGRAPHICS
Age

Onset age: mid childhood

- jLS: mean age of onset is 6.4 to 8.7 years.[6–9] jLS can present at birth.
- jSSc: mean age of onset is slightly older at 8.1 to 11 years. jSSc is very uncommon in children less than 5 years old.[3,10,11]

Gender

Girls are more commonly affected than boys.

- jLS: 70% to 80% girls[6–9]
- jSSc: 76% to 84% girls[3,12]

Race

- jLS is more prevalent in Caucasians (73%–82% of cases)[5,6,8,13]
- Racial predominance is less clear for jSSc
  - No racial predilection identified in a registry of patients from Europe, Asia, and South and North America[10,14]
  - Caucasian predominance (92%) in one US study[3]
  - A North American registry reported 78% Caucasian, 19% African American, 3% Asian[11]
  - In adult SSc, African Americans have a higher prevalence, more severe disease, and higher mortality than Caucasians[15]

MAJOR DIFFERENCES FROM ADULT SCLERODERMA

jLS has overall poorer outcome than adult LS[16]:

- Higher frequency of linear scleroderma, mixed morphea, and pansclerotic morphea subtypes[17]
- More deep tissue involvement

- Higher frequency of extracutaneous involvement[17]
- Longer disease duration[16]

jSSc has overall better outcome than adult SSc[3,10,18]:

- Lower frequency of major visceral organ involvement[3,10,18]
- Lower mortality[3,10,18]

DELAYS IN DIAGNOSIS ARE COMMON FOR BOTH JUVENILE LOCALIZED SCLERODERMA AND JUVENILE SYSTEMIC SCLEROSIS

The median time between initial symptom and diagnosis of jLS is 11 to 13.1 months, with diagnosis delayed for more than 2 years in 20% of patients.[8,19,20] Those with head lesions often have a longer delay; one study reported a median time to diagnosis of 8.9 years, with some not diagnosed for greater than 40 years.[21]

The median delay in jSSc diagnosis is 8 months to 2.8 years, with diagnosis delayed for 2 or more years in greater than 20% of patients.[3,10,11,20]

WHEN TO CONSIDER JUVENILE LOCALIZED SCLERODERMA

jLS should be considered in a child with one or more persistent, unilateral, linear, or oval skin lesions that has erythema, violaceous color, a white or yellow waxy appearance, and/or skin thickening or induration (**Fig. 1**A, B). Lesions often have hyperpigmentation and/or a depressed contour because of atrophy of dermal subcutaneous, and deeper tissues (**Fig. 1**C, **Fig. 2**A). Head lesions may have facial or scalp hair loss (see **Fig. 2**A). Linear lesions follow a specific pattern (Blaschko lines; **Fig. 2**).

HOW JUVENILE LOCALIZED SCLERODERMA PRESENTS

LS encompasses a large spectrum of clinical presentations and severities. A classification schema developed by the Pediatric Rheumatology European Society divides jLS into 5 subtypes (**Fig. 1, Table 1**; see Ref.[22]). Not included are eosinophilic fasciitis, lichen sclerosus et atrophicus (LSA), or atrophoderma of Pasini and Pierini, which are included in some other classification criteria.[17,23]

Most pediatric patients have the linear scleroderma subtype, either alone or as part of mixed morphea.[6,8,9,17] Linear scleroderma can present as individual lesions that later merge to form a continuous long lesion. These lesions follow Blaschko lines, an embryonic pattern that represents genetic mosaicism (see **Fig. 2**).[7,17] Linear lesions often involve underlying subcutaneous tissue and muscle and can become hard and bound down to these tissues, restricting mobility. Atrophy of underlying tissues can result in a depressed contour or groovelike appearance (see **Figs. 1**C and **2**; **Fig. 3**). Linear lesions on the head, known as en coup de sabre (ECDS), can cause alopecia of scalp, eyebrow, or eyelashes, and thinning or depression of the skull (see **Fig. 2**A).[19] The atrophy from the Parry-Romberg syndrome (PRS) form varies from subtle to severe, with overlying skin often normal (**Fig. 4**).

Circumscribed morphea is the most common adult subtype, but only represents about 30% of jLS (see **Fig. 1**A, B).[8] Lesions can be single or multiple. When lesions are larger and involve more body sites, the patient has generalized morphea; these lesions often extend and coalesce, involving large regions. Pansclerotic morphea has widespread, often confluent skin and deep tissue involvement (see **Fig. 1**E). The mixed subtype is a combination of 2 or more subtypes and occurs in 14% to 23% of jLS patients.[6,8,13,24]

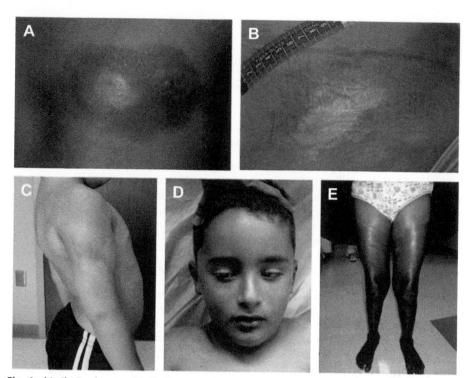

Fig. 1. (*A–E*) LS subtypes. (*A, B*) Circumscribed superficial morphea. (*C*) Linear scleroderma of limb. (*D*) Linear scleroderma of face (ECDS). (*E*) Pansclerotic morphea. (*A*) Active lesion with severe level of erythema and central thickening that has a waxy white appearance. (*B*) Active lesion with violaceous border around waxy center; there is mild epidermal and dermal atrophy with visible venous pattern. (*C*) Linear scleroderma extending along arm from back to fingers, with mild erythema and violaceous color around resolving waxy skin thickening. There is hyperpigmentation and subcutaneous atrophy of mid upper arm. (*D*) Early ECDS, with mild erythema extending from right medial forehead to cheek. (*E*) Pansclerotic morphea affecting both legs with hyperpigmentation and increased skin thickening. There is mild erythema in upper thighs, and severe subcutaneous atrophy of lower legs. ([*A, B*] *From* Li S, Pope E. Localized scleroderma. In: Petty R, Laxer R, Lindsley C, editors. Cassidy's textbook of pediatric rheumatology. 7th edition. Philadelphia: Elsevier; 2016. p. 407; with permission.)

Clinical Features

Cutaneous features

Skin lesions proceed through different stages. Careful assessment for disease activity is essential because immunosuppressive treatment is effective for the active but not the sclerotic phase. Skin scoring measures can help with tracking disease level, with some measures tracking one lesion and others assessing disease level in all affected sites.[25–27] Scored features include skin thickening, erythema, violaceous color, waxy color/texture, and disease extent.[25–27] Tracking activity is often difficult, with skin signs subtle, or obscured by skin damage signs, especially for relapsing disease. In many patients, activity resides primarily in deeper tissues, so it may result in worsening atrophy or contractures without obvious skin activity signs. Imaging (ultrasound, MRI) can help monitor some of these patients, in conjunction with experienced clinical assessment.[28–30]

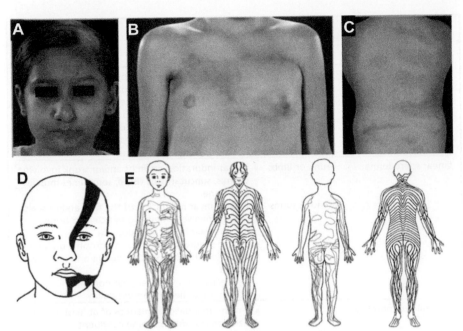

Fig. 2. Blaschko lines. Linear scleroderma lesions follow this embryonic pattern. (*A*) A 10-year-old girl with lesion extending along left side of her face from her scalp to her chin. (*B*, C) Two other patients with linear scleroderma of their chest or back. (*D*) Lesions of patient in (*A*) were plotted on a body chart. (*E*) Red lines show the contours of skin lesions of 31 patients with linear scleroderma, whereas the black lines show Blaschko lines. (*From* Weibel L, Harper JI. Linear morphoea follows Blaschko's lines. Br J Dermatol 2008;159:176; with permission.)

Erythema and violaceous color are early activity signs, with erythema ranging from subtle light pink to deep red (see **Fig. 1**). Additional activity features include waxy white or yellow color (associated with altered skin texture), tactile warmth, and skin thickening, although skin thickening is not exclusively an activity feature.[31] Early skin thickening represents activity from edema or induration, whereas later it represents damage (sclerosis). Because skin thickening varies between anatomic sites, the skin thickening of jLS lesions should be determined in comparison to the contralateral unaffected site. Waxy white or yellow color is an intermediate lesion stage where there is edema, inflammation, and some collagen deposition, causing the skin to become harder and smoother. These lesions are often surrounded by an erythematous or violaceous margin (see **Fig. 1**A, B).[23]

Over time, skin thickening increases and damage features predominate, including dyspigmentation (hyperpigmentation and hypopigmentation) and atrophy. Signs of epidermal and dermal atrophy include shinier or smoother skin, visible veins, loss of hair follicles, and cliff-drop atrophy, whereas subcutaneous tissue atrophy manifests as a deeper, larger, but perhaps less well-demarcated depression of the site. Patients commonly have concurrent signs of both activity and damage (see **Fig. 1**C, E).[32] Evolution of the disease is often slow, with painless enlargement of existing lesions, development of new lesions, and changing lesion features often progressing over months to years before the disease is identified. Lesions may undergo spontaneous softening years later.

Table 1
Preliminary proposed classification of juvenile localized scleroderma

Main Subtype	Subdivision	Description
Circumscribed morphea	Superficial	• Ovoid lesions limited to epidermis and dermis • Referred to as plaque lesions in some criteria • Most on trunk > extremities
	Deep	• Ovoid lesions with deep induration of the skin • Involve subcutaneous tissue, sometimes muscle • Overlying skin can appear normal • Most on trunk > extremities
Linear scleroderma	Trunk or limbs	• Linear induration on limbs and/or trunk involving dermis, subcutaneous tissue, sometimes muscle and bone

	Head: 2 forms	• ECDS. Linear induration of the face and/or scalp
		  ○ May involve underlying muscle and bone
		  ○ Can result in scarring alopecia
		• PRS or progressive hemifacial atrophy; unilateral tissue loss that may involve dermis and underlying tissues
		  ○ Overlying skin may appear normal
		  ○ Skin is mobile, not bound down

Generalized morphea		• 4 or more individual plaques of at least 3 cm in size, lesions often become confluent • Lesions located on at least 2 of the following: head-neck, right or left upper extremity, right or left lower extremity, anterior or posterior trunk • Uncommon in jLS
Pansclerotic morphea		• Circumferential involvement of limb or limbs affecting the skin and underlying tissues • Often widespread involvement of other areas of the body • Rare and the most severe subtype
Mixed Morphea		• Combination of 2 or more of previous subtypes, usually linear and circumscribed, or linear and generalized

Data from Laxer R, Zulian F. Localized scleroderma. Curr Opin Rheumatol 2006;18:606–13, Pediatric Rheumatology European Society Criteria.

Extracutaneous features

Extracutaneous involvement is a major cause of disease morbidity and is associated with all subtypes. It has been reported in 22% to 71% of jLS patients.[13,32–34] The most prevalent type is musculoskeletal, which includes arthralgia, arthritis, joint contractures, myositis, myalgia, muscle spasms, scoliosis, and hemiatrophy.[21,33] Because the disease commonly begins before most children have undergone their major growth spurt, children are at risk of developing severe undergrowth of the affected side (see **Figs. 3** and **4**). Hemiatrophy of the limb can markedly limit function and require surgical intervention, whereas that of the face can impair vision, mastication, and other normal functions.[13,33,35] Growth impairment is common, with studies reporting facial hemiatrophy in half the patients with linear scleroderma of the head, deformity from tissue atrophy and/or muscle bulk reduction in half, and a bone length difference in one-quarter of the patients.[21,32,34]

Patients with head lesions have a higher risk for developing neurologic, oral, dental, and/or ocular extracutaneous morbidity than those who only have lesions on the

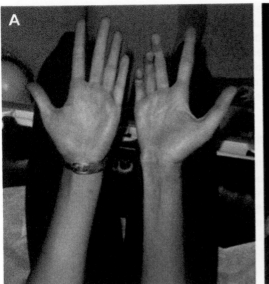
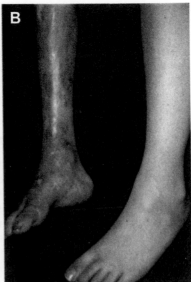

Fig. 3. Musculoskeletal problems from juvenlle LS. (*A*) Linear scleroderma of the right hand resulting in undergrowth and limited extension of several fingers. (*B*) LS of right leg resulting in joint contractures and undergrowth. (*From* [*A*] Li S, Pope E. Localized scleroderma. In: Petty R, Laxer R, Lindsley C, editors. Cassidy's textbook of pediatric rheumatology. 7th edition. Philadelphia: Elsevier; 2016. p. 408; and [*B*] Christen-Zaech S, Hakim MD, Afsar FS, et al. Pediatric morphea (localized scleroderma): review of 136 patients. J Am Acad Dermatol 2008;59(3):390; with permission.)

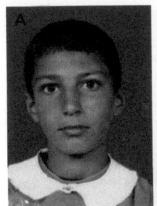
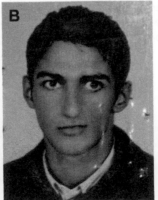
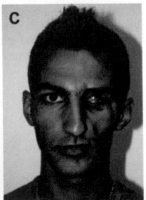

Fig. 4. Progressive PRS of the left side of the face. The patient's appearance at age 8 years (*A*), 16 years (*B*), and 23 years (*C*). Following disease onset at age 6 years, the only treatment of PRS was autologous fat injection at ages 14 and 16 years. Evaluation at age 23 years identified left-sided atrophy of tongue, temporal muscle, zygomatic and maxillary bones, and eye. The patient had displacement of left upper teeth and had lost vision of left eye. (*From* Kaya M, Yilmaz CS, Kurtaran H, et al. Chronologic presentation of a severe case of progressive hemifacial atrophy (Parry-Romberg syndrome) with the loss of an eye. Case Rep Otolaryngol 2014;2014:703017; with permission.)

body (see **Fig. 4**). Neurologic problems include seizures, headaches, cranial nerve palsies, trigeminal and peripheral neuropathy, neuropsychiatric problems, movement disorders, cognitive dysfunction, and other issues.[13,21,33,36] Seizures can be refractory to treatment.[36] Ocular involvement includes fibrotic changes in eyelid or lacrimal gland, anterior segment inflammation (uveitis, episcleritis), hemianopsia, diplopia, ptosis, optic neuritis, keratitis, and strabismus.[33,36] Gastrointestinal, pulmonary, cardiac, and renal problems are rare and not associated with evolution toward jSSc.[13,33,37]

ATYPICAL PRESENTATIONS OF JUVENILE LOCALIZED SCLERODERMA

LS can present at birth or in the toddler age as areas of faint erythema or violaceous color, or atrophy,[38] with colored lesions mistaken for a nevus flammeus or port-wine stain[19] (see **Fig. 12**B, D). Other patients present with extracutaneous involvement, such as arthritis, arthropathy, seizures, or headaches, which can precede the appearance of skin lesions by months to years.[8,36] For 25% to 30% of patients, extracutaneous involvement is remote from the skin lesion site,[33,36] so LS should be considered in the differential of children with unexplained arthropathy, seizures, or other LS-associated problems.

WHEN TO CONSIDER JUVENILE SYSTEMIC SCLEROSIS

jSSc should be considered in a child with moderate to severe Raynaud phenomenon (RP), especially if it is associated with digital ulcers and/or abnormal nailfold capillaroscopy (NFC; **Figs. 7–9**). Other suspicious signs are limited range of finger motion from edema or skin thickening (sclerodactyly) (**Fig. 5**; see **Fig. 10**), and limited oral aperture, especially in a child with poor weight gain or weight loss.

HOW JUVENILE SYSTEMIC SCLEROSIS PRESENTS

Provisional classification criteria for jSSc were developed by the Pediatric Rheumatology European Society and American College of Rheumatology in 2007, which require all subjects to have skin thickening proximal to the metacarpal phalangeal joints, and at least 2 additional (minor) criteria.[39] Minor criteria include several types of organ involvement and certain autoantibodies (**Table 2** see Ref.[39]). Although

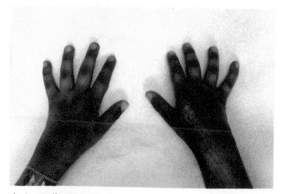

Fig. 5. Hands in early juvenile SSc. Swelling of fingers in a 5-year old girl with SSc. The patient has edema, arthritis, and arthropathy, affecting all fingers and both wrists and both hyperpigmentation and hypopigmentation changes, especially of the right hand and forearm.

Table 2
Provisional classification criteria for juvenile systemic sclerosis

Category	Criteria
Major (required)	Proximal skin sclerosis/induration of the skin
Minor criteria (need at least 2)	
Cutaneous	Sclerodactyly
Peripheral vascular	Raynaud phenomenon (RP) Nailfold capillaroscopy (NFC) abnormalities Digital tip ulcers
Gastrointestinal	Dysphagia Gastroesophageal reflux
Cardiac	Arrhythmias Heart failure
Renal	Renal crisis New-onset arterial hypertension
Respiratory	Pulmonary fibrosis (diagnosed radiologically) Decreased diffusion capacity (DLCO) PAH
Neurologic	Neuropathy Carpal tunnel syndrome
Musculoskeletal	Tendon friction rubs Arthritis Myositis
Serologic	Antinuclear antibodies (ANA) SSc-selective autoantibodies: ACA, ATA, antifibrillarin, anti-PM-Scl, antifibrillin, anti-RNA polymerase I or III

Data from Zulian F, Woo P, Athreya BH, et al. The Pediatric Rheumatology European Society/American College of Rheumatology/European League against Rheumatism provisional classification criteria for juvenile systemic sclerosis. Arthritis Rheum 2007;57(2):203–12.

these criteria were found to have excellent sensitivity and specificity, there is concern that they may miss patients with earlier and/or milder disease, who are potentially better able to respond to current therapies. The adult classification criteria were recently revised to better identify early SSc (**Table 3**[40]). More evaluation is needed to determine if these criteria improve identification of early jSSc.

There are 3 main subtypes of jSSc: diffuse, limited, and overlap[3,18,41]:

- Diffuse cutaneous (dcSSc)
  - Skin affected distal to elbows, knees, and neck, AND
  - Skin of proximal limbs, chest, and/or abdomen affected
  - Rapid skin progression often occurs
  - Major visceral organ involvement: gastrointestinal tract, lung > heart, kidney
  - Antitopoisomerase (ATA) antibody associated
- Limited cutaneous (lcSSc)
  - Skin affected distal to elbows, knees, and neck
  - Vasculopathy is prominent, including RP, pulmonary arterial hypertension (PAH), and renal crisis
  - Anticentromere antibody (ACA) associated
  - Less common in jSSc than adult SSc[3,18]

Table 3

The American College of Rheumatology/European League Against Rheumatism criteria of the classification of systemic sclerosis

Criteria	Subcriteria	Score
Skin thickening of fingers of both hands extending proximal to the metacarpophalangeal (MCP) joints		
Sufficient by itself		9
Skin thickening of fingers		
Only count higher score	Puffy fingers	2
	Sclerodactyly of the fingers (proximal to the proximal interphalangeal and distal to the MCP joints)	4
Fingertip lesions		
Only count higher score	Digital tip ulcers	2
	Fingertip pitting scars	3
Telangiectasia		2
Abnormal NFC		2
Lung involvement		
Only score 1; maximum score = 2	PAH	2
	ILD	2
RP		3
SSc-associated autoantibodies: ACA, ATA I, or anti-RNA polymerase III		3

The total score is calculated by adding the highest score in each category. A score of ≥9 is required for classification as having SSc.

Data from van den Hoogen F, Khanna D, Fransen J, et al. 2013 classification criteria for systemic sclerosis: an American College of Rheumatology/European League against Rheumatism collaborative initiative. Arthritis Rheum 2013;65(11):2737–47.

- Overlap SSc
  - Has features of another rheumatic diseases, most commonly:
    - Dermatomyositis/polymyositis
    - Systemic lupus erythematosus
    - Sjogren syndrome
    - Inflammatory arthritis
  - Can have either a limited or diffuse cutaneous pattern
  - More common in jSSc than adult SSc[3,18]

Clinical Features

Cutaneous features

Skin involvement occurs in nearly all (74%–100%) jSSc patients. Involvement commonly begins in the hands and face and is usually bilateral and symmetric (see **Fig. 5**). The skin transitions through 3 stages: edema, followed by induration and sclerosis, and then atrophy. The induration and sclerosis stage is associated with robust fibrosis causing the skin to become hard, tight, and at times bound down to the underlying subcutaneous tissues.[14,42] Loss of adnexal structures leads to a shinier, smoother appearance, with the face often developing an unwrinkled, immobile, and expressionless appearance with limited oral aperture (**Fig. 6**).[12,14] In the atrophic phase, the skin softens, losing its thickness.[42] Other skin changes include dyspigmentation (hyperpigmentation and hypopigmentation), telangiectasias, and calcinosis

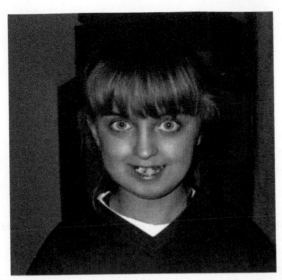

Fig. 6. Smooth facies of SSc. This jSSc patient shows typical facial features with excessively un-wrinkled and smooth skin appearance. She also has limited oral aperture. (*Courtesy of* Jennifer E Weiss, MD, Hackensack, NJ.)

(over extensor and periarticular surfaces), with calcinosis more prominent in limited jSSc.[14]

The modified Rodnan Skin Score is used to track extent and severity of skin thickening in adult SSc. The body is divided into 17 anatomic sites, with skin thickening assessed by gentle wrinkling of the skin with either both thumbs or the thumb and index finger of one hand; a score of 0 represents no increased thickening and 3 immobile, rock-hard skin thickening.[42] Higher scores are associated with a higher likelihood of internal organ involvement and mortality.[42] More study is needed on how to assess skin thickening in children because it is affected by body mass index and Tanner stage, with healthy children found to have elevated scores compared with normal adults.[43]

Raynaud phenomenon

RP is common in jSSc, affecting 74% to 100% of patients.[3,10,18] RP results from transient vasospasm of peripheral arteries and arterioles, often in response to cold or stress. Affected areas show sharply demarcated color changes, with cyanosis indicating blood deoxygenation from stasis, and pallor indicating lack of blood from complete blood vessel closure (**Fig. 7**).[44] With prolonged vasospasm, patients experience numbness or paresthesias and then pain. Pain indicates local ischemia, with prolonged episodes causing tissue infarction that can produce digital pits, ulcers, or gangrene (**Fig. 8**). Ischemic episodes should be reversed quickly and ideally prevented from occurring. RP can be either primary or secondary. The latter refers to RP associated with rheumatic diseases or other identifiable causes, including exposure to certain medications or chemicals, and repetitive local trauma or injury. Primary RP is common in the general population, and unlike secondary RP, not associated with irreversible tissue damage.[45] RP patients at risk for developing scleroderma often have an abnormal NFC pattern. Instead of the normal pattern of thin, linear capillaries that are fairly uniform in dimension, SSc patients and those at risk for developing SSc often have giant vessels ($\geq$2-fold increase in width) associated with a moderate to severe decrease in capillary density, and even avascular regions (**Fig. 9**).[45–47]

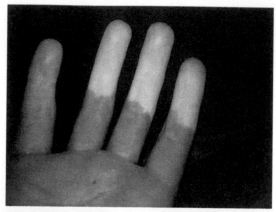

Fig. 7. RP. Sharp demarcation of pallor in this adolescent with RP after cold exposure. (*Courtesy of* Dr J.E. Weiss, Hackensack U. Medical Center, Hackensack, NJ.)

Musculoskeletal problems

Musculoskeletal involvement occurs in 50% to 80% of patients with jSSc and includes arthralgia, joint stiffness, contractures, myalgia, and weakness.[3,11,14,48] Hands commonly have limited range of motion, from edema (puffy fingers), synovitis, and fibrosis of the skin (sclerodactyly), joint, and/or tendon tissues (see **Fig. 5**). The fibrosis and joint destruction can progress to disabling deformity (**Fig. 10**).[48] Muscle involvement is usually symmetric, involving proximal muscles and manifesting as myositis, fibrosis, and atrophy.[14,48,49] Children also develop tapering of the fingertips and shortening of the middle and distal phalanges, possibly from chronic digital ischemia.[3] Tendon friction rubs, a rubbing, squeaking sensation over tendons of the wrists, ankles, and other joints, are associated with severe diffuse skin involvement, internal organ involvement, and higher mortality in adults.[48]

Gastrointestinal disease

Gastrointestinal involvement is found in 42% to 74% of jSSc. Any part of the gut can be affected, with the esophagus affected early.[3,11,41] Heartburn, dysphagia with a sensation of stuck food in the midchest, early satiety, bloating, nighttime cough,

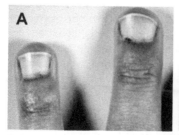
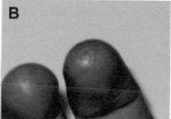
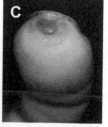

Fig. 8. NFC changes and digital tissue loss associated with RP in SSc. (*A*) The NFC changes in this patient with jSSc can be seen without magnification. (*B*) Mild digital pitting. (*C*) Deep ischemic ulceration in a patient with SSc. (*Courtesy of* Drs. V Smith and M Cutolo on behalf of the EULAR study group on microcirculation in Rheumatic Diseases; *From* Cutolo M, Sulli A, Pizzorni C, Accardo S. Nailfold videocapillaroscopy assessment of microvascular damage in systemic sclerosis. J Rheumatol 2000;27:155–60.)

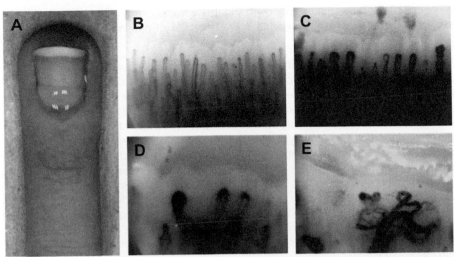

Fig. 9. NFC patterns associated with SSc. Examining the NFC of patients with RP can help identify those at risk for developing SSc. (*A*) NFC can be examined by videocapillaroscopy with immersion oil or lubricating jelly placed over the periungual area of each finger. In the office, an ophthalmoscope set at 10 to 40 Diopters can be used, with the examiner manually zooming in until they can clearly see the NFC. (*B*) Normal capillary pattern with fairly uniform vessels. (*C*) Early SSc changes include capillary dilation, giant vessels ($\geq$50 μm), and hemorrhages. Active (*D*) and late (*E*) scleroderma patterns show capillary loss with avascular areas. There is neoangiogenesis in the late pattern. (*Courtesy of* Drs V. Smith, Ghent University, Gent, Belgium; and M. Cutolo, University Medical School of Genova, Genova, Italy, on behalf of the EULAR study group on microcirculation in Rheumatic Diseases; and *Data from* Cutolo M, Sulli A, Pizzorni C, et al. Nailfold videocapillaroscopy assessment of microvascular damage in systemic sclerosis. J. Rheumatol 2000;27:155–60.)

and pain are common.[49] Constipation and diarrhea also occur.[41] Disease-related problems include esophageal strictures, gastroesophageal reflux disease, gastric antral vascular ectasia, dysmotility and slow motility, malabsorption, intestinal pseudo-obstruction, bacterial overgrowth, and impaired anal sphincter function.[41] A

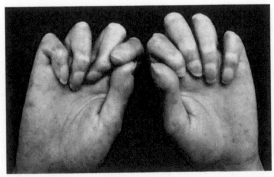

Fig. 10. Severe joint contractures of SSc. Hands of a 27-year-old woman with dcSSc that began in childhood. There was essentially no movement possible in these fingers. (*From* Zulian F. Systemic sclerodermas. In: Petty R, Laxer R, Lindsley C, editors. Cassidy's textbook of pediatric rheumatology. 7th edition. Philadelphia: Elsevier; 2016. p. 400; with permission.)

major concern is malnutrition, so growth should be tracked, monitoring for poor weight gain or weight loss, which is reported in 14% to 18% of patients.[10,11]

Heart and lung disease

Cardiopulmonary disease is a major cause of SSc mortality, with interstitial lung disease (ILD) and PAH the main culprits.[12,50] Lung disease occurs in 34% to 55% of jSSc patients, and heart disease occurs in 4% to 17%.[3,11] Symptoms include nonproductive cough, mild dyspnea on exertion, and fatigue.[12] All patients should be regularly screened with a pulmonary function test (PFT) to look for restrictive disease (decreased forced vital capacity) and/or decreased diffusion capacity of carbon monoxide (DLCO). Patients with abnormal PFTs should be evaluated with a high-resolution computed tomography (HRCT) scan because of its better sensitivity for ILD; signs include ground glass opacities, fibrosis, honeycombing, and traction bronchiectasis (**Fig. 11**).[12] Patients should also be regularly screened for the development of pulmonary hypertension, initially with an echocardiogram. If the echocardiogram is normal but suspicion of early PAH is high, right heart catheterization can be performed for diagnosis.[12] Other problems include pericarditis, arrythmias, ventricular dysfunction, and cardiomyopathy.[10,14]

Other organ Involvement

Scleroderma renal crisis, with rapidly progressive malignant hypertension and renal failure, needs aggressive treatment to prevent mortality. High-dose corticosteroid treatment is associated with increased risk in adults, but this association is less clear in jSSc partly because of the rarity of renal crisis in jSSc (<5%).[3,10] Rapidly progressive skin disease, tendon rubs, and RNA Pol III autoantibodies are other adult risk factors.[41] Neurologic problems are uncommon and include seizures and peripheral and cranial neuropathy.[10,14]

ATYPICAL PRESENTATIONS OF JUVENILE SYSTEMIC SCLEROSIS

A rare presentation is systemic sclerosis sine scleroderma, where the patient has RP and severe internal organ disease typical for SSc, but no skin thickening.[51] A small subset of jSSc patients have a rapidly progressive course, leading to mortality within 1 to 5 years of diagnosis.[50] Potential risk factors for early mortality are raised creatinine level, pericarditis, and signs of fibrosis on chest radiograph (CXR).[50]

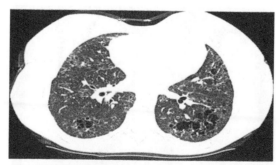

Fig. 11. Lung disease at diagnosis in a 9-year-old patient with SSc. Patient was noted to have blue fingers at age 5 years old, and limited oral aperture by her dentist at age 9 years old. At the craniofacial clinic, she was suspected to have SSc. Her initial lung HRCT scan shows ILD with ground glass opacities, bronchiectasis, cysts, and honeycombing. (*Courtesy of Dr A. Stevens, Seattle Children's Hospital, U. Washington, Seattle, WA.*)

DIFFERENTIAL DIAGNOSIS OR MIMICS OF JUVENILE LOCALIZED SCLERODERMA OR JUVENILE SYSTEMIC SCLEROSIS

A wide range of diseases can be confused with localized or systemic scleroderma, partly related to their varied presentations. Although a skin biopsy may help with diagnosis, for most patients the diagnosis can be made from the history, clinical, and laboratory features. Good diagnostic clues for jLS are atrophy and a Blaschko pattern for linear lesions (see **Fig. 2**), and good diagnostic clues for jSSc are RP and the presence of autoantibodies (**Table 4**).

Active, early jLS lesions may be confused with a bruise, port-wine stain (**Fig. 12**B), insect bite, or a rash related to infection, such as tinea.[32] Two other conditions that follow Blaschko lines are lichen sclerosus et atrophicus (LSA) and atrophoderma of Pasini and Pierini (APP). LSA often coexists with LS and may resemble hypopigmented atrophic lesions.[17] APP can present as depressed erythematous lesions, and in some classification schemes, it is considered a type of LS.[17] Hyperpigmented lesions may resemble granuloma annulare, lichen simplex chronicus, postinflammatory hyperpigmentation, atopic eczema, or a nevus, whereas atrophic lesions may be mistaken for varicose veins or lipoatrophy (**Fig. 12**).[32]

Table 4
Clues to the diagnosis of pediatric scleroderma

	LS	SSc
Pattern of skin involvement	• Unilateral for linear scleroderma (usually) • Bilateral, widespread involvement for generalized or pansclerotic morphea • Discrete areas except for severe generalized or pansclerotic morphea • Linear follows Blaschko lines	• Bilateral, symmetric • On limbs, usually circumferential, contiguous • Back less commonly affected

Skin features	• Skin thickening/hardness
	• Erythema or violaceous color, in lesion or margin
	• Dyspigmentation
	• Telangiectasia
	• Waxy appearance, smooth texture
	• Warmth
	• Atrophy at lesion sites
	  ○ Skin
	  ○ Subcutaneous fat
	• Focal loss of scalp and/or facial hair
		• Skin thickening/hardness
		• May have erythema and pruritis with hand edema
		• Dyspigmentation
		• Telangiectasia
		• Calcinosis
		• Atrophy
		  ○ Diffuse skin atrophy
		  ○ Digital pits, ulcers from RP
		• Color changes of RP
		• NFC changes: scleroderma pattern

Autoantibody findings	• +ANA in about 50% of patients	• +ANA in most patients • Other autoantibodies also present and may be prognostic
Extracutaneous involvement	• Joints common, arthritis can be remote from skin lesion site • Head lesions: higher risk for oral, eye, brain involvement • Neurologic problems: headache, seizures, neuropathy, and other problems	• Joints common, especially fingers • Limited oral aperture • Visceral organ (gut, lung, heart, kidney) involvement common • Neuropathy uncommon

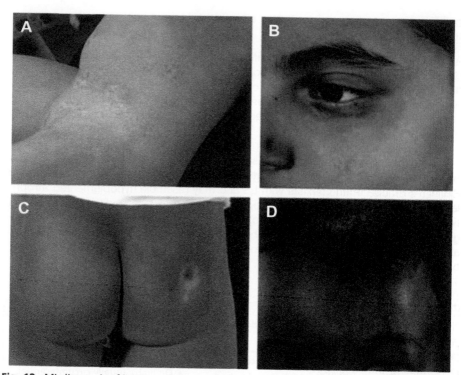

Fig. 12. Misdiagnosis of jLS. Four children whose LS was initially misdiagnosed. All had biopsy-proven disease. (*A*) A 2.5-year-old girl, initial diagnosis telangiectatic nevus, who had a 1 year history of progressive telangiectatic and hypopigmented skin lesions along her left trunk and face associated with atrophy. (*B*) A 6-year-old girl, initial diagnosis port-wine stain, with an 8-month history of persistent erythema of left lower eyelid, with left cheek atrophy. (*C*) A 9-year-old girl, initial diagnosis lipoatrophy, attributed to vaccination, although no history of vaccination at site. She had a 6-month history of progressive right buttock indentation, with dyspigmentation and atrophy of the entire right buttock. (*D*) A 5-year-old girl, initial diagnosis melanocytic nevus, with 7-month history of a unilateral hyperpigmented macule on her left forehead that spread toward her scalp and medial left eyelid. There is hair loss of her scalp and medial left eyebrow. (*From* Weibel L, Laguda B, Atherton D, et al. Misdiagnosis and delay in referral of children with localized scleroderma. Br J Dermatol 2011;165:1310; with permission.)

jLS patients with widespread involvement, such as severe generalized or pansclerotic disease, may be suspected to have jSSc. Other differential diagnoses for widespread jLS or jSSc include extensive eosinophilic fasciitis, mixed connective tissue disease, graft-versus-host disease, progeria, scleroderma-like syndromes induced by environmental factors (ie, eosinophilia-myalgia), scleredema, diabetic cheiroarthropathy, scleromyxedema, and nephrogenic systemic fibrosis.[51,52] Pansclerotic morphea, unlike SSc, can affect the entire back, generally has milder involvement of fingers and hands, and is rarely associated with RP or major internal organ involvement. Eosinophilic fasciitis is associated with more inflammation and less fibrosis than scleroderma. Patients often develop painful swelling of limbs, including hands and feet, followed by progressive thickening and induration in a peau d'orange pattern.[17,23] Scleredema affects primarily the torso, neck, and upper arms, but unlike SSc, generally does not affect the hands or feet.[52] The skin may be smooth or have a peau d'orange texture similar to eosinophilic fasciitis. Scleredema can be associated with infections, poorly controlled diabetes mellitus, or neoplasms.

CAUSE AND PATHOGENESIS

Scleroderma is a complex disease involving derangements in the immune, vascular, and connective tissue systems. LS and SSc share some pathophysiologic processes. Common cytokine and immune cell profiles have been identified,[53] and a shared inflammatory gene expression pattern was identified in LS and SSc skin.[54] However, major differences exist between the diseases, including different HLA allele associations and a higher autoantibody prevalence in SSc, which suggest there are different disease immunophenotypes.[55,56] SSc-specific gene expression profiles have also been identified, including patterns specific to the diffuse or limited subtypes.[54]

Both the innate and the adaptive immune systems are involved, initiating and/or perpetuating inflammation in the vasculature and connective tissue (see Kathleen E. Sullivan's article, "Pathogenesis of Pediatric Rheumatologic Diseases," in this issue for overview of immune problems in rheumatic disease). Proinflammatory and profibrotic cytokines, including transforming growth factor-beta (TGF-β), platelet-derived growth factor, connective tissue growth factor (CTGF), interleukin 6 (IL-6), IL-4, IL-1-alpha, and chemokine ligand 4 (CXCL4), are secreted by immune, endothelial, and fibroblasts.[56,57] Lymphocyte abnormalities include a predominance of profibrotic T-helper 17 (Th17) and Th2 cells, reduced or defective T-regulator cells, and generation of autoreactive B cells producing autoantibodies.[56]

The normal balance in the vasculature is shifted toward vasoconstriction, causing tissue hypoxia, oxidative stress, and vascular damage.[56] Antiendothelial auto-antibodies can cause microvascular inflammation and endothelial cell apoptosis, resulting in the generation of more immunogenic peptides and autoantibodies, further perpetuating the vasculopathy.[56] Vascular repair and angiogenesis are defective.[56] Endothelin-1, one of the key vasoconstrictors, promotes fibrosis as does tissue hypoxia.[56] Tissue hypoxia induces the transition of epithelial cells into mesenchymal cells and stimulates fibroblasts to produce more collagen and profibrotic cytokines (TGF-β, CTGF).[56,57] SSc fibroblasts also appear to be in a prolonged activated state that is shifted toward extracellular matrix synthesis over degradation.[56] The end result of these processes is capillary loss.[57]

The identification of some environmental and genetic factors suggests the disease may be triggered in susceptible individuals.[56] In LS, 13% to 16% of patients were found to have a history of environmental events close to disease onset, with trauma accounting for most of these events.[8,13,58] Trauma included accidental trauma, surgery, injections, insect bites, herpes zoster, and radiation exposure.[8,58] SSc environmental factors include infection (retroviral, latent cytomegalovirus), organic solvents, crystalline silica, estradiol (higher disease prevalence in women), and neoplasm.[56]

LABORATORY AND IMAGING STUDIES FOR DIAGNOSIS AND CARE
Laboratory Studies

There is no single test for making the diagnosis of jLS or jSSc. General screening tests are performed to evaluate for other conditions, to assess if there are markers of inflammation that can be tracked, and as part of safety monitoring for adverse effects from medications. Typical tests for the primary care provider include complete blood cell count, chemistry panel, erythrocyte sedimentation rate, C-reactive protein, and urinalysis. Muscle enzyme (creatinine kinase, aldolase, lactate dehydrogenase) and immunoglobulin levels may be checked in patients with more extensive and/or deeper disease.

Laboratory test abnormalities include elevated white blood count, eosinophilia, elevated acute phase reactants, elevated muscle enzymes, and anemia, which are more common in jSSc than jLS.[10,14] In jLS, they are more likely associated with generalized, pansclerotic, or deep morphea, and among mimics, are more common in eosinophilic fasciitis.[8,13] Anemia in jSSc can represent chronic disease, vitamin deficiency from malabsorption (B12, folate), or iron deficiency from occult blood loss.[14] The serum creatinine levels and urinalysis should be routinely monitored in jSSc for renal disease.

Autoantibodies

Ordering of specific autoantibodies should be left to the pediatric subspecialist.

ANA: Should be performed by indirect immunofluorescence to capture the nucleolar pattern that will always be missed by multiplex bead technique.[41]

- jLS: present in about half the patients[3,10,14,24]
- jSSc: present in 80% to 97%[3,10,14,24]

Other autoantibodies:

- jLS:
  - Uncommon, may represent an epiphenomenon of autoimmunity because LS is associated with a higher prevalence of other autoimmune diseases.[6,13]
  - ATA and ACA are positive in less than 5% of jLS patients
    - ATA and ACA are not associated with evolution toward SSc, so should not be routinely checked in jLS[6,14]
- jSSc:
  - ATA: 20% to 46% of jSSc patients,[3,10,18] associated with dcSSc and severe ILD in adults[41]
  - ACA: Uncommon in jSSc, associated with lcSSc and PAH in adults[41]
  - Anti U1-RNP and Pm-Scl: associated with overlap subtype
  - Anti-RNA polymerase III: associated with dcSSc and scleroderma renal crisis in adults[41]

Imaging

Choice of imaging modality and its interpretation are best left to the rheumatologist. Ultrasound or MRI can help monitor tissue inflammation in jLS, and radiographs can evaluate severity of some musculoskeletal morbidity. Ultrasound is likely more sensitive for superficial to intermediate tissue layers, whereas MRI is better for fascial, deep muscle, and joint evaluation.[28–30] jLS patients with head lesions may warrant an MRI to evaluate for possible brain involvement, although the correlation between imaging abnormalities and clinical disease is limited.[21,36]

For jSSc, a CXR can screen for cardiopulmonary disease, but is less sensitive than HRCT for detecting and monitoring ILD. The CXR may sometimes identify esophageal dilatation. The barium swallow and upper gastrointestinal series with small bowel follow-through are often performed for SSc gastrointestinal evaluation. Imaging of other sites, such as muscles, joints, or brain, depends on symptoms.

Biopsy

Skin biopsies are not needed for routine diagnosis and are discouraged before referral. They can be helpful in the evaluation of atypical skin findings, or occasionally to better assess disease activity. For patients suspected to have eosinophilic fasciitis, a deeper tissue biopsy is needed. The histopathology for jLS and jSSc can be indistinguishable, although jLS lesions are more likely to show inflammatory cells. Early on, there is perivascular, interstitial, and periadnexal inflammation, primarily with lymphocytes, and increased amounts of abnormal collagen.[59] Later, excessive fibrosis predominates, with dense collagen replacing adnexal structures, fat cells, blood vessels, and other normal structures.[17]

HOW JUVENILE SCLERODERMA IS TREATED

A partnership between the pediatric primary care provider and pediatric rheumatologist is important for optimizing care and outcome for children and adolescents with jLS or jSS. The pediatrician serves a critical role in promoting general health, including monitoring growth and development, minimizing infection risk by providing vaccinations (see Gloria C. Higgins' article, "Complications of Treatments for Pediatric Rheumatic Diseases," in this issue), and encouraging healthy lifestyle, including a good diet with adequate calcium and vitamin D, regular exercise, good sleep quality, and stress management (see Sharon Bout-Tabaku's article, "General Nutrition and Fitness for the Child with Rheumatic Disease," in this issue). Because there are no cures for either disease, treatment goals are to improve function, to reduce the risk for, and/or level of serious morbidity, and to enable the child to have normal growth and development. Given that these are rare chronic diseases, which are often difficult to assess, treatment should be initiated by or in consultation with a pediatric rheumatologist or other physician with expertise in their management.

For both diseases, treatment is typically directed toward controlling inflammation to limit fibrosis and vasculopathy, because there are few options for directly controlling those problems. Systemic immunosuppressive medications, as described in the later sections, are commonly used to control inflammation in jSSc and moderate to severe jLS. Although corticosteroids can be helpful in juvenile LS, serious adverse effects are common with long-term use, so steroid-sparing immunosuppressants are favored for long-term treatment. High-dose corticosteroid treatment increases the risk for renal crisis in adult SSc,[60] and even though this complication is very rare in children, corticosteroids are traditionally used sparingly, if at all, in jSSc. Adult SSc recommendations include avoiding corticosteroid use in early dcSSc and in those with anti-RNA polymerase III antibody if possible, and keeping the daily prednisone dose to <15 mg.[60] Potential adverse effects of medications used to treat scleroderma are discussed in Gloria C. Higgins' article, "Complications of Treatments for Pediatric Rheumatic Diseases," in this issue.

Nonpharmacologic management is also important and includes physical and occupational therapy to reduce contractures and improve function. Children should be encouraged to participate in normal activities, including attending school and most extracurricular activities. Because sclerotic skin may have poorer healing, skin protection is important and includes moisturizing affected skin and avoiding/limiting trauma. jSSc patients should avoid activities that may trigger their RP, such as cold exposure from winter sports or swimming in cold water; other triggers include smoking, caffeine, and emotional stress.[45] They should use sun protection, because ultraviolet radiation from the sun can increase the risk of skin cancer and worsen dyspigmentation. jSSc patients need to guard against overheating because sclerotic skin limits their ability to dissipate heat.

Monitoring of weight and height is important, especially for jSSc patients, whose food intake is often limited by gastrointestinal involvement. Head involvement in jLS is associated with a higher frequency of oral and ocular abnormalities, so these patients should get routine evaluation of their teeth and eyes, including slit-lamp examinations. Patients and families may also benefit with support groups for these diseases, with potential resources provided by arthritis and scleroderma foundations in the United States and Canada (US: https://www.arthritis.org, http://www.scleroderma.

org; CA: http://www.arthritis.ca, http://www.scleroderma.ca), and Childhood Arthritis and Rheumatolgy Research Alliance (CARRA) (https://carragroup.org).

Juvenile Localized Scleroderma Treatment

Treatment of jLS is based on disease severity. Disease severity definitions for jLS were generated by a subgroup of a pediatric rheumatology research network (CARRA) as part of their effort to identify optimal jLS therapies. Low severity is defined as circumscribed superficial morphea not associated with subcutaneous atrophy, extracutaneous involvement, or scalp hair loss. Moderate to high-disease severity includes all other subtypes, and patients who have deeper tissue or extracutaneous involvement.[27] Low-severity disease is often treated by dermatologists with topical agents (corticosteroids, tacrolimus, imiquimod, vitamin D analogues) or phototherapy (UVA or UVB).[17] Those with moderate to high-severity disease are at risk for serious morbidity because they commonly have much longer disease durations and extracutaneous involvement. Deeper tissue involvement may not be detectable by clinical examination or may develop later, so long-term monitoring of patients considered to have low severity disease is recommended to monitor for any changes in disease level.

The CARRA group agreed that moderate to high-severity jLS should be treated with systemic immunosuppressive medications.[27] Three methotrexate-based regimens (with or without intravenous or oral corticosteroids) were generated based on best available evidence and consensus agreement among members.[27] There is general agreement among pediatric rheumatologists and dermatologists on stratifying patients and the use of methotrexate to treat moderate to severe jLS.[13,17,32,61,62] A randomized double-blind placebo-controlled trial has shown the efficacy and safety of combined methotrexate and corticosteroid treatment of active jLS, as have several case series.[61] The aim of jLS treatment is to completely suppress inflammation and thereby minimize development of serious morbidity, such as arthropathy, hemiatrophy, neurologic abnormalities, and other extracutaneous manifestations. It is not clear that any of the current treatment strategies can reverse hemiatrophy, but it is possible that early treatment may limit the severity of this problem, as it may do for other extracutaneous involvement.[63] Because the severity of growth differences may not become manifest until the child enters the pubertal growth spurt, careful continual monitoring for signs of activity and corresponding adjustment of treatment is recommended. Once the child is considered to be in remission on medication, most pediatric rheumatologists in North America continue treatment with methotrexate for an additional 1 to 2 years.[64] However, relapses are common, reported in 15% to 53% of jLS patients, so long-term monitoring of patients is needed.[32,62,65] Detection of flares is often difficult because skin damage features such as hyperpigmentation are nearly universal[66] and may mask early recurrence signs such as erythema.

Mycophenolate mofetil has been found beneficial for some patients with jLS who have an inadequate response to or do not tolerate methotrexate.[17,27] Phototherapy with UVA1 or narrowband UVB has been found effective in several adult trials, but effectiveness for extracutaneous involvement and potential adverse effects such as skin cancer and premature aging for pediatric patients are not known.[17] Other immunomodulators, including biologic agents, are being explored as options for nonresponders. Surgery has been used to correct atrophy or other deformities, but because disease can flare following surgery, this should ideally only be considered when the disease is inactive.[13,17]

Juvenile Systemic Sclerosis Treatment

Treatment of jSSc is based on organs affected, with medications based primarily on adult studies because of the lack of jSSc studies. The European League Against

Rheumatism organization recently updated their treatment recommendations for adult SSc manifestations that had sufficient supporting data.[67] Methotrexate is recommended for skin disease; mycophenolate mofetil may also be beneficial.[67] Cyclophosphamide is recommended for ILD, although it has limited efficacy and serious potential adverse effects.[67] Limited studies suggest mycophenolate mofetil and rituximab are potential alternatives for ILD.[41,67] Duration of treatment with any given medication is not known and will be based on clinical and other evaluations. However, jSSc should be considered a lifetime disease. Autologous hematopoietic stem cell transplant has been used for dire cases, but has a 10% treatment-associated mortality risk.[41]

Calcium channel blockers, commonly nifedipine, are recommended to reduce RP episode frequency and severity and promote healing.[45] For those with an inadequate response, phosphodiesterase type 5 (PDE5) inhibitors (sildenafil, tadalafil), endothelin receptor antagonist (bosentan), and nitropaste are used.[45,67] For those at risk of digital infarct, intravenous prostacyclins (iloprost) are given.[41,67] Several of these treatments (endothelin receptor antagonist, PDE5 inhibitors, and intravenous prostacyclins) are also used for PAH.[41,67] PAH patients need aggressive treatment and monitoring, with nonresponders potentially requiring lung transplantation.[41]

Gastroesophageal reflux disease should be treated aggressively with high doses of proton pump inhibitors.[67] Prokinetics (metoclopramide, erythromycin) are given for motility problems (dysphagia, gastroesophageal reflux disease, early satiety, bloating, pseudo-obstruction), and intermittent or rotating antibiotics given for symptomatic small intestinal bowel overgrowth.[41] Conservative strategies include eating frequent small meals with low fiber, avoiding eating before sleep, and elevating the head of the bed.[41] Good dental hygiene and adequate nutrition are important, with supplementation sometimes needed.

Corticosteroids (typically prednisone), methotrexate, and nonsteroidal anti-inflammatory drugs are used for active musculoskeletal problems, with corticosteroid doses kept low because of concern for renal crisis.[14] Routine monitoring of blood pressure (BP) is important. If renal crisis is suspected, the patient should be admitted to a tertiary care center for aggressive treatment with angiotensin converting enzyme inhibitors and other agents to normalize BP.[67]

WHAT IS THE PROGNOSIS FOR JUVENILE SCLERODERMA?
Juvenile Localized Scleroderma Outcome

Most jLS patients who receive timely, appropriate treatment have a favorable prognosis, with most achieving remission on treatment. Deaths are extremely rare and are usually associated with skin ulcer complications (sepsis, squamous cell carcinoma) in pansclerotic morphea.[37] However, because of the long disease course, high relapse rate, and high frequency of extracutaneous involvement, jLS patients have a substantial risk for severe progressive morbidity. Although the superficial circumscribed morphea subtype can go into remission after 2 to 3 years, linear scleroderma can persist for decades.[2,66,68] Functional impairment has been reported in 28% to 38% of patients.[19,66,69] The presence of extracutaneous involvement negatively impacts quality of life and is associated with longer treatment courses and higher disease impact scores.[34,70]

Juvenile Systemic Sclerosis Outcome

jSSc should be considered a lifetime disease. The outcome for jSSc patients is more guarded, although generally better than for adult SSc. The 10-year survival has been reported at 98% for juvenile onset versus 75% for adult onset.[18] Better survival rates are related to the lower frequency of major internal organ involvement.[10,18] However, organ involvement likely accrues, because a study comparing adults with juvenile versus adult onset found no difference in prevalence of internal organ involvement after a mean of 17.6 years of disease in those with juvenile onset.[71]

Morbidity is a major issue for jSSc, with most patients having multiorgan problems. Functional impairment is common (36% in one study)[11] and may result from ILD, arthropathy, myositis, and RP. Gastrointestinal disease is common, associated with poorer quality-of-life scores, higher frequency of pain, and low body mass index.[3,11] jSSc patients require long-term monitoring by a team of specialists to optimize their care and improve outcome.

SUMMARY

Pediatric sclerodermas are rare autoimmune diseases affecting the skin and other tissues, including musculoskeletal and brain for jLS, and musculoskeletal, gastrointestinal, and cardiopulmonary organs for jSSc. jLS and jSSc are distinct diseases, rather than considered on a spectrum of a shared disease continuum, so jLS does not evolve into jSSc. Both jLS and jSSc are chronic diseases, requiring long-term management. Early diagnosis and treatment likely improve long-term outcome, and management with a pediatric rheumatologist is strongly recommended.

REFERENCES

1. Saigusa R, Asano Y, Yamashita T, et al. Systemic sclerosis complicated with localized scleroderma-like lesions induced by Kobner phenomenon. J Dermatol Sci 2018;89(3):282–9.
2. Peterson L, Nelson A, Su W, et al. The epidemiology of morphea (localized scleroderma) in Olmstead County 1960-1993. J Rheumatol 1997;24:73–80.
3. Scalapino K, Arkaschaisri T, Lucas M, et al. Childhood onset systemic sclerosis: classification, clinical and serologic features, and survival in comparison with adult onset disease. J Rheumatol 2006;33:1004–13.
4. Misra R, Singh G, Aggarwal P, et al. Juvenile onset systemic sclerosis: a single center experience of 23 cases from Asia. Clin Rheumatol 2007;2007:1259–62.
5. Herrick A, Ennis H, Bhushan M, et al. Incidence of childhood linear scleroderma and systemic sclerosis in the UK and Ireland. Arthritis Care Res 2010;62:213–8.
6. Leitenberger J, Cayce R, Haley R, et al. Distinct autoimmune syndromes in morphea. Arch Dermatol 2009;145:545–50.
7. Weibel L, Harper JI. Linear morphoea follows Blaschko's lines. Br J Dermatol 2008;159:175–81.
8. Zulian F, Athreya B, Laxer R, et al. Juvenile localized scleroderma: clinical and epidemiological features in 750 children. An international study. Rheumatology 2006;45:614–20.
9. Wu EY, Rabinovich EC, Torok KS, et al. Description of the localized scleroderma subgroup of the CARRAnet [abstract]. Arthritis Rheumatol 2011;63(suppl 10):S787–8.
10. Martini G, Foeldvari I, Russo R, et al. Systemic sclerosis in childhood. Clinical and immunologic features of 153 patients in an international database. Arthritis Rheum 2006;54:3971–8.
11. Stevens B, Torok K, Li S, et al. Clinical characteristics and factors associated with disability and impaired quality of life in children with juvenile systemic sclerosis. Arthritis Care Res (Hoboken) 2018. [Epub ahead of print].
12. Rabinovich C. Challenges in the diagnosis and treatment of juvenile systemic sclerosis. Nat Rev Rheumatol 2011;7:676–80.

13. Christen-Zaech S, Hakim MD, Afsar FS, et al. Pediatric morphea (localized scleroderma): review of 136 patients. J Am Acad Dermatol 2008;59(3):385–96.

14. Zulian F. Scleroderma in children. Pediatr Clin North Am 2005;52:521–45.

15. Gelber AC, Manno RL, Shah AA, et al. Race and association with disease manifestations and mortality in scleroderma: a 20-year experience at the Johns Hopkins Scleroderma Center and review of the literature. Medicine (Baltimore) 2013; 92(4):191–205.

16. Condie D, Grabell D, Jacobe H. Comparison of outcomes in adults with pediatric-onset morphea and those with adult-onset morphea: a cross-sectional study from the morphea in adults and children cohort. Arthritis Rheumatol 2014;66(12): 3496–504.

17. Kreuter A, Krieg T, Worm M, et al. German guidelines for the diagnosis and therapy of localized scleroderma. J Dtsch Dermatol Ges 2016;14(2):199–216.

18. Foeldvari I, Nihtyanova S, Wierk A, et al. Characteristics of patients with juvenile onset systemic sclerosis in an adult single-center cohort. J Rheumatol 2010;37: 2422–6.

19. Weibel L, Laguda B, Atherton D, et al. Misdiagnosis and delay in referral of children with localized scleroderma. Br J Dermatol 2011;165:1308–13.

20. Hawley DP, Baildam EM, Amin TS, et al. Access to care for children and young people diagnosed with localized scleroderma or juvenile SSc in the UK. Rheumatology (Oxford) 2012;51(7):1235–9.

21. Tollefson M, Witman P. En coup de sabre morphea and Parry-Romberg syndrome: a retrospective review of 54 patients. J Am Acad Dermatol 2007;56: 257–63.

22. Laxer R, Zulian F. Localized scleroderma. Curr Opin Rheumatol 2006;18:606–13.

23. Peterson L, Nelson A, Su W. Classification of morphea (localized scleroderma). Mayo Clin Proc 1995;70:1068–76.

24. Wu E, Li S, Torok K, et al. Description of the juvenile localized scleroderma subgroup of the Childhood Arthritis and Rheumatology Research (CARRA) registry. Arthritis Rheumatol 2015;67(Suppl 10) [abstract: 420].

25. Zulian F, Meneghesso D, Grisan E, et al. A new computerized method for the assessment of skin lesions in localized scleroderma. Rheumatology (Oxford) 2007;46(5):856–60.

26. Kelsey CE, Torok KS. The localized scleroderma cutaneous assessment tool: responsiveness to change in a pediatric clinical population. J Am Acad Dermatol 2013;69(2):214–20.

27. Li SC, Torok KS, Pope E, et al. Development of consensus treatment plans for juvenile localized scleroderma: a roadmap toward comparative effectiveness studies in juvenile localized scleroderma. Arthritis Care Res (Hoboken) 2012; 64(8):1175–85.

28. Wortsman X, Wortsman J, Sazunic I, et al. Activity assessment in morphea using color Doppler ultrasound. J Am Acad Dermatol 2011;65(5):942–8.

29. Li SC, Liebling MS, Haines KA, et al. Initial evaluation of an ultrasound measure for assessing the activity of skin lesions in juvenile localized scleroderma. Arthritis Care Res (Hoboken) 2011;63(5):735–42.

30. Schanz S, Fierlbeck G, Ulmer A, et al. Localized scleroderma: MR findings and clinical features. Radiology 2011;260:817–24.

31. Li S, Torok K, Pope E, et al. Development of a clinical disease activity measure for juvenile localized scleroderma. Arthritis Rheum 2011;63(Suppl 10):2453.

32. Weibel L, Sampaio MC, Visentin MT, et al. Evaluation of methotrexate and corticosteroids for the treatment of localized scleroderma (morphoea) in children. Br J Dermatol 2006;155(5):1013–20.
33. Zulian F, Vallongo C, Woo P, et al. Localized scleroderma in childhood is not just a skin disease. Arthritis Rheum 2005;52(9):2873–81.
34. Li SC, Andrews T, Chen M, et al. Extracutaneous involvement is common in juvenile localized scleroderma and associated with a higher level of perceived disease impact [abstract]. Arthritis Rheumatol 2017;69(suppl 10).
35. Kaya M, Sel Yilmaz C, Kurtaran H, et al. Chronologic presentation of a severe case of progressive hemifacial atrophy (Parry-Romberg syndrome) with the loss of an eye. Case Rep Otolaryngol 2014;2014:703017.
36. Kister I, Inglese M, Laxer R, et al. Neurologic manifestations of localized scleroderma. A case report and literature review. Neurology 2008;71:1538–45.
37. Wollina U, Buslau M, Heinig B, et al. Disabling pansclerotic morphea of childhood poses a high risk of chronic ulceration of the skin and squamous cell carcinoma. Int J Low Extrem Wounds 2007;6(4):291–8.
38. Zulian F, Vallongo C, de Oliveira S, et al. Congenital localized scleroderma. J Pediatr 2006;149:248–51.
39. Zulian F, Woo P, Athreya BH, et al. The Pediatric Rheumatology European Society/American College of Rheumatology/European League against Rheumatism provisional classification criteria for juvenile systemic sclerosis. Arthritis Rheum 2007;57(2):203–12.
40. van den Hoogen F, Khanna D, Fransen J, et al. 2013 classification criteria for systemic sclerosis: an American College of Rheumatology/European League Against Rheumatism collaborative initiative. Arthritis Rheum 2013;65(11):2737–47.
41. Young A, Khanna D. Systemic sclerosis: commonly asked questions by rheumatologists. J Clin Rheumatol 2015;21(3):149–55.
42. Khanna D, Furst DE, Clements PJ, et al. Standardization of the modified Rodnan skin score for use in clinical trials of systemic sclerosis. J Scleroderma Relat Disord 2017;2(1):11–8.
43. Foeldvari I, Wierk A. Healthy children have a significantly increased skin score assessed with the modified Rodnan skin score. Rheumatology (Oxford) 2006;45:76.
44. Wigley F, Flavahan N. Raynaud's phenomenon. Rheum Dis Clin North Am 1996;22:765–81.
45. Pain CE, Constantin T, Toplak N, et al. Raynaud's syndrome in children: systematic review and development of recommendations for assessment and monitoring. Clin Exp Rheumatol 2016;34:200–6. Suppl 100(5).
46. Ingegnoli F, Herrick AL. Nailfold capillaroscopy in pediatrics. Arthritis Care Res (Hoboken) 2013;65(9):1393–400.
47. Cutolo M, Sulli A, Pizzorni C, et al. Nailfold videocapillaroscopy assessment of microvascular damage in systemic sclerosis. J Rheumatol 2000;27:155–60.
48. Morrisroe KB, Nikpour M, Proudman SM. Musculoskeletal manifestations of systemic sclerosis. Rheum Dis Clin North Am 2015;41(3):507–18.
49. Torok KS. Pediatric scleroderma: systemic or localized forms. Pediatr Clin North Am 2012;59:381–405.
50. Martini G, Vittadello F, Kasapcopur O, et al. Factors affecting survival in juvenile systemic sclerosis. Rheumatology (Oxford) 2009;48(2):119–22.
51. Fabri M, Hunzelmann N. Differential diagnosis of scleroderma and pseudoscleroderma. J Dtsch Dermatol Ges 2007;5(11):977–84.
52. Nashel J, Steen V. Scleroderma mimics. Curr Rheumatol Rep 2012;14:39–46.

53. Kurzinski K, Torok K. Cytokine profiles in localized scleroderma and relationship to clinical features. Cytokine 2011;55:157–64.
54. Milano A, Pendergrass SA, Sargent JL, et al. Molecular subsets in the gene expression signatures of scleroderma skin. PLoS One 2008;3(7):e2696.
55. Jacobe H, Ahn C, Arnett F, et al. Major histocompatibility complex class I and class II alleles may confer susceptibility to or protection against morphea. Arthitis Rheum 2014;66:3170–7.
56. Stern E, Denton C. The pathogenesis of systemic sclerosis. Rheum Dis Clin North Am 2015;41:367–82.
57. Hunzelmann N, Krieg T. Scleroderma: from pathophysiology to novel therapeutic approaches. Exp Dermatol 2010;19(5):393–400.
58. Grabell D, Hsieh C, Andrew R, et al. The role of skin trauma in the distribution of morphea lesions: a cross-sectional survey of the morphea in adults and children cohort IV. J Am Acad Dermatol 2014;71:493–8.
59. Torres J, Sánchez J. Histopathologic differentiation between localized and systemic scleroderma. Am J Dermatopathol 1998;20:242–5.
60. Young A, Khanna D. Systemic sclerosis: a systematic review on therapeutic management from 2011 to 2014. Curr Opin Rheumatol 2015;27(3):241–8.
61. Zulian F, Martini G, Vallongo C, et al. Methotrexate treatment in juvenile localized scleroderma: a randomized, double-blind, placebo-controlled trial. Arthritis Rheum 2011;63(7):1998–2006.
62. Pequet MS, Holland KE, Zhao S, et al. Risk factors for morphoea disease severity: a retrospective review of 114 paediatric patients. Br J Dermatol 2014;170(4): 895–900.
63. Khan MA, Shaw L, Eleftheriou D, et al. Radiologic improvement after early medical intervention in localised facial morphea. Pediatr Dermatol 2016;33(2):e95–8.
64. Li SC, Feldman BM, Higgins GC, et al. Treatment of pediatric localized scleroderma: results of a survey of North American pediatric rheumatologists. J Rheumatol 2010;37(1):175–81.
65. Zulian F, Vallongo C, Patrizi A, et al. A long-term follow-up study of methotrexate in juvenile localized scleroderma (morphea). J Am Acad Dermatol 2012;67(6): 1151–6.
66. Piram M, McCuaig CC, Saint-Cyr C, et al. Short- and long-term outcome of linear morphoea in children. Br J Dermatol 2013;169(6):1265–71.
67. Kowal-Bielecka O, Fransen J, Avouac J, et al. Update of EULAR recommendations for the treatment of systemic sclerosis. Ann Rheum Dis 2017;76(8):1327–39.
68. Saxton-Daniels S, Jacobe HT. An evaluation of long-term outcomes in adults with pediatric-onset morphea. Arch Dermatol 2010;146(9):1044–5.
69. Wu EY, Li SC, Torok KS, et al. A28: description of the juvenile localized scleroderma subgroup of the CARRA registry. Arthritis Rheumatol 2014;66:S43–4.
70. Ardalan K, Zigler C, Torok K. Predictors of longitudinal quality of life in juvenile localized scleroderma. Arthritis Care Res 2017;69:1082–7.
71. Foeldvari I, Tyndall A, Zulian F, et al. Juvenile and young adult-onset systemic sclerosis share the same organ involvement in adulthood: data from the EUSTAR database. Rheumatology (Oxford) 2012;51:1832–7.

Chronic Nonbacterial Osteomyelitis and Chronic Recurrent Multifocal Osteomyelitis in Children

Yongdong Zhao, MD, PhD[a], Polly J. Ferguson, MD[b],*

KEYWORDS

- Chronic nonbacterial osteomyelitis • Chronic recurrent multifocal osteomyelitis
- DIRA • Majeed syndrome • NSAID • Whole-body MRI

KEY POINTS

- Chronic nonbacterial osteomyelitis (CNO; also known as chronic recurrent multifocal osteomyelitis) is an inflammatory/autoinflammatory bone disease that primarily affects children and adolescents. It is a diagnosis of exclusion.
- Often the diagnosis of CNO in children is delayed because of a lack of awareness and the occult nature of CNO. Prompt referral to pediatric rheumatology can help establish a diagnosis and determine appropriate treatment.
- Imaging studies, especially MRI with short tau inversion recovery, are essential diagnostic tools.
- Whole-body MRI is the gold standard for disease monitoring.
- Long-term treatment and follow-up are needed to prevent complications, such as vertebral compression fractures and leg-length discrepancies.

INTRODUCTION

Chronic nonbacterial osteomyelitis (CNO; **a.k.a., chronic recurrent multifocal osteomyelitis**) is an inflammatory disorder that presents with bone pain arising from sterile osteomyelitis. It is primarily a pediatric disorder but can persist into adulthood or have an adult-onset presentation. The condition is difficult to diagnose, most commonly suspected to be infectious osteomyelitis or malignancy, with milder cases resembling growing pains. Children may have decreased physical function and poor school

Disclosure: Dr Y. Zhao received research funding from CARRA and Bristol-Myers Squibb (IM101-691_ Zhao). Dr P.J. Ferguson's work is supported by R01AR059703 from NIH/NIAMS.
[a] Pediatric Rheumatology, Seattle Children's Hospital, University of Washington, MA 7.110, 4800 Sand Point Way Northeast, Seattle, WA 98105, USA; [b] Department of Pediatrics, University of Iowa Carver College of Medicine, 200 Hawkins Drive, 4038 Boyd Tower, Iowa City, IA 52242, USA
* Corresponding author.
E-mail address: polly-ferguson@uiowa.edu

attendance when bone pain and inflammation are not controlled adequately. Delays in diagnosis can lead to permanent skeletal damage. The cause of the disease remains unknown for most but involves immune dysregulation resulting in inflammation of the bone and sometimes of other tissues, including skin, joints, and the intestine.

NOMENCLATURE

The disease has gone by many names, making nomenclature complicated (**Box 1**). It was first described as a symmetric multifocal osteomyelitis and later given the name chronic recurrent multifocal osteomyelitis (CRMO).[1] However, because the disease may begin or stay unifocal, CRMO may not be an accurate term for these patients. Thus, the term *CNO* has been proposed as an umbrella term.

INCIDENCE AND DEMOGRAPHICS

In 2011, the annual incidence of CNO in Germany was reported to be 0.4 per 100,000 children,[2] as compared with the reported incidence range of infectious osteomyelitis of 10 to 80 per 100,000 children per year.[3] However, during 2004 to 2014 in a single center in Germany, of the 109 children seen for osteomyelitis, 53% were categorized as infectious and 47% as noninfectious, unexpectedly similar proportions.[3] A single center in Britain reported increased patient referral for CNO after a letter was sent to all orthopedic centers to enhance recognition of the disease.[4] Although the actual incidence of CNO is likely to vary from one region to another, these studies suggest that it is more common than previously appreciated and underscore the importance of raising awareness of CNO.[4]

Age

- The average age of disease onset is 9 to 10 years.[2,4–8] Rarely, disease onset occurs before 3 years of age.

Sex

- Girls are more likely to be affected, with a female to male ratio of 2:1.[2,4–8]

Box 1
Reported terms of chronic nonbacterial osteomyelitis

Bone lesions of acne fulminans

Chronic multifocal cleidometaphyseal osteomyelitis

Chronic recurrent multifocal osteomyelitis

Chronic sclerosing osteitis

Chronic symmetric osteomyelitis

Clavicular hyperostosis and acne arthritis

Diffuse sclerosing osteomyelitis

Pustulotic arthro-osteitis

Sclerosing osteomyelitis of Garré

Sternocostoclavicular hyperostosis

Sternoclavicular pustulotic osteitis

Synovitis, acne, pustulosis, hyperostosis osteitis

Race and Ethnicity

- Most reported cases are of European ancestry, although it has been reported in all races.[2,4–8]
- Prevalence among different ethnicities has not been described.

MAJOR DIFFERENCES FROM ADULT CHRONIC NONBACTERIAL OSTEOMYELITIS (ALSO KNOWN AS SYNOVITIS, ACNE, PUSTULOSIS, HYPEROSTOSIS, OSTEITIS)

- Cutaneous involvement in children is not as common as in adults.
- Common bone sites affected are long bones in children compared with the sternum and clavicles in adults.

DELAYS IN DIAGNOSIS ARE COMMON

The median time between initial symptoms and diagnosis of CNO is 2 years.[9] Forty-eight percent of children were not evaluated by a pediatric rheumatologist until at least 12 months after their first symptom occurred. The delay of diagnosis was likely related to the insidious development of pain, minimal findings on clinical examination, relatively normal laboratory studies, and lack of awareness of this condition. A patient survey study discussed delays in diagnosis for 21 patients who had a single symptomatic site and were initially misdiagnosed as bacterial osteomyelitis; 55% of these patients did not have whole-body imaging, and this was hypothesized to contribute to the delay in the diagnosis of CNO.[10]

WHEN TO CONSIDER CHRONIC NONBACTERIAL OSTEOMYELITIS

CNO should be considered in a child who has intermittent or persistent focal bone or joint pain of the lower extremities, clavicle, spine, and/or mandible. The pain is worse at night and may interfere with sleep, and the child usually has point tenderness of the affected site. Children with more superficially affected bones (eg, tibia, fibula, clavicle, and mandible) can also have local swelling and warmth (**Fig. 1**).

HOW CHRONIC NONBACTERIAL OSTEOMYELITIS PRESENTS

CNO typically presents as insidious bone pain with or without systemic features; however, it can also present as acute onset of pain. Young children may stop using an affected limb. Common features of CNO are shown in **Box 2**. Often there are minimal to no objective changes overlying the lesions, but point tenderness is common when the disease is active. The pain often results in reduced physical activities;

A   **B**

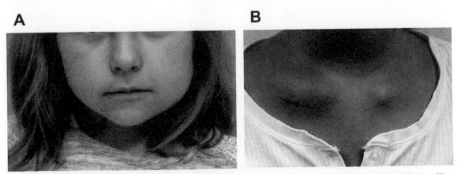

Fig. 1. (*A*) Left mandibular CNO with facial swelling and asymmetry in a child. (*B*) Swelling of right medial clavicle in a child with CNO.

Box 2
Clues to the diagnosis of chronic nonbacterial osteomyelitis

- Point tenderness with or without swelling or warmth
- Pain worse at night
- Limited function/use of affected limb
- Coexisting psoriasis, inflammatory bowel disease, or inflammatory arthritis
- Absence of constitutional symptoms

---

school attendance may be affected, particularly if lower extremities and/or axial bones are involved.

Approximately 40% of patients present with or develop arthritis with their CNO, which is associated with joint swelling and stiffness.[6] These symptoms often occur in joints adjacent to active areas of osteomyelitis of the long bones but can occur in areas without bone involvement. Even without arthritis, many patients have functional limitation of the joints.

Patients may present with constitutional symptoms, such as fever (20%)[7] and weight loss; however, most patients with CNO appear well. Fatigue is common in children with CNO.[9]

Pattern of bone involvement (**Fig. 2**)

- It most commonly affects the metaphyseal regions of long bones.
  - Diaphyseal regions of the long bones are rarely affected.

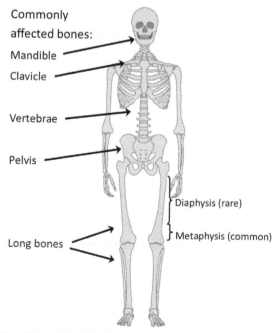

Commonly affected bones:
Mandible
Clavicle
Vertebrae
Pelvis
Diaphysis (rare)
Metaphysis (common)
Long bones

Fig. 2. Common sites affected in CNO. Metaphysis is indicated as the ending of long bones and diaphysis is indicated as the middle part of long bones. (*Adapted from* Vecteezy.com with free license. Accessed February 1, 2018.)

- The commonly affected sites are lower extremity long bones, vertebrae, clavicles, and mandible
  - In these sites, the trabecular bone is enriched and bone turnover is higher.
- There is asymmetric involvement in approximately 60% and symmetric involvement in approximately 40%.[7]
- Unifocal bony involvement at presentation is up to 30%.
  - Over time, most develop multifocal disease (93% in one study after mean of 4 years).[5]
- Clavicular and mandibular lesions are more likely to present as unifocal lesions and remain so throughout the disease course.
- Asymptomatic bone lesions are common.

DISEASE MORBIDITY

The most common complications of CNO are fractures in affected bones (especially of the vertebrae) and deformities due to growth alterations. Kyphosis may occur in patients with multiple vertebral compression fractures. Pathologic fractures in the long bones may occur when there is accelerated bone resorption. Leg-length discrepancy may result after the growth plate is damaged by CNO (**Fig. 3**A) or due to bony overgrowth of the epiphysis from excess inflammation. Angulation of a joint may occur when the growth plate is damaged asymmetrically, and often this complication requires surgical intervention (**Fig. 3**B). Aggressive treatment of patients with physeal damage before closure may reduce the risk of leg-length discrepancy or joint angulation. Untreated or inadequately treated patients may have increasing bony expansion (see **Fig. 3**B). One large study reported that 26% of children with CNO have complications, including localized deformation (particularly of the clavicle) (15%), vertebral fractures (4%), and growth asymmetry (6%).[5]

IMPACT ON QUALITY OF LIFE

CNO causes a significant impact on the quality of life in affected children. School absence due to pain, fatigue, and frequent medical visits are common. Assistive devices may be needed in some children. Inability to participate in desired sports activity because of limited function is frequent. Based on a family survey, most parents reported that their child with CNO was challenged to perform daily tasks or hobbies because of pain, fatigue, and physical limitation.[9] Another family survey study in Germany also reported a negative influence on family life in 80% of children with CNO.[10] Psychosocial support should be considered to improve the quality of life for these children and their families. Nearly half of these families reported a desire to contact other patients/families for mutual support.[10] A pamphlet for families of children with CRMO has been developed by a parent group and can be accessed on the Web site (www.crmoawareness.org). Other sites that allow families to seek further information and connect have been developed (https://www.facebook.com/groups/CRMOawareness, www.kailaskomfort.org).

ASSOCIATED CONDITIONS

In a minority of patients, other coexisting conditions, including psoriasis vulgaris, palmar plantar pustulosis, and inflammatory bowel disease, may occur before, concurrently with, or after the diagnosis of CNO. Psoriasis has been reported in 2% to 17% (**Fig. 4**), palmar plantar pustulosis (PPP) in 3% to 20%, and inflammatory bowel disease (IBD) in 3% to 7% of patients with CNO.[5–8] One proposed diagnostic criterion considers the presence of one of these comorbid conditions to help support

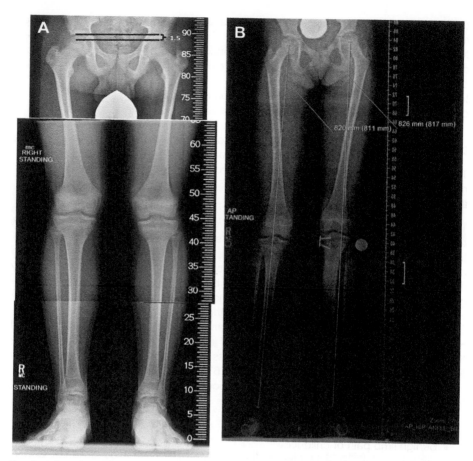

Fig. 3. (A) Radiographs of a child with CNO show a 1.5-cm discrepancy between the total lengths of 2 legs (right > left) due to growth plate damage in left proximal tibia. (B) Radiograph of a child with CNO shows persistent angulation of left knee a year after stapling of the medial proximal tibia.

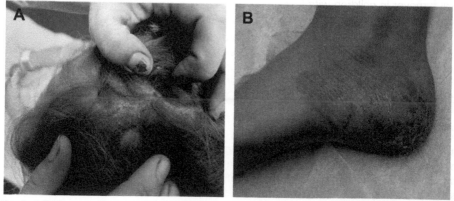

Fig. 4. (A) Plaque psoriasis on the scalp of a child with CNO. (B) Plantar psoriasis on heel of a child with CNO.

the diagnosis of CNO.[7] These comorbid conditions are also present in a high proportion of close relatives of patients with CNO. Up to 50% of patients with CNO have a first- or second-degree family member with psoriasis, PPP, Crohn disease, ulcerative colitis, or inflammatory arthritis. Family history of these diseases increases the positive predictive value of a diagnosis of CNO.[5-7] One category of treatments used for CNO, tumor necrosis factor (TNF)–alpha inhibitors, has also been associated with the development of psoriasis in patients with CNO.[11]

DIFFERENTIAL DIAGNOSIS OR MIMICS

The differential diagnosis of CNO is broad and includes infections of the bone or joint, malignancy, benign bone lesions, metabolic bone disease, amplified pain syndromes, and nutritional deficiencies.

The common differential diagnosis of CNO includes the following

- Leukemia
- Lymphoma
- Langerhans cell histiocytosis
- Primary malignant bone disease
- Benign bone tumor (osteoma, endo-chondroma)
- Infectious osteomyelitis
- Septic arthritis
- Avascular necrosis (osteonecrosis)
- Vitamin C deficiency (scurvy with bony changes)
- Enthesitis-related arthritis
- Psoriatic arthritis
- Amplified musculoskeletal pain syndrome/complex regional pain syndrome
- Hypophosphatasia
- Occult fracture
- Benign limb pain of childhood (growing pains)

A thorough physical examination is essential to help differentiate CNO from malignancy and infection, assessing for the presence of other areas of bone or joint swelling, lymphadenopathy, hepatosplenomegaly, mass, or rash. Lesions in the diaphysis should prompt evaluation for alternative diagnosis, including benign and malignant bone tumors. Lactate dehydrogenase (LDH) and uric acid are useful to screen for increased cell turnover in children with leukemia and lymphoid malignancies. Alkaline phosphatase and serum phosphorus are useful to screen for hypophosphatasia.

Biopsy of multiple bone sites or repeated bone biopsies may need to be performed, especially when there is a concern of a CNO-mimicking disease, such as intraosseous lymphoma.[12] Bone marrow biopsy may also be obtained in patients with strong suspicion of leukemia (cytopenia, episodic pain, nocturnal pain, elevated LDH, raised uric acid). Infectious workup is routinely performed on the biopsied bone samples, and additional blood culture is needed when the concern for infection is high.

Jansson and colleagues[13] developed a scoring system to guide the diagnostic workup based on the presence or absence of 7 components (**Table 1**). This scoring system was intended to distinguish nonbacterial osteomyelitis from infectious osteomyelitis as well as from benign and malignant bone tumor in adults and children. A total score of 28 or less had a negative predictive value of 97% for CNO, whereas a total score of 39 or greater had a positive predictive value of 97% or greater for CNO.

The pattern of pain may also help differentiate CNO from other diseases. Pain is often worse at night and interferes with sleep. This pattern is also seen in children

Table 1
Diagnostic scoring system of chronic nonbacterial osteomyelitis by Jansson and colleagues

Clinical, Laboratory, and Imaging Findings	Points
Normal blood cell count	13
Symmetric lesions	10
Lesions with marginal sclerosis	10
Normal body temperature	9
Vertebral, clavicular, or sternal lesions	8
Radiologically proven lesions $\geq$2	7
C-reactive protein $\geq$1 mg/dL	6

Total possible score is 63. This scoring system was intended to distinguish nonbacterial osteomyelitis from infectious osteomyelitis as well as from benign and malignant bone tumor in adults and children. A total score of 28 or less had a negative predictive value of 97% for CNO, whereas a total score of 39 or greater had a positive predictive value of 97% or greater for CNO.

Data from Jansson AF, Muller TH, Gliera L, et al. Clinical score for nonbacterial osteitis in children and adults. Arthritis Rheum 2009;60:1152–9.

who have growing pains (also known as benign limb pain of childhood, see Jennifer E. Weiss and Jennifer N. Stinson's article, "Pediatric Pain Syndromes and Non-inflammatory Musculoskeletal Pain," in this issue). Episodic severe bone pain with significantly elevated erythrocyte sedimentation rate (ESR) and C-reactive protein (CRP) should raise concerns for osseous infiltration from leukemia or lymphoma. Diffuse body pain and tenderness to touch (allodynia) may be an indication of amplified musculoskeletal pain syndrome (discussed in Chapter 10) rather than active CNO. Some children with CNO may also have amplified musculoskeletal pain syndrome, which can make it challenging to determine if they have active disease; in such cases, MRI can be helpful.[14]

IMAGING, LABORATORY, AND BIOPSY STUDIES FOR DIAGNOSIS IN CARE
Imaging

Whole-body MRI is considered the gold standard imaging modality by experts. Patients almost always have a radiograph taken initially. However, MRI is preferred for its sensitivity and lack of radiation. Typical findings of CNO from each imaging modality are listed next.

Radiographs

- Most common findings
  - Lytic lesion during early phase (**Fig. 5**A)
  - Sclerosis, bony expansion, or mixed picture during later stage (**Fig. 5**B)
  - Normal in 80% of patients
- Other findings
  - Pathologic fracture during acute lytic phase (rare)
  - Compression fracture of vertebrae
    - Can lead to kyphosis or vertebra plana (**Fig. 5**C)
- Advantages
  - Quick
  - Least expensive
- Disadvantages
  - Least sensitive with a high false-negative rate
  - Radiation

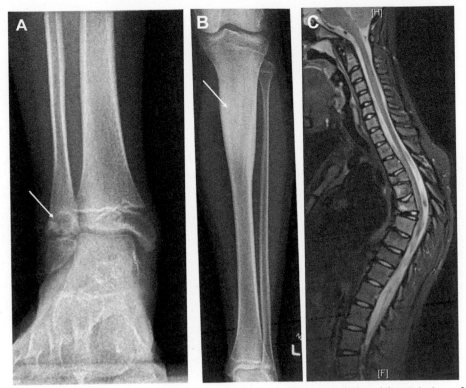

Fig. 5. (*A*) CNO lytic lesion (*arrow*) in fibula. (*B*) Sclerosis (*arrow*) of tibia. (*C*) Height loss of T3 to T6 and plana of T7 due to CNO on MRI, which resulted in 47° of kyphosis.

Computed tomography

- Common findings
  - Lytic lesions, sclerosis, bony expansion, or mixed pattern
- Advantages
  - Three-dimensional rendering of affected bone to guide the biopsy
- Disadvantages
  - Limited use in determining disease activity
  - Radiation

Bone scintigraphy

- Common findings
  - Increased uptake at affected sites (**Fig. 6**)
- Advantages
  - Whole-body level scanning when whole-body MRI is not available
- Disadvantages
  - Not as sensitive as MRI[15]
  - Challenging to distinguish inflamed sites from the physiologic increased uptake at the growth plates
  - Radiation

PET–computed tomography

- Common findings
  - Increased tracer uptake

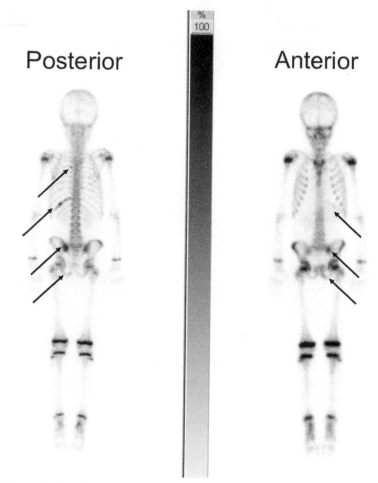

Fig. 6. Bone scintigraphy of a child with CNO reveals increased uptake of radioisotope (*arrows*) in the left third and eleventh ribs, left ilium, and left ischium indicating active inflammation.

- Advantages
  - Correlates with disease activity based on increased metabolism
  - Detailed localization of inflamed sites
- Disadvantages
  - Radiation

MRI

- Common findings
  - Hyperintensity within bone marrow in short tau inversion recovery (STIR) or T2 fat saturation sequences
  - Hyperintensity within surrounding soft tissue in STIR or T2 fat saturation sequences
  - Bony expansion during late stages
- Other findings
  - Physis irregularity or complete bony bar

- o Compression vertebral fracture
- Advantages
  - o Most sensitive in detecting inflamed sites (**Figs. 7** and **8**)
  - o Assesses both disease activity and skeletal damage
- Disadvantages
  - o Requires sedation in young children

Whole body MRI

- Useful protocol of whole-body MRI (**Fig. 9**)[16]
  - o Coronal STIR of total body in 4 to 5 stations
  - o Sagittal STIR of entire spine
  - o Sagittal STIR of feet
  - o Axial STIR of pelvis and knee
- Advantages
  - o Whole-body screening
  - o Most sensitive in detecting inflamed sites
  - o Assesses both disease activity and skeletal damage
- Disadvantages
  - o Requires sedation in young children

Frequency of Imaging monitoring

There is no consensus on how often imaging should be performed to monitor disease activity of CNO. In North America, about half of the surveyed pediatric rheumatologists use imaging regularly, with 54% of them repeating imaging every 6 months and 25% every 12 months.[17] Because of the occult nature of the disease and lack of reliable biomarkers or physical findings, more frequent radiation-free imaging may be necessary to provide an accurate estimate of disease activity in order to guide the treatment. In general, early in the disease, repeating MRI 3 to 6 months after initiation of the treatment is reasonable. In patients who have a completely normal MRI and remain on stable medications or are off medications, repeating MRI every 6 to 12 months is appropriate.

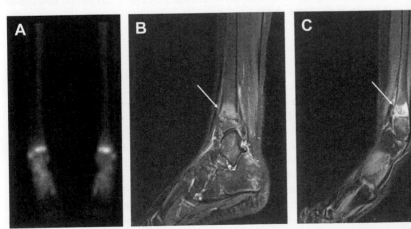

Fig. 7. (A) Normal bone scintigraphy of a child. (B) Abnormal STIR signal (*arrow*) on MRI within left distal tibia of the same child. (C) Abnormal STIR signal (*arrow*) on MRI within right distal fibula of the same child.

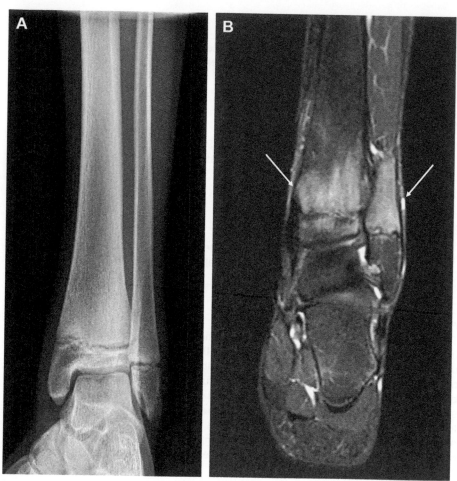

Fig. 8. (*A*) Normal leg radiograph of a child. (*B*) Abnormal STIR signal (*arrow*) on MRI within distal tibia and fibula of the same child.

Laboratory Evaluation

There is no diagnostic test for CNO. Most children have a normal complete blood cell count (CBC) at presentation.[5–7] Because of the broad differential diagnoses for CNO, laboratory tests are most useful to rule out alternative diagnoses. Inflammatory markers, such as ESR and CRP, are elevated in some patients with CNO, but most have normal levels at presentation.[4,7,8,13,18,19] The use of urinary N-terminal telopeptide (NTx) as a disease-monitoring tool in CNO has been reported in a small cohort,[20] with the test found able to identify some children with disease flares. More study is needed to determine the normal range of NTx in healthy children and evaluate the sensitivity and specificity of NTx for screening children for CNO. HLA-B27 positivity and low titer antinuclear antibody positivity have been reported in only a small fraction of these patients.[5,7] Serum TNF-α was increased in 66% of patients in one study.[7] Total immunoglobulin (Ig) G and its subclasses, IgG1, IgG2, IgG3, as well as IgD were elevated in 7% to 33% in one cohort.[7]

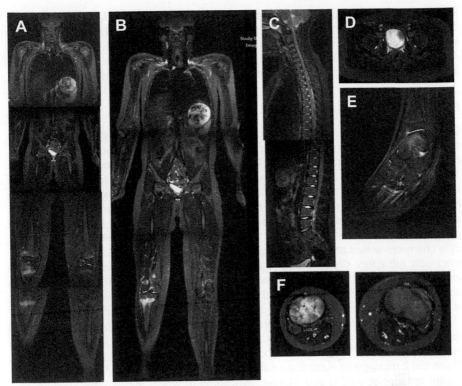

Fig. 9. Whole body MRI of a child with CNO includes coronal STIR of total body in 4 to 5 stations (*A*) with stitched image (*B*), sagittal STIR of entire spine (*C*), axial STIR of pelvis (*D*), sagittal STIR of feet (*E*), and axial STIR of the knee (*F*). It demonstrates active inflammation in right proximal tibia and left talus.

Initial screening laboratory tests in a child with typical chronic nonbacterial osteomyelitis usually show

- Normal CBC; sometimes anemia from chronic disease
- Normal or mildly elevated ESR, CRP
- Normal LDH, uric acid
- Normal serum calcium, phosphorus, alkaline phosphatase

Bone Biopsy

It may be necessary to obtain a bone specimen to exclude infection and malignancy. Most rheumatologists request a bone biopsy when there are constitutional symptoms or a single bone lesion or an atypical presentation. Conversely, patients with the following characteristics may not need a bone biopsy because of the higher confidence in the likelihood of CNO:

- Bone lesion at a typical site (clavicle, metaphysis of long bones, vertebral body) with normal laboratory test results and no constitutional symptoms
- Multiple bone lesions
- CNO-associated conditions (ie, psoriasis or Crohn disease)[4,17]

When indicated, bone biopsy can be obtained via an open biopsy or needle biopsy depending on the affected sites. Usually a decision of how to obtain biopsy is left to the discretion of the surgeon. Common histologic findings include acute and/or chronic inflammation, marrow fibrosis, osteonecrosis or normal bone.[6,7,17,21,22] No specific staining can confirm the diagnosis of CNO but may exclude other diagnoses. Adequate sample should be obtained to allow for pathologic review as well as for an infectious workup including stains and cultures for bacteria, fungi and mycobacteria.

PATHOGENESIS OF CHRONIC NONBACTERIAL OSTEOMYELITIS

CNO is considered an autoinflammatory disease. Components of the innate immune system, including neutrophils, macrophages, monocytes, and associated cytokines, contribute to disease pathogenesis. Increased proinflammatory cytokines, such as TNF-α and interleukin (IL)-6, and decreased antiinflammatory cytokines, especially IL-10, were reported in children with CNO.[23] IL-6 and C-C motif chemokine 11/eotaxin have been shown to sufficiently differentiate patients with CNO from healthy children and those with other inflammatory diseases in a German cohort.[24] Recently, a serum cytokine profile has been proposed as a marker for CNO.[25] Persistently elevated monocyte chemoattractant protein-1, IL-12, and soluble interleukin-2 receptor were associated with refractory CNO in one cohort; but their use as biomarkers needs to be validated.[25] Imbalanced cytokines cause increased osteoclast activity that results in accelerated bone breakdown during the early phase of disease. Overall bone turnover is increased, and excessive bone formation occurs as a response during the later stage.

There is evidence of a genetic component to CNO, including reports of clustering in some families and a reported association of CNO with a rare allele of marker D18S60 on chromosome 18.[26] For a small minority of patients, CNO may be genetically driven. There are 2 monogenic autoinflammatory bone diseases called deficiency of IL-1 receptor antagonist (DIRA) and Majeed syndrome in which sterile osteomyelitis is a prominent phenotype. These two diseases have distinct clinical features, which can aid in diagnosis. DIRA presents as neonatal onset of sterile multifocal osteomyelitis, periostitis, and pustulosis. Clinical symptoms typically start within the first month of life.[27] DIRA is due to recessive mutations in *IL1RN*, which encodes the IL-1 receptor antagonist, a regulatory protein that binds IL-1 receptors on cells and blocks the binding and activity of IL-1. Affected children respond only partially to glucocorticoids and disease-modifying antirheumatic drugs (DMARDs) but respond very well to replacement treatment with recombinant human IL-1 receptor antagonist, anakinra.[27] Majeed syndrome presents with sterile multifocal osteomyelitis with onset in the first 2 years of life and is associated with congenital dyserythropoietic anemia; a few patients with Majeed syndrome also have a neutrophilic dermatosis resembling Sweet syndrome.[28,29] Majeed syndrome is due to recessive mutations in *LPIN2*. Recently a homozygous missense mutation in the gene *FBLIM1* was reported by Cox and colleagues[30] as the cause of CNO and psoriasis in 2 unrelated children.

HOW CHRONIC NONBACTERIAL OSTEOMYELITIS IS TREATED

Nonsteroidal antiinflammatory drugs (NSAIDs) are often used as the first-line treatment of children with CNO.[8,17,31] Naproxen at 10 mg/kg (maximum 500 mg) twice daily is the most commonly used NSAID. Other NSAIDs used for treatment are indomethacin and meloxicam. Based on the study of Beck and colleagues,[8] responders have significant pain relief and a decrease in the number of bone lesions on MRI by as early as 3 months. Patients who have persistent bone pain and hyperintense signal within bone marrow on STIR imaging after 3 months of NSAID treatment are considered NSAID treatment failures. These patients need treatment with a second-line agent.[31,32]

Second-line treatments include methotrexate, TNF inhibitors (TNFi; most commonly monoclonal antibodies), and bisphosphonates.[5–8,17,19,20,22,32–34] Depending on the severity of disease, one or more of the aforementioned medications may be used sequentially or concurrently after a child fails to achieve a favorable response to NSAIDs. Comparative effectiveness studies have not been done to determine relative efficacy. Retrospective studies suggest that nonbiological DMARDs (such as methotrexate or sulfasalazine) have lower efficacy than TNFi and bisphosphonates.[6] When other associated conditions, such as IBD or enthesitis-related arthritis, are present, TNFi with or without DMARDs are more appropriate to treat both CNO and these coexisting conditions. When spinal lesions are present, bisphosphonates may prevent further compression and allow some recovery of vertebral body height.[18,35] Combining TNFi and bisphosphonates has been reported to provide substantial disease control in children with CNO and a poor response to NSAIDs.[19]

There have been limited reports of the use of other biological medications. The IL-1 inhibitor anakinra has been reported to be effective in 2 small cohorts of patients, associated with a decrease in the CRP after 6 to 8 months of treatment.[36,37] Pardeo and colleagues[37] reported a favorable response in 5 of 9 patients who had refractory CNO (failing NSAIDs, glucocorticoids, pamidronate). After 6 months of anakinra at a median dosage of 2 mg/kg/d, 5 of 9 patients had normalized CRP and ESR. The total number of bone lesions detected by bone scintigraphy at baseline decreased from 77 to 35, although 20 new asymptomatic lesions were identified. At a median of 1.7 years of follow-up, 6 of 9 patients maintained a zero or minimal physician global assessment score.

Of note, glucocorticoids are not recommended during the initial workup or as long-term treatment due to adverse long-term side effects and the potential for harm should the child turn out to have a lymphoid malignancy. Short-term use (up to 6 weeks) in patients with a well-established diagnosis of CNO as a transitional medication may be appropriate.[32]

Without treatment guidelines, there is variability in which medications are used for NSAID failures. The selection and dosing of second-line medications differs among rheumatologists. However, consensus treatment plans (CTPs) have been developed based on the best available evidence and current treatment practices of North American pediatric rheumatologists for the treatment of pediatric CNO refractory to NSAIDs and/or with active spinal lesions.[32] These CTPs will allow future comparative effectiveness studies to identify the most effective therapies.

In a CNO cohort, aggressive combination treatment with a TNFi plus methotrexate with or without bisphosphonate induced clinical remission along with significantly decreased active lesions on MRI compared to treatment with NSAIDs.[19] Further study is needed to determine if early aggressive treatment of children with CNO results in better long-term outcomes[19] and to determine the optimal treatment duration.

CLINICAL MONITORING

Different criteria have been reported to define clinical responses to treatments in CNO. Most of these criteria included 3 main components: pain due to CNO, inflammatory markers (ESR and CRP), and imaging findings. Effective treatments may lead to complete resolution of pain and normalized ESR and CRP, which may precede the complete resolution of lesions on MRI. A composite score, PedsCNO score, includes ESR, number of lesions on MRI, physician global assessment of disease activity, patient/parent global assessment of disease activity, and childhood health assessment questionnaire.[8] PedsCNO 30, 50, and 70 were defined as 30%, 50%, and 70% improvement in at least 3 of 5 variables with no more than one of the remaining variables deteriorating by more than 30%, 50%, and 70%. Recently, proposed criteria of treatment failure were suggested[32] as no improvement in more than 50% of available criteria or at least 4 of the following 6 criteria: patient pain; total number of clinically active lesions; total number of radiological lesions by whole body MRI or bone scintigraphy; size and degree of marrow edema of CNO lesions; and/or presence of soft tissue swelling/inflammation related to CNO lesion on imaging, physician global assessment, abnormal ESR, and/or CRP after exclusion of other potential causes.

MANAGEMENT OF CLINICALLY ASYMPTOMATIC LESIONS SHOWN IN MRI

Asymptomatic lesions have often been reported, and their clinical significance has not been fully elucidated.[8,14,37] Currently, most physicians do not make clinical decisions based on asymptomatic lesions unless vertebral bodies are affected, which potentially poses a high risk of spinal fracture.

WHAT IS THE PROGNOSIS FOR CHRONIC NONBACTERIAL OSTEOMYELITIS?

Long-term observational studies have reported an average 40% rate of clinical remission (defined as absence of bone pain) in children with CNO after 1 to 5 years of follow-up.[5–8,34] The only long-term follow-up study done on adult patients with childhood onset of CNO showed a persistent presence of active bone lesions, defined as increased signal intensity on STIR images, in 10 of 17 patients who were available for a median of 15-year follow-up.[14] Among these 10 patients, 6 had ongoing clinical symptoms, whereas the other 4 patients were completely asymptomatic. This study underscores the importance of regular imaging monitoring in patients with CNO and demonstrates that, for some, the disease may persist into adulthood. Pediatric rheumatologists manage these patients in collaboration with other specialists (eg, orthopedic surgeon, oral surgeon, neurosurgeon, dermatologist) and assist these patients in their transition into adult rheumatologists for the optimal care.

Recurrence of disease is very common, with 50% of patients relapsing after a median of 2.4 years in a large German cohort study.[34] The relapse rate was even higher (83%) in a large cohort from North America after a median of 1.8 years of follow-up.[6]

In a large cohort study, factors associated with severe disease and a poor outcome include male sex, multifocal disease, extrarheumatologic manifestations, family history of associated disease, and CRP greater than 1 mg/dL.[5] These patients were more likely to receive bisphosphonates and/or TNFi as a result of refractory disease.

REFERENCES

1. Giedion A, Holthusen W, Masel LF, et al. Subacute and chronic "symmetrical" osteomyelitis. Ann Radiol (Paris) 1972;15:329–42.
2. Jansson AF, Grote V. Nonbacterial osteitis in children: data of a German Incidence Surveillance Study. Acta Paediatr 2011;100:1150–7.
3. Schnabel A, Range U, Hahn G, et al. Unexpectedly high incidences of chronic non-bacterial as compared to bacterial osteomyelitis in children. Rheumatol Int 2016;36:1737–45.
4. Roderick MR, Shah R, Rogers V, et al. Chronic recurrent multifocal osteomyelitis (CRMO) – advancing the diagnosis. Pediatr Rheumatol 2016;14(1):47.
5. Wipff J, Costantino F, Lemelle I, et al. A large national cohort of French patients with chronic recurrent multifocal osteitis. Arthritis Rheumatol 2015;67:1128–37.
6. Borzutzky A, Stern S, Reiff A, et al. Pediatric chronic nonbacterial osteomyelitis. Pediatrics 2012;130:e1190–7.

7. Jansson A, Renner ED, Ramser J, et al. Classification of non-bacterial osteitis: retrospective study of clinical, immunological and genetic aspects in 89 patients. Rheumatology 2007;46:154–60.
8. Beck C, Morbach H, Beer M, et al. Chronic nonbacterial osteomyelitis in childhood: prospective follow-up during the first year of anti-inflammatory treatment. Arthritis Res Ther 2010;12:R74.
9. Oliver M, Lee T, Halpern-Felsher B, et al. Disease burden and social impact of chronic nonbacterial osteomyelitis on affected children and young adults [abstract#82]. Arthritis Rheumatol 2017;69(suppl 4).
10. Silier CCG, Greschik J, Gesell S, et al. Chronic non-bacterial osteitis from the patient perspective: a health services research through data collected from patient conferences. BMJ Open 2017;7:e017599.
11. Zhao Y, Foster SK, Murdock TJ, et al. A rare case of chronic recurrent multifocal osteomyelitis with undifferentiated juvenile idiopathic arthritis, uveitis, and psoriasis. Case Rep Clin Med 2016;5. https://doi.org/10.4236/crcm.2016.57041.
12. Haque SA, Shad A, Ozdemirli M, et al. A thirteen year old female with primary T-cell rich B-cell lymphoma of bone masquerading as chronic recurrent multifocal osteomyelitis. Pediatr Rep 2009;1:e3.
13. Jansson AF, Muller TH, Gliera L, et al. Clinical score for nonbacterial osteitis in children and adults. Arthritis Rheum 2009;60:1152–9.
14. Voit AM, Arnoldi AP, Douis H, et al. Whole-body magnetic resonance imaging in chronic recurrent multifocal osteomyelitis: clinical long-term assessment may underestimate activity. J Rheumatol 2015;42:1455–62.
15. Morbach H, Schneider P, Schwarz T, et al. Comparison of magnetic resonance imaging and technetium-labelled methylene diphosphonate bone scintigraphy in the initial assessment of chronic non-bacterial osteomyelitis of childhood and adolescents. Clin Exp Rheumatol 2012;30:578–82.
16. Khanna G, Sato TSP, Ferguson P. Imaging of chronic recurrent multifocal. Radiographics 2009;29:1159–77.
17. Zhao Y, Dedeoglu F, Ferguson PJ, et al. Physicians' perspectives on the diagnosis and treatment of chronic nonbacterial osteomyelitis. Int J Rheumatol 2017. https://doi.org/10.1155/2017/7694942.
18. Hospach T, Langendoerfer M, von Kalle T, et al. Spinal involvement in chronic recurrent multifocal osteomyelitis (CRMO) in childhood and effect of pamidronate. Eur J Pediatr 2010;169:1105–11.
19. Zhao Y, Chauvin NA, Jaramillo D, et al. Aggressive therapy reduces disease activity without skeletal damage progression in chronic nonbacterial osteomyelitis. J Rheumatol 2015;42:1245–51.
20. Miettunen PM, Wei X, Kaura D, et al. Dramatic pain relief and resolution of bone inflammation following pamidronate in 9 pediatric patients with persistent chronic recurrent multifocal osteomyelitis (CRMO). Pediatr Rheumatol Online J 2009;7:2.
21. Girschick HJ, Krauspe R, Tschammler A, et al. Chronic recurrent osteomyelitis with clavicular involvement in children: diagnostic value of different imaging techniques and therapy with non-steroidal anti-inflammatory drugs. Eur J Pediatr 1998;157:28–33.
22. Girschick HJ, Raab P, Surbaum S, et al. Chronic non-bacterial osteomyelitis in children. Ann Rheum Dis 2005;64:279–85.
23. Hofmann SR, Morbach H, Schwarz T, et al. Attenuated TLR4/MAPK signaling in monocytes from patients with CRMO results in impaired IL-10 expression. Clin Immunol 2012;145:69–76.

24. Hofmann SR, Böttger F, Range U, et al. Serum interleukin-6 and CCL11/eotaxin may be suitable biomarkers for the diagnosis of chronic nonbacterial osteomyelitis. Front Pediatr 2017;5:1–11. Available at: http://journal.frontiersin.org/article/10.3389/fped.2017.00256/full.

25. Hofmann SR, Kubasch AS, Range U, et al. Serum biomarkers for the diagnosis and monitoring of chronic recurrent multifocal osteomyelitis (CRMO). Rheumatol Int 2016;36:769–79.

26. Golla A, Jansson A, Ramser J, et al. Chronic recurrent multifocal osteomyelitis (CRMO): evidence for a susceptibility gene located on chromosome 18q21. 3-18q22. Eur J Hum Genet 2002;10:217–21.

27. Aksentijevich I, Masters SL, Ferguson PJ, et al. An autoinflammatory disease with deficiency of the interleukin-1-receptor antagonist. N Engl J Med 2009;360:2426–37.

28. Ferguson PJ, Chen S, Tayeh MK, et al. Homozygous mutations in LPIN2 are responsible for the syndrome of chronic recurrent multifocal osteomyelitis and congenital dyserythropoietic anaemia (Majeed syndrome). J Med Genet 2005;42:551–7.

29. Majeed H, Kalaawi A, Mohanty M, et al. Congenital dyserythropoietic anemia and chronic recurrent multifocal osteomyelitis in three related children and the association with Sweet syndrome in two siblings. J Pediatr 1989;115:730–4.

30. Cox AJ, Darbro BW, Laxer RM, et al. Correction: recessive coding and regulatory mutations in FBLIM1 underlie the pathogenesis of chronic recurrent multifocal osteomyelitis (CRMO). PLoS One 2017;12(7):e0169687. PLoS One 2017;12:1–22.

31. Hedrich CM, Hofmann SR, Pablik J, et al. Autoinflammatory bone disorders with special focus on chronic recurrent multifocal osteomyelitis (CRMO). Pediatr Rheumatol 2013;11:47.

32. Zhao Y, Wu EY, Oliver MS, et al. Consensus treatment plans for chronic nonbacterial osteomyelitis refractory to nonsteroidal anti-inflammatory drugs and/or with active spinal lesions. Arthritis Care Res (Hoboken) 2017. https://doi.org/10.1002/acr.23462.

33. Simm P, Allen R, Zacharin M. Bisphosphonate treatment in chronic recurrent multifocal osteomyelitis. J Pediatr 2008;152:571–5.

34. Schnabel A, Range U, Hahn G, et al. Treatment response and long-term outcomes in children with chronic nonbacterial osteomyelitis. J Rheumatol 2017;44(7):1058–65.

35. Gleeson H, Wiltshire E, Briody J, et al. Childhood chronic recurrent multifocal osteomyelitis: pamidronate therapy decreases pain and improves vertebral shape. J Rheumatol 2008;35:707–12.

36. Wendling D, Prati C, Aubin F. Anakinra treatment of SAPHO syndrome: short-term results of an open study. Ann Rheum Dis 2012;71:1098–100.

37. Pardeo M, Marafon DP, Messia V, et al. Anakinra in a cohort of children with chronic nonbacterial osteomyelitis. J Rheumatol 2017;44:1231–8.

Pediatric Pain Syndromes and Noninflammatory Musculoskeletal Pain

Jennifer E. Weiss, MD[a],*, Jennifer N. Stinson, RN, PhD[b]

KEYWORDS

- Musculoskeletal pain • Pain amplification syndrome
- Juvenile fibromyalgia syndrome • Hypermobility syndrome • Overuse syndromes

KEY POINTS

- Noninflammatory musculoskeletal pain is common in children and adolescents.
- Chronic musculoskeletal pain (CMP) can have a negative impact on physical, social, and psychological functioning.
- The most common noninflammatory CMP includes amplified musculoskeletal pain, benign limb pain of childhood, hypermobility, overuse syndromes, and back pain.
- A multidisciplinary approach to treatment is necessary to return the child to a functional state.

INTRODUCTION

Noninflammatory musculoskeletal (MSK) pain in children and adolescents is a common reason for pediatric rheumatology referral. Chronic musculoskeletal pain (CMP) is defined as ongoing pain in the bones, joints, and tissues of the body that persists longer than 3 months.[1,2] CMP is the third most prevalent recurrent and persistent kind of pain, behind headaches and abdominal pain.[3] The most common forms of nonarthritic CMP in children include[4]:

- Amplified MSK pain syndromes (AMPS)
- Benign limb pain of childhood (also known as growing pains, benign nocturnal limb pain of childhood)
- Benign joint hypermobility syndromes

Disclosure: The authors have no relevant disclosures.
[a] Pediatric Rheumatology, Seton Hall School of Medicine, Hackensack University Medical Center, 30 Prospect Avenue, Hackensack, NJ 07601, USA; [b] Research Institute, Child Health Evaluative Sciences, Hospital for Sick Children, University of Toronto, 555 University Avenue, Toronto, Ontario M5G 1X8, Canada
* Corresponding author.
E-mail address: Jennifer.Weiss@HackensackMeridian.org

Pediatr Clin N Am 65 (2018) 801–826
https://doi.org/10.1016/j.pcl.2018.04.004
0031-3955/18/© 2018 Elsevier Inc. All rights reserved.

- Overuse syndromes
- Skeletal defects
- Back pain

It is essential that primary and acute care clinicians understand how to recognize and treat these conditions. This article provides an overview of the epidemiology, assessment, and management of the most common nonarthritic CMPs. CMP associated with rheumatic conditions is discussed in Kathleen A. Haines' article, "The Approach to the Child with Joint Complaints," in this issue.

CMP can negatively affect physical, social, academic, and psychological aspects of health-related quality of life (HRQL). In addition, CMP may have a negative effect on families and has a high cost to the health care system (US$19.5 billion/y).[5–10] From 5% to 8% of children with recurrent and persistent pain develop significant pain-related disability.[11] Pain prevalence rates increase with age, and girls report more MSK pain than boys.[11,12] Psychosocial variables affecting pain prevalence include anxiety, depression, low self-esteem, other chronic health conditions, and low socio-economic status.[3] CMP in children is therefore best understood within a context of a biopsychosocial framework.[1,5]

GENERAL APPROACH TO PATIENTS WITH NONARTHRITIC CHRONIC MUSCULOSKELETAL PAIN

A detailed history and physical examination, including joint inspection, palpation, range of motion (ROM), and strength testing, is critical to the effective diagnosis and management of CMP. Kathleen A. Haines's article, "The Approach to the Child with Joint Complaints," in this issue, discusses factors to consider in the evaluation of children with CMP that can help identify those with inflammatory and other serious causes. Although most patients with nonarthritic CMP do not require imaging or other evaluation, it is important to identify those who may have a disorder requiring orthopedic or other management, to minimize their risk for serious complications. Features that suggest more evaluation is needed include persistent limp, neurologic signs, systemic signs (ie, fever, weight loss, severe fatigue), and worsening focal pain.

An important part of the evaluation is the assessment of the patient's pain, daily functioning, and HRQL (**Fig. 1, Table 1**). When assessing pain, it is critical to consider pain as a multidimensional experience that comprises sensory, affective, and evaluative components.[8] Sensory components include the quality, intensity, location, and duration of pain, whereas affective components reflect the emotional impact of pain. Evaluative components address pain interference with physical, psychological, and social functioning.

The main approaches to measuring pain intensity in children are self-report and observation. For children 3 to 7 years of age, a simple pain word self-report scale should be used (ie, no pain, a little pain, a medium amount of pain, a lot of pain). For children 5 to 12 years of age there are several well-validated face pain scales (Faces Pain Scale Revised and the Wong Baker Faces Pain Scale) that are scored on a common metric of 10. For children more than 7 years of age a numerical rating scale (0 = no pain to 10 = worst pain possible) should be used. Observational (behavioral) pain tools should be used with children and adolescents with CMP who are (1) less than 4 years of age; (2) too distressed to self-report their pain; (3) communicatively or cognitively impaired; or (4) providing self-report ratings considered to be exaggerated, minimized, or unrealistic.[13] The Revised FLACC (facial expression, leg movement, activity, cry, and consolability) is a behavioral tool that uses the indicators listed in the acronym to assess pain.[14,15]

1. *Evaluate child with chronic MSK pain*

- Complete medical and pain history
- Assess pain intensity, location, onset, duration, quality, variability, aggravating and alleviating factors
- Assess associated disability including impact of pain on daily life, such as sleep, school, social, emotional, and physical activities
- Physical and neurological examination, including appearance, posture, gait, growth parameters, and vital signs
- Complete appropriate diagnostic tests

2. *Diagnose the primary and secondary causes*

- Current nociceptive and neuropathic components
- Attenuating physical symptoms
- Contributing psychological factors, social factors, and biological processes

3. *Select appropriate therapies to improve overall functioning* and quality of life

Pharmacological
- Acetaminophen
- NSAIDs
- Adjunct analgesics (for CRPS)
- Opioid analgesics; consult subspecialist if required

Physical
- Graded exercise program
- Regular daily activity (eg, walking, swimming, stretching)
- Pacing
- Heat, ice, massage, TENS

Psychological
- Relaxation strategies
- CBT
- School reintegration
- Sleep hygiene
- Teach parents adaptive responses to child's pain

4. *Implement pain management plan*

- Provide pain diagnosis, feedback on causes and contributing factors
- Provide rationale for integrated treatment program
- Develop mutually agreed upon treatment goals
- Measure child's pain and functional improvement regularly
- Evaluate effectiveness of treatment plan
- Revise plan as necessary

Fig. 1. Treatment algorithm for chronic musculoskeletal pain. CBT, cognitive behavior therapy; CRPS, complex regional pain syndrome; NSAIDs, nonsteroidal antiinflammatory drugs; TENS, transcutaneous electrical nerve stimulation. (*From* Stinson J, Reid K. Chronic pain in children. In: Twycross A, Bruce L, Stinson J, editors. Pain in children: a clinical guide. 2nd edition. London: Blackwell Science; 2013. p. 201; with permission.)

In addition to pain intensity, a more comprehensive pain assessment (associated symptoms, temporal variations, functional impact, triggers) is often necessary (see **Table 1**). It is important to assess pain intensity and pain interference regularly (routine visits) to determine effectiveness of treatments. For those with more complex pain,

Table 1
Pain history questions for children with chronic pain and their parents/carers

Description of pain	Type of pain: is the pain recurrent or chronic (eg, there all the time)
	Onset of pain: when did the pain begin? What were you doing before the pain began? Was there any initiating injury, trauma, or stressors?
	Duration: how long has the pain been present? (eg, hours/days/weeks/months)
	Frequency: how often is pain present? Is the pain always there or is it intermittent? Does it come and go?
	Location: where is the pain located? Can you point to the part of the body that hurts?
	Does the pain go anywhere else? (eg, radiates up or down from the site that hurts)
	Intensity: what is your pain intensity at rest? What is your pain intensity with activity? (Use a developmentally appropriate intensity assessment tool)
	Over the past week, what is the least pain you have had? What is the worst pain you have had? What is your usual level of pain?
	Unpleasantness: how unpleasant/bothersome is the pain right now? (Use a developmentally appropriate unpleasantness assessment tool)
	Over the past week, what is the least unpleasant/bothersome your pain has been? What is most unpleasant/bothersome your pain has been? How unpleasant/bothersome is it usually?
	Quality of pain: school-aged children can communicate about pain in more abstract terms.
	Describe the quality of your pain (eg, word descriptors such as sharp, dull, achy, stabbing, burning, shooting, or throbbing)
	Word descriptors can provide information on whether the pain is nociceptive or neuropathic or a combination of both
Associated symptoms	Are there any other symptoms that go along with or occur just before or immediately after the pain (eg, nausea, vomiting, light-headedness, tiredness, diarrhea, or difficulty ambulating)?
	Are there any changes in the color or temperature of the affected extremity or painful area? (These changes most often occur in children with conditions such as complex regional pain syndromes)
Temporal or seasonal variations	Is the pain affected by changes in seasons or weather?
	Does the pain occur at certain times of the day (eg, after eating or going to the toilet)?
Impact on daily living	Has the pain led to changes in daily activities and/or behaviors (eg, sleep disturbances, change in appetite, decreased physical activity, change in mood, or a decrease in social interactions or school attendance)?
	What level would the pain need to be so that you could do all your normal activities (ie, tolerability)? What level would the pain need to be so that you would not be bothered by it? (Rated on same developmentally appropriate scale as pain intensity)
	What brings on the pain or makes the pain worse (eg, movement, deep breathing and coughing,)?
Pain-relief measures	What has helped to make the pain better?
	Have you taken medication to relieve your pain? If so, what was the medication and did it help? Were there any side effects?
	It is important to also ask about the use of physical, psychological, and complementary and alternative treatments tried and how effective these methods were in relieving pain
	The degree of pain relief (or change in pain intensity) after a pain-relieving treatment/intervention should be determined

having patients track their pain and function over time can help to identify triggers that increase pain that can then be targeted for treatment (eg, poor sleep, not pacing activities). **Table 2** outlines multidimensional pain self-report measures. Real-time data collection methods using electronic diaries have been developed for children with CMP.[16,17] A tool currently freely available is PainQuILT (http://painquilt.com), which can be used to track pain over time (for 2–4 weeks).[18,19]

General Treatment Strategies for Patients with Nonarthritic Chronic Musculoskeletal Pain

Patients with some types of skeletal defects need orthopedic management, but most patients with nonarthritic CMP can be treated conservatively with reassurance, education on the diagnosis, and pain-relieving strategies such as rest, ice, heat, and analgesics such as acetaminophen or nonsteroidal antiinflammatory drugs (NSAIDs). Some patients may benefit from physical therapy (PT), relaxation exercises, and cognitive behavior therapy (CBT) (see **Fig. 1**).

AMPLIFIED MUSCULOSKELETAL PAIN SYNDROMES
When to Consider Amplified Musculoskeletal Pain Syndromes

Consider AMPS in a child with CMP who has pain of variable intensity without complete remission even for a short time. Children with AMPS may report pain on contact with clothing (allodynia) or an exaggerated response to a mildly painful stimulus (hyperalgesia) such as normal joint examination palpation. They may show hypervigilance toward the affected area with guarding and fear of movement. These patients may have new onset of physical limitations or disability, dystonic position of extremities, mood changes, social dysfunction, and sleep disturbances.[4] AMPS should also be considered in adolescent girls reporting severe, widespread joint and muscle pain with several other symptoms (fatigue, sleep disturbance, mood difficulties, and recurrent headaches and abdominal pain; see **Fig. 2**).

Overview

There are 2 types of AMPS: localized AMPS/complex regional pain syndrome (CRPS) and diffuse AMPS/juvenile fibromyalgia syndrome (JFMS) (see **Fig. 2**). There can be overlap of these two syndromes.[4]

Incidence and prevalence:

- CRPS: estimated to have an incidence of 1.2/100,000 in children 5 to 15 years old[20]
- Diffuse AMPS/JFMS: estimated that 2% to 6% of children have JFMS[21]

Demographics:

- Age:
  - 10 to 15 years old, mean 12 years old.
  - Less common in children less than 10 years old and rare in children less than 5 years old[22]
  - JFMS is most frequent in adolescent girls.[21]
- Gender:
  - More common in girls in both conditions
- Race and ethnicity:
  - In JFMS it is estimated that ~ 80% are white in study samples from the United Sates.[23] There are no data for CRPS.

Table 2
Three self-report pain tools

Tool	Components	Considerations
Adolescent Pediatric Pain Tool Savedra et al,[96] 1989	Pain intensity measured using: • A 0–100 mm word graphic rating scale • Body outline to describe location of pain • Word descriptors	• Originally developed for children and adolescents with postoperative pain; has been used in children with acute and chronic disease-related pain (eg, cancer, sickle cell disease, arthritis) • Intended for use in children aged 5–16 y; used in children aged 4–18 y • Well-established evidence of reliability, validity, and ability to detect change • Easy to use, well liked and requires minimal training, and takes 3–6 min to complete
Pediatric Pain Assessment Tool Abu-Saad et al,[97] 1990	Pain intensity measured using: • 0–10 cm VAS • Body outline (number of body areas marked) • 32-word descriptors	• Initially developed for acute medical and postoperative pain; has also been used with recurrent pain (headaches) and chronic pain (arthritis) • Intended for use in children aged 5–16 y; used in children up to 17 y • Well-established evidence of reliability and validity and some evidence of ability to detect change • Child, parent, and health care professional forms • Easy to use and takes 5–10 min to complete
Pediatric Pain Questionnaire Varni et al,[98] 1987	Pain intensity measured using: • 0–10 cm VAS anchored with happy and sad faces for present and worst pain • Gender-neutral body outline to describe location of pain (number of body areas marked) • Pain intensity (choosing 4 of 8 colored crayons to represent various levels of pain intensity, including none, mild, moderate, and severe) • 46 word descriptors to assess the sensory, affective and evaluative qualities of pain	• Originally developed for children and adolescents with recurrent and chronic pain (eg, juvenile arthritis) • Intended for use in children aged 5–16 y; used in children 4–18 y • Child, adolescent, and parent versions • Children younger than 7 y usually need to be read the instructions to complete the VAS and body outline. Young children seem to be able to complete the tool without issue (Benestad et al, 1996)[99] • Well-established evidence of reliability and validity and some evidence of ability to detect change • Minimal training and takes 10–15 min to complete • Web site: www.pedsgl.org

Abbreviation: VAS, visual analog scale.
Data from Refs.[96–98]

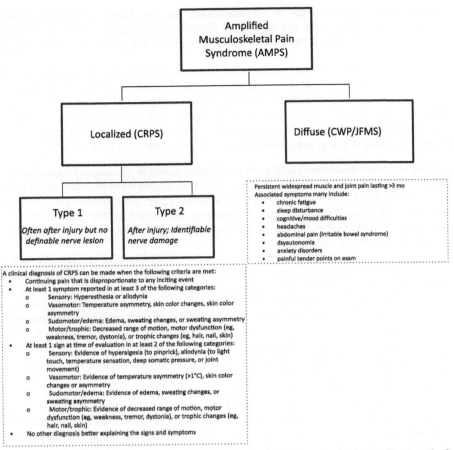

Fig. 2. Criteria for the diagnosis of AMPS. CWP, chronic widespread pain; JFMS, juvenile fibromyalgia syndrome.

Localized amplified musculoskeletal pain syndromes/complex regional pain syndrome

Localized AMPS/CRPS is characterized by constant pain that increases with movement. Fear of moving the affected site can result in profound disability, including the complete loss of the ability to ambulate independently. Pain descriptors include burning, shooting, stabbing, or electrical. Patients may have muscle weakness and atrophy that varies from mild to severe from disuse. Autonomic findings can include swelling and edema, temperature changes (affected limb is cooler), hyperhidrosis, changes in skin color, cyanosis, cold sensitivity, and mottled dry skin. Trophic skin changes may be seen with time. Motor involvement is most often limited to decreased ROM but might include tremors or jerks. Contracture can develop if symptoms are allowed to persist without intervention.[24] There are 2 types of localized AMPS/CRPS (see **Fig. 2**):

- Type 1 (previously called reflex sympathetic dystrophy) usually follows an injury (minor trauma, limb immobilization, surgery, or minor medical procedure) without a definable nerve lesion. However, in many cases there is no direct physical injury.
- Type 2 (rare in children) occurs following damage to an identifiable nerve.

Diagnostic criteria include those developed by the International Association for the Study of Pain, and the Budapest Criteria; however, they are not concordant.[25] The median interval between symptom onset and diagnosis is 2 months (range 1–12 months).[20]

CRPS is considered to be a multifactorial syndrome of neuropathic pain with central and peripheral nervous system sensitization, inflammation, and altered somatosensory representation in the brain.[26–28] Small fiber changes and genetic factors may also be a mechanism of disease.[29–31] Psychological factors, including emotional distress, stressful life events, wanting to excel academically, and parental enmeshment,[32] can play a role in the development and progression of CRPS.[33,34]

Diffuse amplified musculoskeletal pain syndromes/juvenile fibromyalgia syndrome

Diffuse AMPS/JFMS is thought to represent a more severe form of CMP, with higher levels of pain and functional impairment.[21] Reports of pain tend to be in the moderate to severe range (>6/10) and can be incongruent with affect showing no or minimal discomfort. Patients often have a poor sleep pattern and nap during the day; thus, school attendance can be affected.[21]

The diagnosis of diffuse chronic widespread pain/JFMS remains controversial in part because it is a purely symptom-based diagnosis. In addition, there is debate about which classification criteria should be used.[21,35] The Yunus and Masi[36] classification system includes the hallmark symptom of widespread muscle and joint pain lasting more than 3 months with associated symptoms of fatigue, sleep difficulty, anxiety, and painful tender points on examination.[35] The 2010 American College of Rheumatology fibromyalgia questionnaire is brief[35] (<5 minutes) and should be used as a screening tool to aid early diagnosis and treatment (**Fig. 3**). Clinicians may use the label chronic widespread pain rather than fibromyalgia because of the stigma and poor prognosis of fibromyalgia syndrome in the adult population.

Understanding of the mechanisms in JFMS is limited. Emerging evidence in the study of adult fibromyalgia points toward abnormal pain processing, with potential neurologic, biochemical, inflammatory, and/or genetic factors, along with psychosocial and environmental components.[21,37,38]

How Localized Amplified Musculoskeletal Pain Syndromes/Complex Regional Pain Syndrome and Diffuse Amplified Musculoskeletal Pain Syndromes/Juvenile Fibromyalgia Syndrome Are Treated

The goal of treatment of AMPS is to return the child to a functional state that will enable them to participate in daily activities, return to school, and see friends. A multidisciplinary, multimodal approach that incorporates the 3 Ps (physical, psychological, and pharmacologic interventions) is most likely to be effective (**Table 3**). Management should involve patient and family education and focus on nonpharmacologic therapies.[39] Goals of treatment include restoring function with relief of pain as a secondary outcome. The standard of care is intensive PT, with the goal of working up to 30 minutes of vigorous exercise 2–3 times per week, and psychological therapies (counseling, CBTs). Physical therapists should be familiar with these conditions so they can provide individualized graded strength training.[40,41] However, long-term adherence and motivation for regular exercise can be poor, especially for children with diffuse AMPS.

For children with CRPS, patients start with desensitization followed by weight-bearing and ROM exercises. Patients with CRPS may develop depression, anxiety, or posttraumatic stress disorder, all of which heighten the perception of pain and make rehabilitation efforts more difficult. Most beneficial is a comprehensive

WIDESPREAD PAIN INDEX (WPI)

A Have you had pain in the following location(s) in the last week?

Shoulder, right	Shoulder, left	Upper arm, right	Upper arm, left
Lower arm, right	Lower arm, left	Hip (buttock), right	Hip (buttock), left
Upper leg, right	Upper leg, left	Lower leg, right	Lower leg, left
Jaw, right	Jaw, left	Chest	Abdomen
Upper back	Lower back	Neck	

Part A Score = Total number of areas marked yes

SYMPTOM SEVERITY (SS)

B How much of a problem have the following been for you during the past week?

	No problem	Slight/Mild problem, generally mild or intermittent	Moderate, Considerable problem, often present	Severe, pervasive, continuous, life-disturbing problem
Fatigue	0	1	2	3
Waking Still Feeling Tired	0	1	2	3
Concentration or Memory Problems	0	1	2	3

Part B Score: Total of all domains

C Have you had problems with any of the following during the past three months?

Muscle pain	Headache	Sun sensitivity	Chest pain
Muscle weakness	Dizziness	Blurred vision	Hair loss
Numbness/tingling	Shortness of breath	Loss/changes in taste	Fever
IBS	Nervousness	Hearing difficulties	Thinking problem
Abdominal pain/cramps	Depression	Ringing in ears	Dry mouth
Diarrhea	Fatigue/tiredness	Easy bruising	Dry eyes
Constipation	Insomnia	Frequent urination	Itching
Heartburn	Loss of appetite	Bladder spasms	Wheezing
Vomiting	Rash	Painful urination	Oral ulcers
Nausea	Hives/welts	Seizures	Raynaud's

Part C Score: 0 = No symptoms, 1= Few symptoms, 2 = Moderate number of symptoms, 3 = A great deal of symptoms

WPI = A Score

SS = B Score + C Score

Fibromyalgia if: WPI ≥7 and SS ≥5 OR WPI 3 –6 and SS ≥9

Fig. 3. 2010 American College of Rheumatology adult fibromyalgia criteria. (*From* Ting TV, Barnett K, Lynch-Jordan A, et al. 2010 American College of Rheumatology adult fibromyalgia criteria for use in an adolescent female population with juvenile fibromyalgia. J Pediatr 2016;169:182.e1; with permission.)

CBT program directed at identifying and eliminating trigger factors that affect the child's pain and disability, and educating the family about CRPS and how to manage it.

Patients not responding need further therapies tailored to their specific needs which may include sleep hygiene (see National Sleep Foundation at www.sleepfoundation. org), pharmacotherapy, and/or a multimodal intensive rehabilitation program for those severely disabled.[40] Kashikar-Zuck and colleagues[42] have shown that an 8-week CBT

Table 3
Three Ps approach to managing chronic musculoskeletal pain in children

Pharmacologic	Physical	Psychological
Simple analgesics (NSAIDs and acetaminophen)	Exercise	Education (about pain diagnosis and coping)
Opioid analgesics (tramadol with or without acetaminophen, hydrocodone with or without acetaminophen, oxycodone, morphine, and fentanyl)	Thermal stimulation (heat, cold, desensitization)	Sleep hygiene (good sleep habits)
	Physiotherapy	Relaxation
	Occupational therapy	Biofeedback
	Massage	Behavioral therapies
Anticonvulsant medications (pregabalin or gabapentin)	Transcutaneous electrical nerve stimulation	Cognitive therapies
Antidepressant medications (amitriptyline, nortriptyline, and duloxetine)	Acupuncture	Cognitive behavior therapies (imagery, distraction, and relaxation)
Antiarrhythmic medications		Acceptance and commitment therapy
Anxiolytics		Mindfulness therapy
Nerve blocks		Family therapy
Topical local anesthetic creams and patches (lidocaine)		Psychotherapy
Bisphosphonates		
Botulinum toxin injections		
N-methyl-D-aspartate receptor antagonists (dextromethorphan, ketamine)		

Adapted from Stinson J, Reid K. Chronic pain in children. In: Twycross A, Bruce L, Stinson J, editors. Pain in children: a clinical guide. 2nd edition. London: Blackwell Science; 2013. p. 196; with permission.

program was superior to education alone in reducing functional disability in teens with JFMS.

Medications may allow children to fully participate in PT. However, few of the medications prescribed are licensed for use in children,[43] with the clinical indications and use extrapolated from research and clinical practice in adults with chronic pain. There is limited research supporting their use in children.[19] A recent systematic review found no evidence that regional anesthesia is effective compared with placebo for managing CRPS.[44] If the provider is considering opioid use, the authors recommend sending the patient to a pediatric chronic pain team for help with management. For disturbed sleep, consider low-dose amitriptyline, cyclobenzaprine, or pregabalin at night.[37]

What Is the Prognosis for Localized Amplified Musculoskeletal Pain Syndrome/Complex Regional Pain Syndrome 1 and Diffuse Amplified Musculoskeletal Pain Syndrome/Juvenile Fibromyalgia Syndrome

Most children with localized AMPS/CRPS 1 have complete resolution of symptoms with noninvasive treatment; a small proportion (20%) continue to have pain and pain-related disability or relapse. Early recognition and treatment offer the best prognosis.[45]

In early community-based studies of patients with diffuse AMPS/JFMS who were not seeking treatment, long-term prognosis was fairly positive with approximately 70% of children no longer meeting AMPS criteria after 2 years.[46,47] However, more recent studies of those seeking treatment at a tertiary pediatric rheumatology clinic found a high likelihood of continued symptoms into young adulthood.[48]

BENIGN JOINT HYPERMOBILITY SYNDROME
When to Consider Benign Joint Hypermobility Syndrome

Consider benign joint hypermobility syndrome (BJHS) in any school-aged child who complains of joint pain, usually of the lower extremities, especially the knees, and who has a normal examination except for joint laxity.[49] Patients often complain of pain in the evening or during periods of increased activity. The patient may wake during the night with pain but should be asymptomatic with a normal gait in the morning.

Background

BJHS is one of the most common causes of joint pain in school-aged children (most common <8 years) affecting 13% to 20% of children in some populations.[50,51] It is generally more common in girls. BJHS is a heritable disorder of connective tissue characterized by generalized joint hypermobility and laxity, musculoskeletal pain, and potentially injury.[49,50,52–55] Joint pain has been positively correlated to joint laxity; however, not all patients with joint laxity complain of pain.[56] Adolescents with hypermobility have a 2-fold increase in shoulder, knee, ankle, and foot pain,[49] and obesity causes an even greater risk for knee pain.

How to Diagnose Benign Joint Hypermobility Syndrome

BJHS is a clinical diagnosis made in children presenting with joint pain and identified by either the Beighton score or the Brighton scale (validated in patients ≥16 years old) (**Box 1, Tables 4** and **5**).[52,55] To calculate the Beighton score,[52] patients gain 1 point (for right or left side) for the ability to perform each of the movements in **Box 1**. The Brighton Diagnostic Criteria (**Table 6**) use the Beighton score as one of the criteria. Hypermobility may be associated with genetic syndromes such as Marfan, Ehlers-Danlos (ED), Stickler, or Williams syndrome; osteogenesis imperfecta; and trisomy 21, making it important to assess for signs of other organ system involvement, especially of the cardiovascular system. BJHS and ED hypermobile type are clinically indistinguishable from each other.[53] Pacey and colleagues[53] found the most common manifestations, present in greater than 40% of patients with BJHS, are soft skin, recurrent joint instability in 3 or more joints, chronic pain in 4 or more joints, and easy bruising. Pes planus and genu recurvatum may be associated with BJHS.

How Benign Joint Hypermobility Syndrome Is Treated

The patient should be advised to wear comfortable, properly fitting shoes with good arch support. PT is useful for conditioning, strengthening the periarticular muscles,

---

Box 1
Beighton criteria for benign joint hypermobility syndrome

Passive dorsiflexion of fifth finger beyond 90°

Passive apposition of thumb to the flexor aspects of the forearms

Elbow hyperextension beyond 100°

Knee hyperextension beyond 100°

Forward flexion of the trunk, with knees straight, so palms rest on the floor

Beighton criteria: score 1 point for each item, count right and left sides separately.
    Adapted from Beighton P, Solomona L, Soskolne CL. Articular mobility in an African population. Ann Rheum Dis 1973;32:413–8.

Table 4
Brighton diagnostic criteria for benign joint hypermobility syndrome

Major Criteria	Minor Criteria
Generalized joint hypermobility (Beighton score ≥4 out of 9 points)	Beighton score ≤4 out of 9 points (See **Box 1**)
	Arthralgia in 1–3 joints, or back pain ≥ 3-mo, or spondylolysis/spondylolisthesis
Pain in ≥4 joints for ≥3 mo	Dislocation/subluxation in >1 joint, or in 1 joint more than once
	Soft tissue rheumatism ≥3 lesions (tenosynovitis)
	Marfanoid habitus
	Abnormal skin (striae, hyperextensibility)
	Eye signs (drooping eyelids)
	Varicose veins, hernia, or uterine/rectal prolapse

Using the revised Brighton criteria for BJHS, patients must have 2 major criteria, or 1 major and 2 minor, or 4 minor criteria.

Adapted from Grahame R, Bird HA, Child A. The revised (Brighton 1998) criteria for the diagnosis of benign joint hypermobility syndrome (BJHS). J Rheumatol 2000;27(7):1777–9.

and improving joint proprioception.[57] Soft braces or taping can help with joint stability. A short course of analgesics may help.

BENIGN LIMB PAIN OF CHILDHOOD
When to Consider Benign Limb Pain of Childhood

A school-aged child who reports intermittent, bilateral shin, calf, thigh, or posterior knee pain, and who has a normal physical examination, may have benign limb pain of childhood (BLPC).[56] Pain descriptors include deep, achy, and severe, and pain may cause nocturnal awakening producing fatigue.[58] The pain usually resolves with rest. If the patient has nocturnal awakening caused by pain with symptoms of night sweats, fevers, weight loss, or lymphadenopathy, malignancy should be considered.

Background

BLPC is self-limited lower extremity pain of unknown cause affecting up to 49% of children (commonly 4–14 years old).[56,58–60] Studies have found that there may be a familial component and that affected patients may have a decreased pain threshold or decreased bone density.[58,61,62] Overuse, emotional disturbance, family stress, and hypermobility may also be associated with BLPC.[58]

How to Diagnose Benign Limb Pain of Childhood

The diagnosis is based on a consistent history and normal examination findings.[58] Laboratory and imaging results are often normal and should be ordered judiciously.

How Benign Limb Pain of Childhood Is Treated

The patient and parents should be educated on the self-limited nature of BLPC. Massage offers some relief but can become a maladaptive coping mechanism. Patients with hypermobility or pes planus may benefit form PT and shoe inserts.[63]

COMMON OVERUSE INJURIES AND SKELETAL DEFECTS
Background

Skeletally immature athletes are at risk for developing sports-related pain and injuries, and certain skeletal defects (**Fig. 4**; see **Tables 5** and **6**). Children now train more

Table 5
Common osteochondroses

Disease	Location	Age (y) Gender	Triggering Activity or Presentation Pattern	Pathology
Little league shoulder	Shoulder	11–16	Pitching curveballs and sliders: baseball	Traction on the proximal physis of the humerus
Little league/ golfer's elbow	Elbow	8–12	Throwing baseball, golf	Medial epicondylitis
Panner disease	Elbow	4–10	Lateral elbow pain	Abnormal ossification and necrosis of capitellum humeri
Tennis elbow/ Wiiitis	Elbow	Any	Backhand tennis, Wii	Lateral epicondylitis
Gymnast's wrist	Wrist	12–14 (girls)	Tumbling, vaulting	Radial epiphysitis
Madelung deformity	Wrist	8–13 (girls)	Volar translation of the wrist and hand, often bilateral and painless	Distal radial epiphysis, genetic defect
Legg-Calvé-Perthes	Hip	3–9 (boys>girls)	Hip pain, 10% bilateral, 25% painless limp	Abnormal ossification and necrosis of epiphysis of femoral head
Iliac crest apophysitis	Hip	<15, but up to 25	Gymnastics, sprinting	Iliac crest apophysitis; avulsion can occur
Anterior superior iliac spine	Hip	Up to late teens	Kicking, "soccer hip"	Anterior superior iliac spine apophysitis
Sinding-Larsen-Johansson	Knee	10–12	Running, cutting, jumping Soccer, basketball, ballet	Apophysitis of the inferior pole of patella
Osgood-Schlatter	Knee	10–15 (boys) 8–13 (girls)	Cutting and jumping Soccer, basketball, volleyball	Tibial tubercle apophysitis
Freiberg disease	Foot	Adolescents	Painful forefoot in dancers	Ossification disorder of second metatarsal head
Köhler disease	Foot	2–8 (boys>girls)	Midfoot pain and limp	Navicular osteonecrosis
Sever disease	Foot	7–10	Jumping, running, basketball, soccer, track	Calcaneal apophysitis
Scheuermann disease	Back	10–12	Back pain and deformity hump-back	Anterior vertebral body wedging, end-plate irregularity

Adapted from Weiser P. Approach to the patient with noninflammatory musculoskeletal pain. Pediatr Clin North Am 2012;59:471–92.

aggressively at a younger age, putting increased strain at the tendon attachment sites (apophyses), joint surfaces (articular cartilage), and growth plates (physes).[64] The epiphyseal plates and apophyses are the weakest components in the pediatric musculoskeletal system so, during periods of skeletal maturation, overuse and

Table 6
Selected skeletal defects

Disease	Location	Age (y)/Gender	Presentation	Pathology
Slipped capital femoral epiphysis	Hip	7–15 (obese boys)	Limp, hip, groin, and knee pain (referred)	Displacement of proximal femoral epiphysis
Meyer dysplasia	Hip	≤5, boys>girls	Hip pain mimics Legg-Calvé-Perthes on radiograph	Dysplasia epiphysis, capitis femoris
Patellofemoral syndrome (runner's knee)	Knee	Adolescents	Pain with keeping knees flexed, squatting, going upstairs	Lateral tracking of the patella, chondromalacia patellae
Osteochondritis dissecans	Knee, elbow, other sites	Adolescents	Persistent knee pain 20%–30% bilateral Elbow: lateral elbow pain with swelling	Osteonecrosis of lateral aspect of the medial condyle Elbow: flattening of capitellum, articular surface defects, and loose bodies
Spondylolysis/ spondylolisthesis	Back	Adolescents	Back pain Sports with hyperextension, runners, gymnasts, ballet, dance, martial arts, weight lifters	Pars Interarticularis defect L4–5

Adapted from Weiser P. Approach to the patient with noninflammatory musculoskeletal pain. Pediatr Clin North Am 2012;59:471–92.

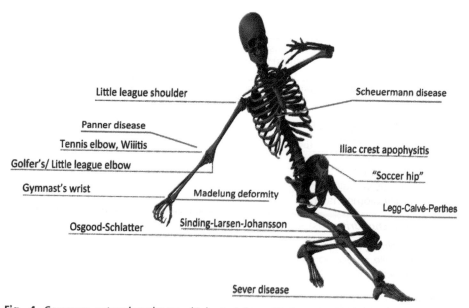

Fig. 4. Common osteochondroses. (*Adapted from* Weiser P. Approach to the patient with noninflammatory musculoskeletal pain. Pediatr Clin North Am 2012;59:471–92; with permission.)

repetitive microtrauma can lead to inflammation (apophysitis), or derangement of the epiphyseal ossification center (osteochondrosis).[65] Although most osteochondroses (see **Table 5**) are self-limited, some, such as Legg-Calvé-Perthes and Scheuermann disease, can result in permanent disability.

Girls are more likely to have lower extremity overuse injuries.[64] Girls' sports associated with the highest frequency of overuse injury include track and field, lacrosse, and field hockey.[64]

Prevention is the most important form of management of overuse injuries; however, once diagnosed they need to be treated promptly and effectively. Left untreated, these injuries can lead to CMP, decreased HRQL, and osteoarthritis.[64] Symptomatic treatment includes analgesics and ice. Most patients benefit from PT. Some of the more common overuse injuries and skeletal defects are discussed later.

LOWER EXTREMITY PAIN
Patellofemoral Pain Syndrome

When to consider patellofemoral pain syndrome
Patellofemoral pain syndrome (PFPS; runner's knee) should be suspected in patients, especially adolescent girls, reporting knee pain while running, ascending/descending stairs, squatting, or sitting with knees flexed (so-called theater sign) (see **Table 6**).

Background
PFPS is one of the most common causes of anterior knee pain in pediatrics.[6] Imbalances in the forces controlling patellar tracking during knee flexion and extension result in retropatellar or peripatellar pain.[66] Risk factors include overuse, trauma, muscle dysfunction, patellar hypermobility, and poor quadriceps flexibility.[66]

How to diagnose patellofemoral pain syndrome
The patient's lower extremities should be assessed for ROM, pain/tenderness, muscle atrophy, and joint swelling, because full ROM and absence of atrophy and swelling are expected.[66] Gait should be observed.[66] Positive examination findings may include pain with squatting to 80°; lateral deviation of the patella with ROM from flexion to extension (J sign); or a positive grind, patella apprehension, or compression test.[66] Patients may have pes planus, genu valgum, tight hamstrings, or weak quadriceps. Crepitus is nonspecific. Imaging should be ordered if there is no improvement after 4 to 6 weeks of conservative therapy.[67]

How patellofemoral pain syndrome is treated
High-impact activities should be avoided. PT with use of elliptical trainers and stationary bikes is helpful.[66] Quadriceps strengthening with leg lifts can be done at home. Some patients benefit from patella bracing and taping.[67] Orthotics can assist those who have excessive calcaneovalgus foot and pes planus to correct and improve their lower extremity biomechanics.[66,67]

Juvenile Osteochondritis Dissecans

When to consider juvenile osteochondritis dissecans of the knee
Consider juvenile osteochondritis dissecans (JOCD) in teenage patients complaining of knee pain with locking, popping, and/or catching.[68]

Background
JOCD is an idiopathic disorder of bone necrosis affecting subchondral bone and its overlying articular cartilage (see **Table 6**).[67–70] Trauma (microtrauma and macrotrauma), family history, endocrinopathies, and vascular insufficiency have all been

reported as contributing factors to developing JOCD.[67–69] One study showed that patients aged 12 to 19 years had 3 times the risk of osteochondritis dissecans (OCD) of the knee compared with 6 to 11-year-olds.[70,71] Boys are more often affected than girls (4:1).[67,71] The knee is most often affected (medial femoral condyle > lateral femoral condyle, patellofemoral joint), but JOCD can also develop in the elbow (capitellum) and ankle (talus) of athletes involved in overhand throwing or weight bearing.[66,67,72] Lesions can break off, resulting in loose bodies in the joint space with pain, locking, and further destruction.[69]

How to diagnose juvenile osteochondritis dissecans
Patients have focal tenderness and joint effusion at the affected site. Anteroposterior and lateral radiographs of the knee may miss an OCD lesion, so tunnel and Merchant views should be ordered.[68] A typical radiograph finding is an expanding concentric lesion at the margin of an otherwise normal epiphysis.[73,74] MRI helps determine lesion stability and the presence of loose bodies.[68]

How juvenile osteochondritis dissecans is treated
Treatment is based on the lesion stage and stability. Skeletally immature patients with stable lesions have the best prognosis and can be treated with restricted/modified activity, patellar taping, and PT.[67] Arthroscopy with removal of any loose bodies may be indicated for patients with unstable lesions, stable lesions that have not healed after 6 months, or mechanical symptoms, and for skeletally mature patients with stable lesions.[68,69,74]

Slipped Capital Femoral Epiphysis

When to consider slipped capital femoral epiphysis
Consider slipped capital femoral epiphysis (SCFE) in overweight adolescents or pre-adolescent children (7–15 years old), especially boys, who present with groin, lateral or posterior hip, medial thigh, or knee pain that is worsened by walking or climbing and improved by rest (see **Table 6**). SCFE can also occur in older, nonobese, and short patients, especially if they have endocrine disorders. Initially, the pain may be low level, later developing into dull, aching, or boring pain.

Background
During the growth spurt, patients with SCFE have widening of their femoral physis, which, coupled with the normal developmental rotation of the angle of the femoral physis, puts the physis at risk for shearing and displacement with a mechanical overload. Risk factors include obesity and endocrine disorders (hypothyroidism, growth hormone deficiency, and panhypopituitarism).[75] A higher incidence of SCFE is also found in African Americans, Hispanic people, and Pacific Islanders.[75] Bilateral disease occurs in a third or more of patients, most within 18 months of the first slip, with higher rates in those with endocrine disorders.[75]

How to diagnose slipped capital femoral epiphysis
Patients often have an antalgic, waddling, or Trendelenburg gait, with externally rotated foot.[75] Hip ROM is limited, especially for internal rotation and flexion. Diagnosis is often delayed in children who present only with knee pain, so the ipsilateral hip should always be examined in children presenting with knee pain, comparing ROM with the contralateral hip. Anteroposterior (AP) and frog-leg-view radiographs show a widened and irregular physis and displacement of the proximal femoral metaphysis anterolaterally and superiorly. Radiographs may miss the diagnosis in early SCFE, so other imaging studies may help identify some SCFE-related abnormalities.[75]

The greater the displacement of the slip, the worse is the long-term prognosis, with a higher risk of osteonecrosis.[75]

How slipped capital femoral epiphysis is treated
Prompt orthopedic referral is vital to minimize the risk for chondrolysis and osteonecrosis of the femoral epiphysis. Patients need surgical intervention to stabilize the epiphysis, with those unable to bear weight on the affected hip even with crutches (unstable slip) needing urgent intervention because of their higher risk for osteonecrosis.[75]

Osteochondrosis and Apophysitis

When to consider osteochondrosis or apophysitis
Consider these disorders of bone and tendon in athletes complaining of joint pain, especially of the hip, knee, foot, elbow, or back that is exacerbated by movement.[4,76,77] Although most osteochondroses are fairly benign, Legg-Calvé-Perthes and Scheuermann disease can cause more serious growth disturbances and are discussed separately later.

Background
Osteochondroses and apophysitis result from a combination of abnormal development, ischemic injury, or overuse or trauma of the growth plate and surrounding ossification centers.[76,77] Reports of a pop should raise concern for an avulsion fracture. Sever disease (SD) or calcaneal apophysitis, and Osgood-Schlatter disease (OSD) or tibial tuberosity apophysitis, are the most common areas of lower extremity involvement; other affected sites are shown in **Fig. 4** and **Table 5**.[64] Pathology reveals minor avulsions at the site and subsequent inflammatory reaction, resulting in patellar tendinitis, multiple subacute fractures, and irregular ossification of underlying bone.[78,79]

How to diagnose osteochondrosis and apophysitis
These disorders typically present with tenderness and swelling of the affected site (see **Fig. 4**). OSD occurs most commonly in active adolescents, who may have pain that worsens with resisted knee extension; these patients may have tight hamstrings or quadriceps as well as swelling, tenderness, and enlargement of the tibial tubercle.[80–82] Pain may be aggravated by kneeling, jumping, or stair climbing and improve with rest.[66] Boys commonly present between 12 and 15 years old and girls between 8 and 12 years old[80] OSD is bilateral in 20% to 30% of patients.[83]

SD is the most common form of heel pain (unilateral or bilateral) in growing athletes, with a reported incidence of 3.7/1000 children.[84] Patients may have mild swelling and tenderness at the Achilles insertion onto the calcaneus.[70] Ankle dorsiflexion is limited and painful.[70,85] Pain may be elicited on squeezing the lateral and medial calcaneus (positive squeeze test).[85] Boys present between 8 and 15 years of age and girls between 8 and 13 years of age.[66] Patients report heel pain with running or jumping, and after activity.[70] Children with obesity, greater waist circumference, increased height, pronated feet, and tight Achilles tendons may be predisposed to SD.[86]

Imaging for osteochondrosis or apophysitis in a typical location with typical physical findings is not usually needed and is most often done to diagnose avulsion fracture or exclude other disorders.

How osteochondrosis and apophysitis are treated
Most patients with osteochondrosis or apophysitis have self-limiting disease that resolves with rest and modified activity. Treatment of SD with rest, a heel raise inlay,

or PT can significantly reduce symptoms.[87] Permanent resolution occurs with closure of the growth plate.[79]

Legg-Calvé-Perthes Disease: An Osteochondrosis with More Serious Consequences

When to consider Legg-Calvé-Perthes disease

Any young boy of approximately 3 to 9 years of age presenting with a limp with hip, thigh, and/or knee pain, especially if there is a family history, should be suspected of having Legg-Calvé-Perthes disease (LCPD). The pain may be mild and intermittent, only occurring during activity. The pain may initially occur in the groin, radiate into the thigh or knee, or only occur in the knee. As with SCFE, diagnosis is often delayed in children who present only with knee pain; it is vital that the ipsilateral hip is examined in children presenting with knee pain.

Background

LCPD is an osteochondrosis associated with necrosis of the of the epiphysis of the femoral head, resulting in impaired ossification (see **Fig. 4**, **Table 5**) and potentially in collapse of the femoral head and the presence of bone fragments within the joint. It most commonly affects boys during early childhood, with possible causes including vascular insufficiency, hypercoagulability, delayed skeletal maturity, and also repetitive microtrauma because it is found most commonly in hyperactive children.[88] Use of corticosteroids may increase risk of LCPD because they can cause a degenerative process and also inhibit repair.[89] Factors associated with a poor prognosis include being overweight, female sex, age greater than 6 years, and lack of hip abduction.[90]

How to diagnose Legg-Calvé-Perthes disease

Common findings are a limping gait and pain with passive ROM of the hip joint accompanied by limitation of abduction and internal rotation. About 10% to 15% of children have bilateral disease, although usually not simultaneously. There may be a leg length difference because of hip contracture or collapse of the epiphysis.[88] AP and frog-leg radiographs are needed to make the diagnosis and assess the stage of the disease, the containment of the femoral head in the acetabulum, and the extent of involvement.[80] MRI is more sensitive and can detect earlier changes.

How Legg-Calvé-Perthes disease is treated

A pediatric orthopedist should manage the patient. If less than 50% of the femoral head has necrosis, and depending on associated findings, the patient may be managed expectantly with rest, analgesics, and PT. The need for a surgical intervention is based on the percentage of femoral head necrosis.[80] Prognosis depends on stage, and the orthopedist should advise on sports participation. After the lesion heals, later surgical interventions may be needed to help correct leg length discrepancy and malalignment, and to reduce hip pain or dysfunction.

UPPER EXTREMITY PAIN
Upper Extremity Overuse Injuries

When to consider upper extremity overuse injuries

Consider overuse injuries in athletes presenting with elbow or shoulder pain, especially those who play overhead sports such as baseball/softball, tennis, swimming, gymnastics, and golf.[64]

Background

The most common upper extremity sites of involvement are the proximal humeral epiphysis (Little League shoulder [LLS]), and the medial epicondylar apophysis of the elbow (golfer's elbow, Little League elbow [LLE]) (see **Fig. 4, Table 5**).[64,83] LLS is most common in male baseball pitchers but can occur in girls, other baseball players, and tennis players.[65,81] Concomitant elbow pain is present in up to 13% of patients.[85] Almost one-quarter of competitive swimmers have shoulder pain (swimmer's shoulder) from the higher peak torques in internal shoulder rotation.[65]

How to diagnose upper extremity overuse injuries
In patients complaining of shoulder pain, examination findings may reveal pain with ROM, tenderness on palpation of the anterolateral proximal humerus, and pain and weakness with shoulder rotation and abduction.[64,65] Patients with LLE have tenderness on palpation of the medial epicondyle,[64] whereas patients with tennis elbow have lateral epicondyle pain (see **Fig. 4**).

How upper extremity overuse injuries are treated
Patients with most types of upper extremity overuse injuries should be treated with a 3-month period of rest followed by a training program using proper mechanics, a preseason strengthening program, and education on prevention.[84,86] After rest and PT, symptoms may recur in some patients (7%) after return to sports.[64] Pitchsmart@ usabaseball.com has a useful table showing the number of days of rest a child should have based on age and number of pitches thrown to try to minimize injury.

Upper Extremity Skeletal Defects and Osteochondroses

When to consider upper extremity skeletal abnormalities
Consider skeletal abnormalities of the elbow in athletes presenting with elbow pain that worsens with activity. Both osteochondrosis of the capitellum (Panner disease; see **Fig. 4, Table 5**) and capitellar OCD (see **Table 6**) can present as pain, tenderness, and swelling over the lateral elbow; there can be limited extension of the elbow joint.[80,91] Patients with Panner disease can complain of elbow stiffness, whereas those with OCD can have elbow locking or catching.

Background
Skeletal abnormalities of the upper extremity are uncommon. Two of them, Panner disease and capitellar OCD, are more likely in overuse situations. Both Panner disease and capitellar OCD are more common in boys, with Panner disease affecting younger boys (4–12 years old) and OCD adolescent boys (11 years and older). In contrast, Madelung deformity, an osteochondrosis of the distal radial epiphysis, has a genetic basis (see **Fig. 4, Table 5**).[80,84,91] This deformity affects girls 8 to 13 years old.[91]

How to diagnose upper extremity skeletal abnormalities
Both Panner disease and capitellar OCD can present as lateral elbow pain with limited extension.[80,91] Because OCD can lead to degenerative changes, adolescent boys with lateral elbow pain should get radiographs to evaluate for OCD.[92] Similar to knee OCD, standard radiographs may miss the abnormality; an AP view with the elbow in 45° flexion can help, but computed tomography (CT) or MRI may be needed.[92] Radiograph findings include flattening of the capitellum, articular surface defects, and loose bodies.[92] Patients with Madelung deformity present with volar translation of the wrist and hand, decreased extension, pronation, and supination, and sometimes pain.[84]

How upper extremity osteochondroses are treated
Capitellar OCD should be monitored by orthopedics because unstable lesions need surgery, and may have a poor prognosis.[92] Most patients with Panner disease improve with rest and refraining from activities that increase valgus stress, although the optimal

duration is not known.[80] Madelung deformity may need surgical correction, although splinting may be helpful to decrease symptoms in mild cases.

Back Pain

Background

Back pain is a common complaint in children, increasing in frequency with age. Less than 10% of children aged 10 years and younger report having back pain, but by mid to late adolescence most have had at least 1 episode of back pain, with a lifetime prevalence of 70% to 80% by 20 years of age[82] Girls have a higher incidence than boys.[82] Back pain may be idiopathic, or caused by mechanical abnormalities, infection, inflammatory disorders, congenital abnormalities, hypermobility, and malignancy. Younger children are more likely to have infectious causes, such as discitis of lumbar vertebrae (L3–L4), whereas adolescents are more likely to have mechanical and rheumatic causes. For most adolescents, back pain is nonspecific and self-limiting with an organic cause rarely found.[82]

Yang and colleagues[93] identified the most common causes of chronic low-back pain (LBP) in patients aged 10 to 19 years after 1 year of follow-up. Approximately 80% of the patients were categorized as having unspecified LBP. The most common subsequent diagnoses and some of their characteristics are:

- Sprain, strain, or muscle spasm (8.9%).[64,93] Overuse can also cause back pain from sprains or strains, especially for adolescent athletes. There is often localized tenderness, with pain worsened by activity and improved by rest, and pain may be referred to buttock or upper thigh.

- Scoliosis (4.6%).[93] In most cases, scoliosis is idiopathic and does not cause pain. If scoliosis is associated with severe pain or neurologic findings, additional evaluation is needed for more serious problems, including tumor.

- Spondylolysis (defect in the pars interarticularis, usually affecting L4 or L5) (<1%) (see **Table 6**). Athletes who do hyperextension exercises, such as gymnasts or dancers, and those who play soccer, lacrosse, and football, may fracture the pars interarticularis of one of the lumbar vertebrae. They may have a mild to moderate aching pain in the lower back that worsens with extension and flexion and is improved by rest. They may have paraspinal tenderness in the L5 to S1 region, buttock pain, or pain that radiates to the thighs or buttocks.[64,82]

- Spondylolisthesis (0.9%)[89] results when the vertebrae affected by spondylolysis slips anteriorly (see **Table 6**). Pressure on the nerve roots and spinal cord can cause radiculopathy, and bladder and bowel problems.

- Scheuermann disease (0.2%)[94] is a juvenile osteochondrosis of the vertebrae, usually of the thoracic or thoracolumbar spine[88] (see **Fig. 4**, **Table 5**). The ring apophysis becomes avascular and the vertebral body becomes wedge shaped, resulting in a kyphotic deformity of the thoracic spine.[94] Children may present because of a round-shouldered appearance rather than for pain, and some also develop scoliosis. Onset is usually around age 8 to 12 years, with deformity worsening during the growth spurt. Girls and boys are equally affected.[80] Patients may complain of aching pain in the middle or lower back, worsened by prolonged sitting, standing, or activity, with pain often worse later in the day.

- Infectious or noninfectious osteomyelitis. Infectious osteomyelitis is rare during adolescence.[93] It can have an insidious course before presenting with severe back pain, muscle spasms, spine tenderness, limping, and fever. Noninfectious osteomyelitis is discussed in Kathleen A. Haines' article, "The Approach to the Child with Joint Complaints," in this issue.

Evaluation of chronic back pain

Children with back pain accompanied by systemic signs such as fever or weight loss, or who have nighttime pain, neurologic signs, or who refusal to walk, need evaluation for serious causes such as infection, tumor, or spinal cord compression. Patients with chronic back pain who have worsening pain, failure to respond to conservative treatment, new-onset scoliosis, rigid spine, or spinal point tenderness warrant radiographs and possibly other imaging for evaluation.

In spondylolysis, an oblique radiograph can identify the pars defect, and MRI may reveal impending spondylolistheses. In Scheuermann disease, radiographs may reveal vertebral wedging, irregularity of the vertebral endplates, and Schmorl nodes.[94] MRI or CT may be needed based on radiograph findings or poor response to treatment.

How chronic back pain is treated

Most patients with nonspecific back pain, overuse, spondylolysis, mild spondylolisthesis, and mild Scheuermann disease respond to conservative treatment.[64,95] Treatment of moderate Scheuermann disease includes rehabilitation and bracing, with surgery needed for severe degrees of kyphosis.[80] The earlier the start of treatment of Scheuermann disease, the better the outcome.[94] Patients with severe spondylolisthesis may need surgery. Patients with nonspecific LBP that fails to improve with rest and NSAIDs are likely to benefit from PT.

ACKNOWLEDGMENTS

The authors wish to acknowledge Cynthia Nguyen, BSc (Honours), CCRP, MPH, for her help with preparation of this article.

REFERENCES

1. American Pain Society. Assessment and management of children with chronic pain: a position statement from the American Pain Society. Available at: www.ampainsoc.org/advocacy/downloads/aps12-pcp.pdf. Accessed September 1, 2012.
2. Booth J, Moseley GM, Schiltenwolf M, et al. Exercise for chronic musculoskeletal pain: a biopsychosocial approach. Musculoskeletal Care 2017;15(4):1–9.
3. King S, Chambers CT, Huguet A, et al. Epidemiology of chronic pain in children and adolescents revisited: a systematic review. Pain 2011;152:2729–38.
4. Weiser P. Approach to the patient with noninflammatory musculoskeletal pain. Pediatr Clin North Am 2012;59:471–92.
5. Anthony KL, Schanberg LE. Pediatric pain syndromes and management of pain in children and adolescents with rheumatic disease. Pediatr Clin North America 2005;52:611–39.
6. Clinch J, Eccleston C. Chronic musculoskeletal pain in children: assessment and management. Rheumatology 2009;48:466–74.
7. Friedrichsdorf SJ, Giordano J, Dakoji KD, et al. Chronic pain in children and adolescents: diagnosis and treatment of primary pain disorders in head, abdomen, muscles and joints. Children 2016;3(42):1–26.
8. Lalloo C, Stinson JN. Assessment and treatment of pain in children and adolescents. Best Pract Res Clin Rheumatol 2014;28(2):315–30.

9. Lewandowski A, Palermo T, Stinson J, et al. Systematic review of family functioning in families of children and adolescents with chronic pain. J Pain 2010; 11(11):1027–38.

10. Groenewalkd CB, Essner BS, Wright D, et al. The economic costs of chronic pain among a cohort of treatment-seeking adolescents in the United States. The J Pain 2014;15:925–33.

11. Huguet A, Miró J. The severity of chronic pediatric pain: an epidemiological study. The J Pain 2008;9:226–36.

12. Zernikow B, Wager J, Hechler T, et al. Characteristics of highly impaired children with severe chronic pain: a 5-year retrospective study on 2249 pediatric pain patients. BMC Pediatr 2010;12(1):54–66.

13. Stinson J, Jibb L. Pain assessment. In: Twycross A, Bruce L, Stinson J, editors. Pain in children: a clinical guide 2nd edition. London: Blackwell Science; 2013. p. 112–39.

14. Malviya S, Voepel-Lewis T, Burke C, et al. The revised FLACC observational pain tool: improved reliability and validity for pain assessment in children with cognitive impairment. Pediatr Anaesth 2006;16:258–65.

15. Merkel SI, Voepel-Lewis T, Shayevitz JR, et al. The FLACC: a behavioral scale for scoring postoperative pain in young children. Pediatr Nurs 1997;23(3):292–7.

16. Stinson JN, Petroz GC, Stevens BJ, et al. Working out the kinks: testing the feasibility of an electronic pain diary for adolescents with arthritis. Pain Res Manag 2008;13:375–82.

17. Connelly M, Anthony KK, Sarniak R, et al. Parent pain responses as predictors of daily activities and mood in children with juvenile idiopathic arthritis: the utility of electronic diaries. J Pain Symptom Manage 2010;39(3):579–90.

18. Lalloo C, Stinson JN, Brown SC, et al. Pain-QuILT™: assessing clinical feasibility of a web-based tool for the visual self-report of pain in an interdisciplinary pediatric chronic pain clinic. Clin J Pain 2014;30:934–43.

19. Weismann R, Uziel U. Pediatric complex regional pain syndrome: a review. Pediatr Rheumatol Online J 2016;14:29.

20. Abu-Arafeh H, Abu-Arafeh I. Complex regional pain syndrome in children: incidence and clinical characteristics. Arch Dis Child 2016;101(8):719–23.

21. Kashikar-Zuck S, Ting TV. Juvenile fibromyalgia: current status of research and future developments. Nat Rev Rheumatol 2014;10:89–96.

22. Wilder RT, Berde CB, Wolohan M, et al. Reflex sympathetic dystrophy in children. Clinical characteristics and follow-up of seventy patients. J Bone Joint Surg Am 1992;74:910–9.

23. Tran ST, Guite JW, Pantaleao A, et al. Preliminary outcomes of a cross-site cognitive-behavioral and neuromuscular integrative training intervention for juvenile fibromyalgia. Arthritis Care Res 2017;69(3):413–20.

24. Agrawal SK, Rittey CD, Harrower NA, et al. Movement disorders associated with complex regional pain syndrome in children. Dev Med Child Neurol 2009;519(7): 557–62.

25. Harden RN, Bruehl S, Perez RS, et al. Validation of proposed diagnostic criteria (the "Budapest Criteria") for complex regional pain syndrome. Pain 2010;150(2): 268–74.

26. Cohen SP, Mao J. Neuropathic pain: mechanisms and their clinical implications. BMJ 2014;348:7656.

27. Lebel A, Becerra L, Wallin D, et al. fMRI reveals distinct CNS processing during symptomatic and recovered complex regional pain syndrome in children. Pain 2008;13:1854–79.

28. Erpelding N, Sava S, Simons LE, et al. Habenula functional resting state resting state connectivity alterations in complex regional pain syndrome. PLoS One 2013;8(2):1–14.

29. Oaklander AL, Fields HL. Is reflex sympathetic dystrophy/complex regional pain syndrome type 1 a small-fiber neuropathy? Ann Neurol 2009;65(60):629–38.

30. Higashimoto T, Baldwin EE, Gold JI, et al. Reflex sympathetic dystrophy: complex regional pain syndrome type 1 in children with mitochondrial disease and maternal inheritance. Arch Dis Child 2008;93(5):390–8.

31. Bruehel S. An update on the pathophysiology of complex regional pain syndrome. Anesthesiology 2010;113:713–25.

32. Sherry DD, Weisman R. Psychological aspects of childhood reflex neurovascular dystrophy. Pediatrics 1998;81(4):572–8.

33. Cruz N, O'Reilly J, Slomie BS, et al. Emotional and neuropsychological profiles of children with complex regional pain syndrome type-1 in an inpatient rehabilitation setting. Clin J Pain 2011;27(1):27–34.

34. Logan DE, Williams SE, Carullo CP, et al. Children and adolescents with complex regional pain syndrome: more psychologically distressed than other children with pain. Pain Res Manag 2013;18(2):87093.

35. Ting TV, Barnett K, Lynch-Jordan A, et al. 2010 American College of Rheumatology adult fibromyalgia criteria for use in an adolescent female population with juvenile fibromyalgia. J Pediatr 2016;169:181–7.e1.

36. Yunus MB, Masi AT. Juvenile primary fibromyalgia syndrome. A clinical study of thirty-three patients and matched normal controls. Arthritis Rheum 1985;28: 138–45.

37. Zernikow B, Gerhold K, Burk G, et al. Definition, diagnosis and therapy of chronic widespread pain and so-called fibromyalgia syndrome in children and adolescents. Schmerz 2012;26(3):318–30.

38. Arnold LM, Coy E, Clauw DJ, et al. Fibromyalgia and chronic pain syndromes. A white paper detailing current challenges in the field. Clin J Pain 2016;32:737–46.

39. Garcia DA, Nicolas M, Hernandez S. Clinical approach to fibromyalgia: synthesize of evidence-based recommendations: a systematic review. Reumatol Clin 2016;12(2):65–71.

40. McFarlane GJ, Kronisch C, Dean LE, et al. EULARE revised recommendations for the management of fibromyalgia. Ann Rheum Dis 2017;76:318–28.

41. Nelson NL. Muscle strengthening activities and fibromyalgia: a review of pain and strength outcomes. J Bodyw Mov Ther 2015;19:370–6.

42. Kashikar-Zuck S, Ting TV, Arnold LM, et al. Cognitive behavioral therapy for the treatment of juvenile fibromyalgia. A multisite, single blind, randomized controlled clinical trial. Arthritis Rheum 2012;64:297–305.

43. Grégoire MC, Finley GA. Why were we abandoned? Orphan drugs in paediatric pain. Paediatr Child Health 2007;12(2):95–6.

44. Perez RS, Zollinger PE, Dijkstra PU, et al. Evidence based guidelines for complex regional pain syndrome type 1. BMC Neurol 2010;10(20):1–14.

45. Tan EC, Zijlstra B, Essink M, et al. Complex regional pain syndrome type 1 in children. Acta Peaediatrica 2008;97:875–9.

46. Buskila D, Neumann L, Hershman E, et al. Fibromyalgia syndrome in children: an outcome study. J Rheumatol 1995;26:525–8.

47. Mikkelssojn M. One year outcome of preadolescents with fibromyalgia. J Rheumatol 1999;26:674–82.

48. Kashikar-Zuck S, Cunningham N, Sil S, et al. Long-term outcomes of adolescents with juvenile-onset fibromyalgia in early adulthood. Pediatrics 2014;133(3): e592–600.
49. Tobias JH, Deere K, Palmer S, et al. Joint hypermobility is a risk factor for musculoskeletal pain during adolescence: findings of a prospective cohort study. Arthritis Rheum 2013;65(4):1107–15, 2013.
50. Vougiouka O, Moustaki M, Tsanaktsi M. Benign hypermobility syndrome in Greek schoolchildren. Eur J Pediatr 2000;159(8):628.
51. Sperotto F, Brachi S, Vittadello F, et al. Musculoskeletal pain in schoolchildren across puberty: a 3-year follow-up study. Pediatr Rheumatol Online J 2015;13:16.
52. Beighton P, Solomona L, Soskolne CL. Articular mobility in an African population. Ann Rheum Dis 1973;32:413–8.
53. Pacey V, Tofts L, Adams RD, et al. Quality of life prediction in children with joint hypermobility syndrome. J Paediatr Child Health 2015;51(7):689–95.
54. Fikree A, Aziz Q, Grahame R. Joint hypermobility syndrome. Rheum Dis Clin North Am 2013;39(2):419–30.
55. Grahame R, Bird HA, Child A. The revised (Brighton 1998) criteria for the diagnosis of benign joint hypermobility syndrome (BJHS). J Rheumatol 2000;27(7): 1777–9.
56. Uziel Y, Philip J, Hashkes PJ. Growing pains in children. Pediatr Rheumatol 2007; 5:5.
57. Ferrell WR, Tennant N, Sturrock RD, et al. Amelioration of symptoms by enhancement of proprioception in patients with joint hypermobility syndrome. Arthritis Rheum 2004;50:3323–8.
58. Peterson H. Growing pains. Pediatr Clin North Am 1986;33(6):1365–72.
59. Evans AM, Scutter SD. Prevalence of "growing pains" in young children. J Pediatr 2004;145:255–8.
60. Mohanta MP. Growing pains: practitioner's dilemma. Indian Pediatr 2014;51: 379–83.
61. Hashkes P, Friedland O, Jaber L, et al. Children with growing pains have decreased pain threshold. J Rheumatol 2004;31:610–3.
62. Friedland O, Hashkes PJ, Jaber L, et al. Decreased bone strength in children with growing pains as measured by quantitative ultrasound. J Rheumatol 2005;32: 1354–7.
63. Naish JM, Apley J. Growing pains: a clinical study of non-arthritic limb pains in children. Arch Dis Child 1951;26:1134–40.
64. Wu M, Fallon R, Heyworth BE. Overuse injuries in the pediatric population. Sports Med Arthrosc Rev 2016;24(4):150–8.
65. Paz DA, Chang GH, Yetto JM, et al. Upper extremity overuse injuries in pediatric athletes: clinical presentation, imaging findings, and treatment. Clin Imaging 2015;39(6):954–64.
66. Dixit S, DiFiori JP, Burton M, et al. Management of patellofemoral pain syndrome. Am Fam Physician 2007;75(2):194–202.
67. Seto CK, Statuta SM, Solari IL. Pediatric running injuries. Clin Sports Med 2010; 29(3):499–511.
68. Bauer KL, Polousky JD. Management of osteochondritis dissecans lesions of the knee, elbow and ankle. Clin Sports Med 2017;36:469–87.
69. Detterline AJ, Goldstein JL, Rue JPH, et al. Evaluation and treatment of osteochondritis dissecans lesions of the knee. J Knee Surg 2008;21(2):106–15.
70. Yen YM. Assessment and treatment of knee pain in the child and adolescent athlete. Pediatr Clin North Am 2014;61(6):1155–73.

71. Kessler JI, Nikizad H, Shea KG, et al. The demographics and epidemiology of osteochondritis dissecans of the knee in children and adolescents. Am J Sports Med 2014;42(2):320–6.
72. Kessler JI, Weiss JM, Nikizad H, et al. Osteochondritis dissecans of the ankle in children and adolescents: demographics and epidemiology. Am J Sports Med 2014;42(9):2165–71.
73. Bradley J, Dandy DJ. Osteochondritis dissecans and other lesions of the femoral condyles. J Bone Joint Surg Br 1989;71(3):518–22.
74. Uppstrom TJ, Gausden EB, Green DW. Classification and assessment of juvenile osteochondritis dissecans knee lesions. Curr Opin Pediatr 2016;28(1):60–7.
75. Georgiadis AG, Zaltz I. Slipped capital femoral epiphysis: how to evaluate with a review and update of treatment. Pediatr Clin North Am 2014;61(6):1119–35.
76. Atanda A Jr, Shah SA, O'Brien K. Osteochondrosis: common causes of pain in growing bones. Am Fam Physician 2011;83(3):286–91.
77. Launay F. Sports-related overuse injuries in children. Orthop Traumatol Surg Res 2015;101:S139–47.
78. Patel DR, Villalobos A. Evaluation and management of knee pain in young athletes: overuse injuries of the knee. Transl Pediatr 2017;6(3):190–8.
79. Circi E, Atalay Y, Beyzadeoglu T. Treatment of Osgood-Schlatter disease: review of the literature. Musculoskelet Surg 2017;101(3):195–200.
80. Doyle SM, Monahan A. Osteochondroses: a clinical review for the pediatrician. Curr Opin Pediatr 2010;22:41–6.
81. Heyworth BE, Kramer DE, Martin DJ, et al. Trends in the presentation, management, and outcomes of little league shoulder. Am J Sports Med 2016;44(6): 1431–8.
82. Jones GT, Macfarlane GJ. Epidemiology of low back pain in children and adolescents. Arch Dis Child 2005;90:312–6.
83. Marshall KW. Overuse upper extremity injuries in the skeletally immature patient: beyond little league shoulder and elbow. Semin Musculoskelet Radiol 2014;18(5): 469–77.
84. Arora AS, Chung KC, Otto W. Madelung and the recognition of Madelung's deformity. J Hand Surg 2006;31A:177–82.
85. Wiegerinck JI, Yntema C, Brouwer HJ, et al. Incidence of calcaneal apophysitis in the general population. Eur J Pediatr 2014;173:677–9.
86. Zaremski JL, Krabak BJ. Shoulder injuries in the skeletally immature baseball pitcher and recommendations for the prevention of injury. PM R 2012;4(7): 509–16.
87. Wiegerinck JI, Zwiers R, Sierevelt IN, et al. Treatment of calcaneal apophysitis: wait and see versus orthotic device versus physical therapy: a pragmatic therapeutic randomized clinical trial. J Pediatr Orthop 2016;36(2):152–7.
88. Nelitz M, Lippacher S, Krauspe R, et al. Perthes disease: current principles of diagnosis and treatment. Dtsch Arztebl Int 2009;106(31–32):517–23.
89. Kerachian MA, Cournoyer D, Harvey EJ, et al. New insights into the pathogenesis of glucocorticoid-induced avascular necrosis: microarray analysis of gene expression in a rat model. Arthritis Res Ther 2010;12(3):R124.
90. Rampal V, Clement JL, Solla F. Legg-Calvé-Perthes disease: classifications and prognostic factors. Clin Cases Miner Bone Metab 2017;14(1):74–82.
91. Panner HJ. An affection of the humeral capitellum resembling Calvé-Perthes disease of the hip. Acta Radiol 1927;8:617–8.
92. van Bergen CJA, van den Ende K, Brinke B, et al. Osteochondritis dissecans of the capitellum in adolescents. World J Orthop 2016;7(2):102–8.

93. Yang S, Werner BC, Singla A, et al. Low back pain in adolescents: a 1-year analysis of eventual diagnoses. J Pediatr Orthop 2017;37(5):344–7.
94. Palazzo C, Sailhan F, Revel M. Scheuermann's disease: an update. Joint Bone Spine 2014;81(3):209–14.
95. Leonidou A, Lepetsos P, Pagkalos J, et al. Treatment for spondylolysis and spondylolisthesis in children. J Orthop Surg (Hong Kong) 2015;23(3):379–82.
96. Savedra MC, Tesler MD, Holzemer WL, et al. Pain location: validity and reliability of body outline markings by hospitalized children and adolescents. Res Nurs Health 1989;12(5):307–14.
97. Abu-Saad HH, Kroonen E, Halfens R. On the development of a multidimensional Dutch pain assessment tool for children. Pain 1990;43:249–56.
98. Varni JW, Thompson KL, Hanson V. The Varni/Thompson pediatric pain questionnaire: I. Chronic musculoskeletal pain in juvenile rheumatoid arthritis. Pain 1987; 28:27–38.
99. Benestad B, Vinje O, Veierod MD, et al. Quantitative and qualitative assessments of pain in children with juvenile chronic arthritis based on the Norwegian version of the pediatric pain questionnaire. Scandinavian Journal of Rheumatology 1996; 25(5):293–9.

Complications of Treatments for Pediatric Rheumatic Diseases

Gloria C. Higgins, MD, PhD

KEYWORDS

- Pediatric rheumatic disease • Treatment • Complications • Side effects • Infections
- Immunizations • Childhood lupus • Juvenile idiopathic arthritis

KEY POINTS

- Biologic response modifiers (BRMs), which target specific mediators or cells involved in immunity and inflammation, have improved outcomes in childhood rheumatic diseases; they may be used in combination with nonsteroidal anti-inflammatory drugs, disease-modifying antirheumatic drugs, or glucocorticosteroids.
- Physicians caring for children with rheumatic disease should be aware of possible toxic, metabolic, neoplastic, and infectious side effects of these different medications.
- Children on antirheumatic treatment are susceptible to unusual and opportunistic infections, and usual childhood infections, for which they should receive the usual immunizations with non-live vaccines.
- Medical care providers should consult with the rheumatologist immediately for potentially serious illness, which could represent a complication of treatment, disease flare, or both.

INTRODUCTION

The medications typically prescribed to treat various childhood rheumatic diseases have been discussed in previous articles in this issue. As a group, these medications are associated with risks for noninfectious and infectious side effects. Naturally, parents and patients worry about the possible side effects of medications[1] but do not always sufficiently appreciate the entire spectrum and severity of consequences of undertreated or untreated rheumatic disease. Nor do they always appreciate that, despite possible side effects, most medications prescribed for childhood rheumatic disease by pediatric rheumatologists have an acceptable to excellent benefit/risk ratio. Primary care providers (PCPs) are often consulted about the advisability of taking medications recommended by subspecialists. Along with emergency physicians and hospitalists, the PCP may be the first medical care provider who sees the rheumatic

Disclosures: The author has no relevant disclosures.
Pediatric Rheumatology, Nationwide Children's Hospital, 700 Children's Drive, Columbus, OH 43205, USA
E-mail address: gloria.higgins@nationwidechildrens.org

Pediatr Clin N Am 65 (2018) 827–854
https://doi.org/10.1016/j.pcl.2018.04.008
0031-3955/18/© 2018 Elsevier Inc. All rights reserved.

disease patient with a possible medication side effect. These providers are likely not well acquainted with all risk factors and potential toxicities associated with disease and medications. This article provides an easy-to-read reference on these morbidities. It consists of three parts:

1. First there is a general discussion of possible medication side effects and the potential difficulties in assignment of causality in individual children with rheumatic diseases.
2. The second section discusses potential side effects of medications individually and is organized by category of medications rather than by disease. This arrangement was chosen because the same medications may be used for treatment of more than one disease, and potential side effects are generally similar among children irrespective of their specific rheumatic disease. In this section, toxic/metabolic and infection-related side effects are discussed.
3. Finally, of special interest to the PCP, individual immunizations are discussed relative to contraindications, timing, and likelihood of protective response.

MEDICATION SIDE EFFECTS
Association Versus Causality

Large population studies can measure the incidence of various signs and symptoms in patients who take a medication versus those who do not. However, it can be difficult to determine the cause of a new symptom in an individual child or adolescent with rheumatic disease, particularly if it is a common symptom, such as rash, abdominal discomfort, headache, or behavioral change. There may be little information available to decide if the symptom is a new manifestation of the disease itself, a treatment side effect, or something unrelated. In the labeling information for medications, the designation of certain signs and symptoms as "associated" speaks to the difficulty of assigning causality. In an individual patient, sometimes a careful interval history can tease out the cause. Other times, it may be safe to stop a medication and later restart it to demonstrate correlation with signs and symptoms, providing evidence of causality.

Degree and Type of Risks

It is important to understand that for any one patient, the absolute risk of any adverse event caused by any medication can be difficult to determine. Type and degree of risk are related not only to the mechanism of action of an individual drug but also to medication dose and duration, concomitant use of other medications or substances, the disease for which it is given, age, lifestyle, and hereditary factors. Side effects of medications used to treat rheumatic diseases can be generally divided into metabolic, toxic, neoplastic, and infectious. The metabolic adverse effects include conditions like weight gain, fatigue, and decreased bone density. Toxic side effects result in injury to tissues and organs (eg, skin, liver, kidney). These types of side effects are more common with older, less specific treatments, such as nonsteroidal anti-inflammatory drugs (NSAIDs), glucocorticosteroids (GCS), and nonbiologic disease-modifying antirheumatic drugs (DMARDs). Infection is almost never a side effect of NSAIDS, but is of concern, to varying degrees, with GCS, DMARDSs and biologic response modifiers (BRMs). Neoplasms have also been associated with DMARDs and BRMs. The categories of neoplastic and infectious risks are discussed in more detail next.

More about risk for neoplasms

Because immunosuppressive medications can interfere with immune surveillance, neoplasms are on the list of possible side effects of some medications used for rheumatic diseases. However, it has been shown that children with juvenile idiopathic arthritis (JIA) have an increased baseline risk of malignancy related to their autoimmune disease alone, irrespective of treatment.[2–4] It is likely that other childhood rheumatic diseases also confer increased baseline risk of neoplasms.

Many DMARDs currently used for rheumatic diseases were originally developed to suppress immune responses to transplanted organs, or for cancer chemotherapy. Some nonbiologic DMARDs, such as cyclophosphamide, are known to increase the risk of certain cancers in the long term, especially at the higher doses used for chemotherapy. However, such potent medications are typically used when the children are at risk for severe organ damage or death because of rheumatic disease, situations that clearly affect the benefit/risk ratio. BRMs are the newest type of antirheumatic medications, and have fewer and less frequent side effects in general compared with many DMARDs.[5] Because it has been less than 20 years since the first BRM (etanercept, a tumor necrosis factor [TNF] inhibitor) was approved for children with polyarticular JIA in North America, and because there are several different kinds of BRMs available for treatment of children currently, their effects on cancer risk have not been clearly quantified. However, in the case of TNF inhibitors (TNFi), their contribution to cancer risk seems to be small.[3]

More about risk for infections

Because virtually all rheumatic diseases are associated with overactive immunity against self, and/or dysregulated inflammation (see Kathleen E. Sullivan's article, "Pathogenesis of Pediatric Rheumatologic Diseases," in this issue), most treatments are intended to suppress and control these processes. Given that the immune system is responsible for defending against pathogens, the frequency and severity of certain infections is increased as a result of immunosuppression. However, it is clear that rheumatic diseases themselves confer a baseline increased risk of infection, unrelated to treatment, in adults and children[6–8] Even patients with polyarticular JIA, whose routine laboratory tests typically reveal little to no laboratory evidence of immune dysfunction, have a disease-related component of infection risk. Using a nationwide Medicaid database, an increased baseline risk for serious bacterial infections was reported for patients with JIA *not* treated with either methotrexate (MTX) or BRMs, with a hazard ratio (HR) for serious bacterial infection of 2.0 (95% confidence interval [CI], 1.5–2.5) compared with the general population of children of similar age.[8] Lupus patients with active disease also have an increased baseline risk of infections even before immunosuppressive treatment.[7,9]

How can autoimmunity cause an increased risk for infection? Simplistically, one could imagine that immune and inflammatory pathways are focused on attacking parts of one's own body, so the machinery may be "working beyond capacity" or "fail to recognize" microbial invaders. Alternately, the immune system itself may be a target of autoimmunity. This concept is perhaps best understood by thinking about certain common features of active lupus, such as autoimmune lymphopenia and neutropenia, aberrant white blood cell functioning, and low complement levels caused by consumption (see Stacey E. Tarvin and Kathleen M. O'Neil's article, "Systemic Lupus Erythematosus, Sjögren Syndrome, and MCTD in Children and Adolescents," in this issue). In such situations, immunosuppressive medications that allow the patient's own immune system to function more normally may not always cause increased infection risk.

Most infections in children treated for rheumatic disease are usual childhood infections of usual severity. However, GCS, certain DMARDS (eg, cyclophosphamide), and perhaps certain BRMs confer some risk of greater severity of typical childhood infections, and of infection by unusual or opportunistic organisms. In an acutely ill patient with rheumatic disease, both infection and disease flare should always be considered. Suspicion should be heightened for unusual or opportunistic infections, such as mycobacterial and fungal diseases (tuberculosis [TB], histoplasmosis, *Pneumocystis jiroveci*, cryptococcosis, blastomycosis, and coccidiomycosis) based on possible exposure history and prevalence in the local environment. In addition, previous infections in a latent phase can be reactivated (eg, cytomegalovirus, hepatitis B, TB, varicella, and herpes simplex).

Laboratory Monitoring for Medication Side Effects and Disease Activity

Patients with rheumatic disease typically have laboratory tests checked regularly to monitor for medication side effects. Difficulties with attribution can occur in interpreting these results, whether in the presence or absence of new symptoms. For example, in a patient with lupus the complete blood count may show new onset of cytopenias because of disease flare or incipient macrophage activation syndrome (MAS) (see Stacey E. Tarvin and Kathleen M. O'Neil's article, "Systemic Lupus Erythematosus, Sjögren Syndrome, and MCTD in Children and Adolescents," in this issue), or suppression by a common viral infection, or a medication side effect. As a second example, in several rheumatic diseases elevation of transaminases (aspartate aminotransferase [AST], alanine aminotransferase [ALT]) might be caused by damage from autoimmune liver disease, or a viral hepatitis, or medication. Consultation with the patient's rheumatologist helps other physicians caring for the patient to differentiate the cause. It is also important to cast the net widely when looking for causes of laboratory abnormalities. For example, AST and ALT (common on general chemistry profiles) are not strictly liver enzymes because they are also released from inflamed or damaged muscle. In a patient with elevated transaminases who has had, or could develop, muscle inflammation or damage based on their rheumatic disease, an infection, or their physical activities, it is next appropriate to check creatine kinase (CK, from muscle) and γ-glutamyltransferase (from liver) to help differentiate the source.

Response to Signs and Symptoms Perceived to Be Medication Side Effects

In general, for mild to moderate signs and symptoms that seem to be caused by medications, dosage can often be adjusted to allow ongoing use of antirheumatic medications. However, in the case of patients on long-term systemic GCS, the possibility of adrenal insufficiency should be considered and caution should be exercised in reducing dosage abruptly.

Because of their impaired immunity, rheumatic disease patients can sometimes become sick quickly from infections, or their disease may suddenly flare in association with infection. Their other medical caregivers should promptly discuss with the patient's rheumatologist, or an on-call rheumatologist, any illness that seems unusual or more severe than expected, and any possible changes to rheumatic disease treatment regimen. If there is a high likelihood of a serious infection or medication reaction, some or all anti-rheumatic medications may be held. When a serious infection is suspected, following collection of appropriate samples for pathogen identification, it is seldom wrong to treat empirically with antimicrobials based on clues from history and physical examination. Transfer to a tertiary center (particularly one where the patient's rheumatologist has privileges) should be considered on a case-by-case basis.

POSSIBLE SIDE EFFECTS ACCORDING TO MEDICATION

Tables 1 and **2** list individual drugs or groups of drugs, some potential adverse effects, and recommended safety monitoring. These tables are intended more as handy

Table 1
Common and rare potential side effects and safety monitoring of medications for childhood rheumatic disease

Category: Drug Intervals, Routes	Frequent or Serious Potential Side Effects (from Package Inserts)	Monitoring, Precautions (from Package Insert or References)
NSAIDs Oral, interval depending on drug, or as needed	GI: nausea, vomiting, diarrhea, ulcerations Liver: injury Kidney: injury Skin: rash, photosensitivity Hematologic: platelet inhibition (bruising, bleeding) Neuropsych: behavior changes	CBC, diff, plts, Cr, AST, ALT q 3 mo[27] Consider antacid, PPI or H_2 blocker for GI complaints

Glucocorticosteroids
  Oral q d, q od.
  i.v. pulse various intervals
Intermittent intra-articular steroids have minimal side effects when injected properly
	GI: ulcerations, nausea, hyperphagy
	Growth: obesity, short stature
	Bone: osteopenia, osteoporosis, fractures, osteonecrosis
	Liver: fat accumulation
	Muscle: weakness
	Skin: fragility, striae, purpura
	Metabolic: hypertension, dyslipidemia, atherosclerosis
	Endocrine: adrenal suppression, hypertension, hyperglycemia, diabetes
	Ophthalmologic: cataracts, glaucoma
	Neuropsych: mood and behavior changes, psychosis
	Immune: serious infections (signs/symptoms may be masked)
		Bone mineral density baseline and up to yearly for chronic use, preferably by DXA using pediatric protocol and comparing to pediatric norms
		Monitor height velocity, weight
		Lipid panel baseline, 1 mo, and q 6–12 mo
		Fasting glucose yearly and prn
		Eye examination yearly and prn[13]

DMARD
  Methotrexate
  Oral or subcutaneous, once weekly
	GI: nausea, vomiting, oral ulcerations
	Liver: injury
	Bone marrow: cytopenias
	Skin: hair loss, rash, photosensitivity
	Reproductive: teratogenicity
	Neuropsych: anticipatory nausea
	Constitutional: fatigue
	Immune: serious infections
		CBC, diff, plts, Cr, AST, ALT; 1 mo from start, then q 3 mo[27]
		Supplement folic acid
		Avoid alcohol ingestion
		Limit sun exposure
		Hold for serious infections
		Negative pregnancy test at start, reliable birth control, hold DMARD for late menses

DMARD
  Lefunomide
  Oral, weekly
	GI: nausea, oral ulceration
	Liver: injury
	Bone marrow: cytopenias
	Skin: rash, hypersensitivity reaction
	Reproductive: teratogenicity
	Metabolic: long persistence in tissues; toxicity or pregnancy may require "wash out" with cholestyramine
	Respiratory: interstitial lung disease (mainly adults)
	Immune: serious and opportunistic infection especially TB reactivation, Pneumocystis jiroveci, aspergillus
		CBC, diff, plts, Cr, AST, ALT q mo × 6 at start or dose increase, then q 6–8 wk
		Avoid alcohol ingestion
		Hold for serious infections
		Pregnancy precautions as for MTX; continue birth control until after "wash-out" with cholestyramine

(continued on next page)

Table 1 (continued)		
Category: Drug Intervals, Routes	**Frequent or Serious Potential Side Effects (from Package Inserts)**	**Monitoring, Precautions (from Package Insert or References)**
DMARD Sulfasalazine Oral, twice daily	GI: nausea, ulceration Liver: injury Hematologic: cytopenias, hemolytic anemia (unusual) with G6PD deficiency Skin: rash, photosensitivity, hypersensitivity reactions Kidney: injury	CBC, diff, plts, Cr, AST, ALT, UA at start, q 2 wk × 3 mo, then q 4 wk × 3 mo, then q 3 mo Contains sulfa and salicylate moieties; avoid if sulfa allergy
DMARD Hydroxychloroquine Oral, daily	Eye: retinal deposition and toxicity (dose related), vision changes Skin: photosensitivity, hyperpigmentation, other rashes Hematologic: hemolytic anemia with G6PD deficiency GI: nausea, abdominal pain Muscle: weakness	New recommendations[35]: full ophthalmology examination before 1 y of treatment, then electroretinography or spectral domain optical coherence tomography (see text for schedule)
DMARD Azathioprine Oral, q d or bid	GI: nausea, diarrhea Liver: injury Hematologic: cytopenias, perhaps more severe with low TPMT activity Reproductive: teratogenicity Immune: serious infections *Neoplastic: lymphoma, skin cancer*	CBC, diff, plts q wk x 1 mo, then q 2 wk × 2 mo, then q mo AST, ALT, alk phos, bili "periodically" Check TPMT activity or alleles Limit sun exposure Avoid alcohol ingestion Hold for serious infections Negative pregnancy test at start, reliable birth control, hold DMARD for late menses
DMARD Mycophenolate mofetil, mycophenolic acid Oral or i.v. bid	GI: naurea, diarrhea, vomiting Skin: rashes Hematologic: cytopenias Reproductive: teratogenicity, decreases effectiveness of oral contraceptives Immune: serious infections (especially herpes reactivation, CMV), *opportunistic infections, very rare PML* *Neoplastic: lymphoma, lymphoproliferative disorders, skin cancer*	CBC, diff, plts q wk x 1 mo, q 2 wk × 2 mo, then q mo Limit sun exposure Avoid alcohol ingestion Hold for serious infections Negative pregnancy test at start, abstinence or 2 methods of birth control concurrently 4 wk before start (if possible) and for 6 wk after stopping med, hold DMARD for late menses
DMARD Calcineurin inhibitors: Cyclosporine A Tacrolimus Oral or i.v.	Endocrine, renal: nephrotoxicity, severe hypertension GI: nausea, vomiting Liver: damage CNS: headaches Skin: hirsutism, gum dysplasia Metabolic: hypomagnesemia, hyperkalemia Reproductive: prematurity, complicated pregnancy Immune: serious infections	BUN, Cr at start, then q 2 wk for 3 mo, then q mo Potassium, AST, ALT, magnesium q mo Timed drug levels Monitor blood pressure Limit sun exposure Hold for serious infections Multiple drug interactions Avoid pregnancy

(continued on next page)

Table 1
(continued)

Category: Drug Intervals, Routes	Frequent or Serious Potential Side Effects (from Package Inserts)	Monitoring, Precautions (from Package Insert or References)
	Opportunistic infections: P jiroveci, CMV, rare PML *Neoplastic: Lymphomas (especially in organ transplant patients)*	
DMARD: Cyclophosphamide, i.v. q mo to q 3 mo, oral daily	Kidney, urinary tract: injury, hemorrhagic cystitis Hematologic: cytopenias GI: nausea, vomiting, mucositis Skin: rashes, hair loss Reproductive: infertility (may be irreversible), teratogenicity, fetal loss Immune: serious and opportunistic infections *Neoplastic: leukemia, lymphoma, sarcomas, carcinomas (especially bladder cancer)*	CBC, diff, plts predose and at nadir (1–2 wk postdose) for i.v., or q mo for oral Lytes, BUN, Cr, UA "frequently" Take orally in morning with copious fluids, give i.v. with fluids and MESNA to protect bladder PJP oral prophylaxis Hold for serious infections Females: avoid pregnancy, consider IM leuprolide q mo; may protect from infertility Males: consider sperm banking
DMARD Tofacitinib, oral twice daily	Not approved, but being studied, for poly and systemic JIA In adults with RA: GI: diarrhea, nausea Hematologic: cytopenias Metabolic: hyperlipidemia CNS: headache Immune: serious and *opportunistic infections (TB, cryptococcus, P jiroveci, CMV, varicella zoster)* *Neoplastic: malignancies including lymphomas*	CBC, diff, plts at start, 4–8 wks, then q 3 mo Lipids at start, then 3–6 mo TB test at start, and periodically Hold for serious infections Avoid pregnancy
Biologic response modifiers See **Table 2** for individual medications	Infusion or injection site reactions, hypersensitivity *Immune: serious infections, opportunistic infections* *Neoplastic: various malignancies*	See **Table 2** for details regarding individual medications

Note: (1) Not all potential side effects are listed. In some cases, association does not signify causality. For more information, consult package inserts (available online) or references provided in table or text. Common potential side effects that can range from mild to severe are listed in plain text. *Rare potential side effects that are typically serious, and may be associated with disease itself, are listed in italics.* (2) Risk of side effects and severity are related to dose of medication, duration of treatment, concomitant use of other medications that can cause the same or related side effects, environmental exposures, and pre-existing conditions. Stop medication for suspicion of serious side effects except under special circumstances (eg, steroids and adrenal suppression). (3) Safety monitoring listed is the minimum required, assuming that no signs or increased risk of toxicity are present.

Abbreviations: ALT, alanine aminotransferase; AST, aspartate aminotransferase; BUN, blood-urea-nitrogen; CBC, complete blood count; CMV, cytomegalovirus; CNS, central nervous system; Cr, creatinine; DXA, dual X-ray absorptiometry; GI, gastrointestinal; i.v., intravenously; JIA, juvenile idiopathic arthritis; PJP, *Pneumocystis jiroveci* pneumonia; plts, platelets; PML, progressive multifocal leukoencephalopathy; PPI, proton pump inhibitor; RA, rheumatoid arthritis; TB, tuberculosis; TPMT, thiopurine S-methyltransferase; UA, urinalysis.

Table 2
Common and rare potential side effects and safety monitoring of biologic response modifiers for childhood rheumatic disease

Target – Medication	Route, Frequency	Typical Uses (Diseases)	Associated Infections and Other Risks (TB, Varicella, Hepatitis B, Fungal and Opportunistic Infections for All)	Monitoring and Precautions (TB Test, and Serology for Varicella and Hepatitis B for All, Before Initiating Treatment)
TNF-α Etanercept, Adalimumab, Infliximab, Golimumab	Subcu 1–2 times weekly; Subcu q 2 wk; Subcu/i.v. q 4 wk; I.v. infusion being studied for JIA	Polyarticular JIA; Extended oligoarticular JIA; Psoriatic arthritis; Spondyloarthropathy; Uveitis; Some autoinflammatory diseases	*Serious bacterial infections, lymphoma, other cancers*	Routine laboratory studies only as indicated for disease and other medications
IL-1 receptor Anakinra	Subcu daily	Systemic JIA; MAS	Neutropenia; *Serious bacterial infections*	CBC, diff, plts q mo × 3, then q 3 mo
IL-1α Canakinumab	Subcu q 4 wk	Systemic JIA; Some autoinflammatory diseases	*Serious bacterial infections*	Routine laboratory studies only as indicated for disease and other medications
IL-6 receptor Tocilizumab	IV infusion monthly, or subcu q wk–2wk	Polyarticular and systemic JIA; MAS	Cytopenias, hepatic injury; Hyperlipidemias; *Serious bacterial infections*	CBC, diff, plts, AST, ALT, cholesterol, triglycerides 4–8 wk after start, then q 3 mo
T-cell costimulation Abatacept	IV infusion monthly, or subcu weekly	Polyarticular JIA; Extended oligoarticular JIA	*Serious bacterial infections*	Routine laboratory studies only as indicated for disease and other medications
CD20 B cells Rituximab	IV infusion, various intervals	Lupus; Severe vasculitis	Serious bacterial infections; Fungal infections; Mucocutaneous reactions; Renal toxicity; *PML caused by JC virus*	CBC, diff, BUN, Cr before and at intervals after dosing; Quantitative immunoglobulins, B cells and subsets as indicated
B-lymphocyte stimulator Belimumab	IV infusion or subcu; various intervals	Lupus	Serious bacterial infections; Fungal infections; Depression; *PML caused by JC virus*	CBC, diff, before and at intervals after dosing; Quantitative immunoglobulins, B cells and subsets as indicated

Note: (1) Not all potential side effects are listed. In some cases, association does not signify causality. For more information, consult package inserts (available online) or references provided in text. All intravenous and subcutaneous medications can cause infusion or injection site reactions. Common potential side effects that can range from mild to severe are listed in plain text. *Rare potential side effects that are typically serious, and may be associated with disease itself, are listed in italics.* (2) Risk of side effects and severity are related to dose of medication, duration of treatment, concomitant use of other medications that can cause the same or related side effects, environmental exposures, and pre-existing conditions. Stop medication for suspicion of serious side effects including infection. (3) Safety monitoring listed is the minimum required, assuming that no signs or increased risk of toxicity are present.
Abbreviations: IL, interleukin; MAS, macrophage activation syndrome; PML, progressive multifocal leukoencephalopathy; subcu, subcutaneous.

reference in the context of patient care, than as text to read through. They list potential side effects that are common (plain text), and those that are rare but serious (italics). Even though the tables do not list every possible side effect of medication, the number and variety listed for some medications may still seem alarming. However, most children taking these medications for rheumatic disease do not experience serious side effects. The most common medications used for pediatric rheumatic disease patients, and some relevant possible side effects, are discussed individually in more detail next. (Also see **Table 1**).

Nonsteroidal Anti-inflammatory Drugs

Long the mainstay of childhood chronic arthritis treatment, chronic NSAIDs are now being used less frequently, and for shorter time periods, because of much more effective treatment of disease by other medications. They are still useful for relief of pain and stiffness, but they do little to retard joint or tissue damage.[10] Their major mode of action is to block cyclooxygenases, thereby inhibiting prostaglandin synthesis. This action is related to the favorable result of analgesia, but also the unfavorable result of gastrointestinal (GI) irritation or damage (abdominal pain, nausea, diarrhea, peptic ulcer disease), and to hepatic and renal toxicity, which are less common in children than adults. Taking these medications with food, staying well hydrated, and avoiding ingestion of other substances with similar effects reduces such problems. Prescribing a gastroprotective agent, such as an antacid, H_2 blocker, or proton pump inhibitor,[11] is a strategy used to reduce GI side effects of NSAIDs. Acute kidney injury is a possible side effect of NSAIDs in children, especially in the setting of dehydration, but is much less common than in adults.[12] NSAIDs do not increase risk of infections.

Glucocorticosteroids

Steroids alter the production of a myriad of proteins involved in immunity and inflammation, and metabolism and growth; therefore, they have widespread effects. Their powerful, broad-spectrum suppression of immune and inflammatory processes has been used to treat a multitude of allergic, rheumatic, autoimmune, and other diseases. Intravenous, oral, and topical GCS are used for rheumatic diseases. Systemic GCS are life-saving for initial treatment of severe disease and can hold inflammation at bay until other medications have had time to work. However, chronic use of systemic GCS in supraphysiologic doses is well known to be associated with numerous toxic and metabolic side effects including excessive weight gain, growth retardation, adrenal insufficiency, osteoporosis, avascular necrosis of bone, skin fragility and striae, atherosclerosis, hyperlipidemia, hypertension, hyperglycemia or steroid-induced diabetes, fatty liver, gastritis, cataracts, mood disorders, and psychosis, in addition to significantly increased incidence of infections.[8,13–16]

Because of their many side effects, long-term systemic dosing should be avoided if possible, or kept as low as possible if required for disease control. Changing oral dosage (prednisone, prednisolone) from daily to alternate day, resulting in lower risk of side effects, can sometimes be effective in patients with less active rheumatic disease.[17] Intermittent intravenous steroid (methylprednisolone) pulses may be associated with fewer metabolic and growth side effects than daily oral steroids. Tapering of systemic steroids should be done only by or with the guidance of a child's rheumatologist because tapering too rapidly may precipitate adrenal crisis or flare of rheumatic disease.

Intra-articular injections of long-acting depot corticosteroids are often used for JIA, with possible side effects of local infection, avascular necrosis of bone, and tissue atrophy. However, such side effects are rare with use of good technique.[18] Systemic effects of intra-articular injection are rare. Many kinds of autoimmune eye disease (eg, uveitis/iritis, scleritis, episcleritis, keratitis), whether idiopathic or a manifestation of systemic rheumatic disease, are treated with topical steroids. Possible side effects of prolonged ocular steroids include glaucoma and cataracts.[19] Refractory eye disease and optic neuritis may require systemic medications.

Nonbiologic Disease-Modifying Antirheumatic Drugs

Nonbiologic DMARDs are chemical compounds that have a wide array of possible metabolic and immunologic effects. Among the most commonly used in pediatric rheumatology are MTX, azathioprine, mycophenolate mofetil/mycophenolic acid, and cyclophosphamide. They are often used initially in combination with systemic corticosteroids to treat serious rheumatic disease manifestations. Some DMARDs are used for ongoing treatment or maintenance of remission.

Methotrexate

MTX is the DMARD used most frequently for childhood rheumatic diseases and is discussed in detail here. Like many other DMARDs, MTX was borrowed from cancer chemotherapy, but it is used in much lower doses and is only dosed intermittently (typically once weekly) for rheumatic diseases, such as JIA, psoriatic arthritis, dermatomyositis, lupus, sclerodermas, and autoimmune eye disease. Because of the comparatively decreased doses, it is not considered chemotherapy when used for rheumatic diseases.

When used in high doses for cancer chemotherapy, MTX is an antimetabolite. By inhibiting the enzyme tetrahydrofolate reductase, it causes a severe deficiency of folic acid needed for purine synthesis and cell proliferation.[20] However, in the doses used to treat rheumatic diseases, this effect does not seem to be the major mechanism of action, and supplementary folic acid is given to counteract symptoms of folate deficiency without altering efficacy. Supplemental folic acid reduces the incidence or severity of possible MTX side effects such as nausea, oral ulcerations, anemia, leukopenia, and hair loss.[20] One important mechanism of MTX in rheumatic diseases is to increase levels of adenosine, which downregulates several pathways of inflammation. Some other side effects of MTX, such as fatigue and possibly the rare occurrence of hepatic fibrosis in children, are likely caused by increased adenosine.[21]

Subcutaneous dosing of MTX results in more reliable absorption and drug levels, sometimes with fewer GI complaints, compared with the oral route,[22] although children often prefer the oral route to injections. Despite individual patient experiences of better disease control on subcutaneous MTX,[22] in a retrospective registry review from 2005 to 2012, patients with JIA taking oral versus subcutaneous MTX had a comparable clinical response and an insignificant difference in the number of adverse events.[23]

Risk of new infections or reactivation of old infections (including varicella zoster) does not seem to be increased in adults taking MTX for rheumatoid arthritis (RA), according to systematic literature reviews.[6,24] Likewise, most children taking MTX in doses used for rheumatic disease do not seem to be at increased risk for infections. In a US Medicaid database over a 5-year period, patients with JIA taking MTX, or taking no DMARD, had similar rates of hospitalized bacterial infections.[8] Opportunistic infections occur occasionally in children taking MTX at rheumatic disease doses, but not with sufficient frequency to know if they are more related to immune suppression from rheumatic diseases themselves, or MTX treatment.

In patients taking high-dose MTX for lymphomas and other malignancies, there is a variable risk of secondary malignancies, particularly secondary lymphomas, depending on many other factors. However, MTX treatment of childhood rheumatic diseases does not appear to further increase the known increased baseline risk of cancers.[2] Rare cases of lymphoproliferative disorders that regress after discontinuing MTX have been reported in children taking this medication for rheumatic disease.[25]

There are other particularly important side effects of MTX that medical care providers should know about. It is a teratogen and should be stopped before pregnancy. Females of reproductive age should have a negative pregnancy test before starting MTX. Adequate birth control (which can include abstinence) must be practiced, and the drug should be held for suspicion of pregnancy. Alcohol ingestion, which increases the potential for liver damage from MTX, should be avoided. Although it has been reported that concomitant administration of MTX and the antibiotic trimethoprim sulfamethoxazole (TMP-Sx) can result in a serious increase in MTX toxicity, particularly cytopenias, there was no significant risk to rheumatic disease patients taking MTX with the lower doses of TMP-Sx used routinely for P jiroveci prophylaxis.[26]

The American College of Rheumatology has published a schedule of regular laboratory monitoring (see **Table 1**) recommended for children taking MTX for JIA, and guidelines for reducing dose, holding, and discontinuing MTX treatment based on laboratory results.[27] Usually, laboratory abnormalities resolve with holding doses and/or reducing the weekly dose of MTX. Although transaminases are monitored for potential hepatotoxicity, one study found that AST and ALT elevations greater than twice the upper limit of normal were rare in JIA, similar in frequency whether or not patients were taking MTX, and generally attributable to other causes, such as infections or systemic antibiotics.[28] Routine liver biopsies are no longer performed in adults[29] or children taking MTX for rheumatic disease because of the low incidence of hepatic fibrosis.

Leflunomide

As listed in **Table 1**, leflunomide is an inhibitor of pyrimidine synthesis, which seems to have efficacy similar to MTX for treatment of JIA[30] and is sometimes used in place of MTX. It has a similar side effect profile, including teratogenicity. Leflunomide has not been studied or used in children as extensively as MTX. Guidelines for use are similar to those for MTX, but persistence in tissues is a unique problem.

Sulfasalazine and hydroxychloroquine

The generally weaker DMARDs sulfasalazine and hydroxychloroquine are considered to be immunomodulators rather than immunosuppressants, and increased risk for infection is not considered to be a side effect. Sulfasalazine is most often used for RA in adults[31] and is occasionally used for JIA. It contains a salicylate and a sulfa moiety, and is contraindicated in patients with sulfa allergy.[32] Hydroxychloroquine is used to treat skin disease in lupus and juvenile dermatomyositis (JDM). In children, it is most commonly used to reduce the risk of flares in patients with lupus while other, more toxic, medications are being tapered, and for maintenance of remission.[33] It is considered first-line immunomodulatory therapy for Sjögren syndrome[34] and is also used in combination therapy for adults with for RA.[33] Hydroxychloroquine has potential cumulative retinal toxicity, which is minimized by appropriate dosing and timely recognition with appropriate ophthalmologic examinations.[35,36] Recent new guidelines for toxicity monitoring include a full ophthalmology examination before the end of 1 year of treatment, followed by electroretinography or spectral domain optical coherence tomography every 1 to 5 years based on risk for the next 5 years, and then yearly thereafter.[35]

Azathioprine and mycophenolates

The immunosuppressive drugs azathioprine, mycophenolate mofetil, and mycophenolic acid are used mainly for systemic lupus, vasculitic diseases including polyarteritis nodosa and anti-neutrophil cytoplasmic antibody (ANCA)-associated vasculitis, idiopathic inflammatory myopathies, and scleroderma. Mycophenolates may be superior to azathioprine in maintenance of lupus remission.[37,38] However, mycophenolates are teratogenic and must be avoided during pregnancy, whereas azathioprine is not known to harm the developing fetus.[39,40] Thiopurines, such as azathioprine and its product 6-mercaptopurine, are associated with an increased rate of malignancy in children with inflammatory bowel disease (IBD).[3,41]

Cyclosporine A and tacrolimus
The calcineurin inhibitors cyclosporine A and tacrolimus are sometimes used for treatment of autoimmune renal disorders, severe vasculitis, and macrophage activation syndrome (MAS), but use is often limited by hepatotoxicity,[42] and renal toxicity manifesting as severe hypertension.[43]

Cyclophosphamide
The alkylating agent cyclophosphamide is a strong chemotherapeutic and immunosuppressive medication. It preferentially kills cells that have low levels of aldehyde dehydrogenase, the enzyme that inactivates the drug. Cyclophosphamide binds to, and cross-links, DNA in susceptible cells, causing cell death. Leukocytes, especially T lymphocytes, are susceptible to this effect, which explains how it works to suppress the immune system, and why a major side effect is leukopenia.[44] Cyclophosphamide is used primarily for severe lupus nephritis or lupus cerebritis, for severe vasculitis of other types including central nervous system vasculitis, and for pulmonary disease in systemic sclerosis. Doses are lower than those used for cancer chemotherapy, but secondary malignancy from a variety of cancers is still a concern.[45,46] It is given intravenously at intervals of several weeks to months, or in smaller doses by mouth daily. In pediatrics, intravenous dosing is almost always used, with vigorous hydration, plus medications to reduce nausea and bladder toxicity. Cyclophosphamide treatment is associated with a higher rate of infection than mycophenolate mofetil or azathioprine in patients with lupus,[14] which is further increased by concomitant treatment with GCS, as is used for severe disease.

Cyclophosphamide can cause infertility in males and females. Gonadotropin-releasing hormone analogues may protect against premature ovarian failure in young women receiving cyclophosphamide therapy for lupus,[47] and sperm banking has been recommended for adolescent and adult male patients.[48] Despite the concerns about fertility, pregnancy can occur in females taking cyclophosphamide, but should be avoided because of high risk of teratogenicity.

New nonbiologic disease-modifying antirheumatic drugs
New nonbiologic DMARDs that inhibit specific pathways involved in autoimmunity have recently been developed for rheumatic and other related diseases, such as psoriasis. These medications are not to be confused with BRMs, another new class of medications discussed next. So far, the new nonbiologic DMARDs are only approved in North America for treatment of rheumatic diseases in adults. One new class is the phosphodiesterase inhibitors (eg, oral apremilast, which is currently used for psoriasis and has been effective in adults with psoriatic arthritis in clinical trials).[49] Another new class of DMARDs is Janus kinase (JAK) inhibitors, including oral tofacitinib. This medication has been approved in North America for adults with RA and is being studied internationally in children with polyarticular JIA[50] (https://clinicaltrials.gov/ct2/show/NCT02592434) and systemic JIA (https://clinicaltrials.gov/ct2/show/NCT03000439).

Biologic Response Modifiers
GCS and strong immunosuppressive drugs have widespread effects on cells involved in immunity and inflammation, and on other kinds of cells.[5,51] In contrast, the newer BRM medications exhibit greater specificity for suppression of individual types of

cells, or inhibition of their immune or inflammatory mediators, and generally have less frequent side effects (See **Table 2**).[5]

BRMs are technically DMARDs, because they are powerful in modifying the course of rheumatic disease, but they are considered a separate class of medications. They differ from traditional DMARDs because they are proteins that are synthesized by living cells in culture, then highly purified, and sometimes chemically modified. They are monoclonal antibodies, soluble receptors, or chimeric proteins that bind specific cytokines or other proteins that are part of immune and inflammatory pathways, and inhibit their function (see Kathleen E. Sullivan's article, "Pathogenesis of Pediatric Rheumatic Diseases," in this issue). More than one BRM should not be used concurrently, because of higher risk for infection without obvious efficacy benefit, as described in the prescribing information (package inserts) for these drugs. However, a BRM is sometimes used in conjunction with certain of the nonbiologic DMARDS, especially MTX. The advent of BRMs brought the expectation that more targeted immune modulation would result not only in better treatment, but also in fewer toxic side effects. When BRMs are used as monotherapy, the prediction of decreased organ toxicity has certainly been correct. In general, health care plans require patients to fail treatment with traditional DMARDs before the much more expensive BRMs will be covered. Because of previous or concomitant use of other DMARDs, it is not necessarily easy to assign a degree of risk conferred by BRMs alone. After 18 years of experience with TNFi, the first type of BRM approved for children, initial concerns about possible increased rates of infection and malignancy have been reduced (discussed next).

Tumor necrosis factor inhibitors: Etanercept, adalimumab, infliximab
In 1999, etanercept was the first BRM approved for the treatment of polyarticular JIA in the United States and Canada. It works by binding to TNF-α, a proinflammatory cytokine that participates in a multitude of inflammatory pathways. Etanercept-bound TNF is prevented from binding to its cellular receptors and activating immune or inflammatory pathways (see Kathleen E. Sullivan's article, "Pathogenesis of Pediatric Rheumatic Diseases," in this issue). Unlike many BRMs, etanercept is not an anticytokine antibody. Instead, it is a fusion protein composed of two naturally occurring soluble TNF receptor moieties (which bind TNF-α), covalently linked to the constant (nonantigen-binding) region of IgG1. Monoclonal antibody TNFi that are also used for children, especially those with JIA, are adalimumab (monoclonal human anti-TNF-α), and infliximab (a mouse-human chimeric anti-TNF-α, not US Food and Drug Administration [USFDA] approved for children with JIA). Another human monoclonal anti-TNF antibody, golimumab, is currently being studied for use in children.[52] TNFi BRMs, especially adalimumab, are used off-label for treatment of JIA-associated uveitis.[53]

Infection risk with tumor necrosis factor inhibitors Because of the much larger number of adults taking BRMs for rheumatic disease (eg, for RA, psoriatic arthritis, and ankylosing spondylitis), the data on infection risk in adults are more robust. However, these studies may not be entirely applicable to children because of differences in comorbidities and risk factors.

In an analysis of children in a US Medicaid database, the rate of hospitalized (serious) infections in 8459 patients with JIA taking various medications was determined over the course of 5 years. Patients with JIA taking neither MTX nor TNFi had an increased rate of hospitalization for infection compared with age-matched control subjects with attention deficit hyperactivity disorder (without JIA), with an adjusted hazard ratio (HR) of 2.0 (CI, 1.5–2.5). These results demonstrated increased risk of infection on the basis JIA itself. JIA patients taking MTX alone had a similar rate of hospitalized infection compared with those taking neither medication (HR, 1.2; CI, 0.9–1.7). Patients taking TNFi (with or without MTX) had a similar serious infection rate (HR, 1.2; CI, 0.8–1.8). Not surprisingly, those taking GCS (dose $\geq$10 mg/d of prednisone or equivalent) had an increased rate of serious infection as compared with those not taking GCS (HR, 3.1; CI, 2.0–4.7).[8] In a registry of patients with JIA in the United Kingdom, those treated with etanercept with or without MTX had similar rates of serious (hospitalized) infection compared with those treated with MTX alone, but higher rates of "significant" infection (not defined, but as designated by their medical providers).[54]

These results differ from an analysis of the German Biologics in Pediatric Rheumatology Registry, the largest registry of children taking TNFi for JIA. In this study, risk of serious (hospitalized) infections in patients taking TNFi was increased compared with those taking MTX only. Serious infections occurred in 21 of 1720 patients (1.2%) taking etanercept, 2 of 177 patients (1.1%) taking adalimumab (1.1%), and 5 of 1453 patients (0.3%) taking MTX alone. Relative risk of infection in those taking etanercept alone was 3.3 (95% CI, 0.95–11.3), and in those taking etanercept plus MTX was 6.1 (95% CI, 2.2–16.7), compared with MTX therapy alone. Previous or concomitant steroids at baseline across the entire registry increased the relative risk of serious infection by approximately two-fold.[55] In this study, the risk of serious infections also correlated with the level of disease severity at start of treatment, suggesting possible confounding by indication. This study was not designed to compare the risk of infection with that of healthy children.

Comparison of the previously mentioned studies on serious infection is difficult, because of their different methodologies. Lacking further evidence, available studies disagree on whether patients with JIA taking TNFi alone have a similar[8,56] or higher[55] rate of serious infections compared with those taking MTX alone, and those taking MTX plus TNFi may have similar[8,56] or a higher[55] rate of infection compared with those taking MTX alone. In the two studies in which it was compared, the addition of concomitant GCS resulted in increased infection rates.[8,55] In all three studies, the absolute rates of serious infection were low. There are insufficient data to compare infection risks in children taking any other BRMs versus traditional DMARDs for other rheumatic diseases.

Cancer risk with tumor necrosis factor inhibitors As summarized by Pisetsky,[57] TNF was so named following its identification in the 1970s as a substance capable of killing tumor cells in mice. Although the doses needed for effective chemotherapy in humans were found to be too toxic, its role as a mediator of inflammation was eventually elucidated. It was found to be the same molecule as a substance produced by activated macrophages causing, among other inflammatory responses, cachexia; hence, its other name "cachexin."[57] Eventually, inhibitors of TNF were developed, tested, and approved by regulatory agencies for treatment of inflammation in autoimmune diseases: RA, ankylosing spondylitis (AS), and Crohn disease in adults, and later for polyarticular JIA (etanercept 1999, adalimumab 2008) and childhood Crohn disease (infliximab 2006). Because data suggested an increased risk of certain malignancies, especially lymphoma, in adults treated with TNFi, the USFDA started collecting cases, including those from the initial clinical trials. The 2009 analysis of these data in children[58] revealed 48 cases of malignancy and their associations with use of TNFi: 31 following infliximab use (mainly for Crohn disease), 15 following etanercept use (for JIA and AS), and two following adalimumab use. Both cases involving adalimumab use were confounded by previous use of nonbiologic DMARDs and infliximab. Patients taking infliximab had a higher reported rate than the childhood average rates of lymphoma and of all malignancies, and those taking etanercept had a higher reported rate than the childhood average rate of lymphoma, but not of all malignancies taken together. As a result, TNFi have a black box USFDA warning about possible increased rates of malignancies.

It had already been shown that adults with RA, especially those with severe disease, have an elevated rate of lymphoma compared with the general adult population. Similarly, Nordstrom and colleagues,[4] using a health plan database, found that biologics-naive children diagnosed with JIA between 1998 and 2007 had a nearly three-fold risk of cancer compared with a matched cohort of children without JIA. A meta-analysis of seven prospective studies in adults with RA showed no evidence of increased malignancies in those treated with TNFi compared with those who were not.[59] Similarly, the recent study of Beukelman and colleagues[3] examined cancer rates among children with JIA, IBD, and juvenile psoriatic arthritis from Medicaid and another US insurance database over a period of 14 years. There was a two-fold higher cancer incidence in the children with these autoimmune diseases, as compared with children in general. A small, statistically insignificant increase in cancer risk was associated with treatment with TNFi (infliximab, etanercept, and adalimumab.) Comparing among subgroups, the only significant increase in cancer was found among children with IBD treated with both a thiopurine (azathioprine or 6-mercaptopurine) plus a TNFi, consistent with a previous report in children.[41] In summary, current evidence does not show an increased cancer risk for children taking TNFi for JIA, above their already increased risk resulting from the disease itself. However, for children with all rheumatic diseases, ongoing surveillance for possible treatment-related side effects is essential.

Abatacept

This novel BRM is approved for treatment of polyarticular JIA. It is a fusion protein composed of the extracellular domain of human CTLA-4 covalently linked to the IgG1 Fc (constant region) domain. The CTLA-4 moiety binds to CD 80/86 on antigen presenting cells, preventing CD 80/86 from binding CD28 on T cells (a process required for T-cell activation). Therefore, abatacept is known as a T-cell costimulation inhibitor. Because activated T cells contribute to production of autoantibodies and stimulation of macrophages to make proinflammatory cytokines, abatacept suppresses immune responses and reduces autoimmunity. Given subcutaneoulsy or intravenously, it has been shown to be effective in biologic-naive patients with JIA, and those who have had poor response to DMARDs or other BRMs.[60] It has also been used off-label for JIA-associated uveitis.[61] Its general side effect profile seems to be similar to other BRMs.

Canakinumab and tocilizumab

Two BRMs, canakinumab and tocilizumab, have transformed treatment of systemic JIA (sJIA), allowing for the use of significantly less or no corticosteroids. Canakinumab (human monoclonal antibody against interleukin-1β [IL-1β]) is given subcutaneously every 4 weeks, and is indicated for use in children with systemic JIA,[62] cryopyrin-associated periodic fever syndromes, and some other autoinflammatory syndromes (see Kathleen E. Sullivan's article, "Pathogenesis of Pediatric Rheumatologic Diseases," in this issue). Tocilizumab (human monoclonal anti-IL-6 receptor) is given subcutaneously or intravenously, and is indicated for children with systemic JIA and polyarticular JIA.[63] It has also been successfully used off-label for severe JIA-associated uveitis refractory to TNFi.[64] In clinical trials, MAS (a known severe complication of systemic JIA, see Jennifer J.Y. Lee and Rayfel Schneider's article, "Systemic Juvenile Idiopathic Arthritis (JIA), in this issue) occurred in patients with sJIA treated with each of these medications. Expert opinion is that these occurrences were most likely caused by underlying sJIA and often by concurrent infections (known provokers of MAS) rather than directly by the treatments themselves.[65,66] Both of these medications are known to attenuate certain symptoms of MAS, making it more difficult to identify.[67]

Anakinra

The other marketed inhibitor of IL-1 activity, anakinra, is not a monoclonal antibody; it is a nonglycosylated recombinant version of the naturally occurring regulatory protein, IL-1 receptor antagonist. It competitively inhibits binding of IL-1 to cell-surface IL-1 type I receptors but does not transduce an IL-1 signal. Originally developed and approved as a medication for adults with RA, it was later approved for treating children with cryopyrin-associated periodic syndromes (see Kathleen E. Sullivan's article, "Pathogenesis of Pediatric Rheumatologic Diseases," in this issue). In North America, it is used off-label for treatment of systemic JIA, and for MAS in children and adults. It seems to have similar efficacy to canakinumab and tocilizumab for systemic JIA.[68] Because of its short half-life anakinra must be administered at least once daily, and subcutaneous injection is painful. Treatment of MAS with anakinra typically requires significantly higher than standard doses, but can be life-saving.[69,70] Clinical trials of anakinra are underway for treatment of MAS (https://clinicaltrials.gov/ct2/show/NCT02780583) and for treatment of sJIA and adult-onset Still disease (https://clinicaltrials.gov/ct2/show/NCT03265132).

Sekukinumab

A human monoclonal antibody against IL-17A, sekukinumab, is approved for adults with psoriasis, psoriatic arthritis, and ankylosing spondylitis. It is mentioned here because it is currently being studied for children with juvenile psoriatic arthritis and enthesis-related arthritis (see Pamela F. Weiss and Robert A. Colbert's article, "Juvenile Spondyloarthritis: A Distinct form of Juvenile Arthritis," in this issue) (https://clinicaltrials.gov/ct2/show/NCT03031782).

Rituximab

This chimeric mouse-human anti-CD-20 monoclonal antibody depletes CD-20 positive B lymphocytes through antibody-mediated cytotoxicity. Rituximab (RTX) was initially developed for treatment of certain lymphomas and leukemias bearing CD-20. In rheumatology, its therapeutic effect is to deplete B lymphocytes including those that would differentiate into plasma cells inappropriately secreting autoantibodies. Although RTX does not directly affect antibody-secreting plasma cells (which lack CD-20), it still confers an increased risk of infection[71] related to general depletion of B cells. It is given by intravenous infusion, and it is approved for treatment of severe refractory RA and ANCA-associated vasculitis in adults. It has been studied and used off-label in severe cases of lupus in adults and children, and other autoantibody-mediated diseases, such as Sjögren syndrome and systemic sclerosis. A trial of RTX in idiopathic inflammatory myositis, involving adults and children, did not reach its primary or secondary end points. However, most patients had a favorable response and it was found effective for refractory skin involvement.[71] Other anti-CD20 monoclonal antibodies that have been used much less frequently for rheumatic diseases are not discussed here.

Belimumab

Excess soluble B lymphocyte stimulating factor (BlyS) is believed to allow survival of autoreactive B cells, contributing to lupus activity. Belimumab, a human monoclonal antibody against Blys, has been shown to decrease lupus activity.[72] It is approved in North America for adult lupus patients refractory to conventional therapy, and has been used off-label in children with severe lupus. It also decreases CD-20 cells, but not as extensively as RTX.[73] Both RTX and belimumab have shown considerable steroid-sparing effects in patients with lupus.[74]

Unusual events associated with biologic response modifiers
Antidrug antibodies Because the adaptive immune system makes antibodies to foreign proteins, one might expect that patients would make antibodies against chimeric human-mouse BRMs. Indeed, anti-drug antibodies (ADAs) against infliximab (a chimeric mouse-human monoclonal antibody TNFi), also known in this situation as human antichimeric antibodies, were first identified during clinical trials.[75] It seems not so surprising that fusion proteins, which are combinations of parts of two or more different human proteins (eg, the TNFi etanercept) could take on unusual configurations that would stimulate the formation of ADAs. Even monoclonal antibodies with fully human protein sequence, because they lack glycosylation in the normal locations, (eg, the TNFi adalimumab) can stimulate ADAs. In a recent meta-analysis of 68 studies of ADAs against the TNFi currently marketed in North America involving greater than 14,000 adult patients, it was calculated that overall approximately 13% of adults taking TNFi develop ADAs which may cause a decrease or loss of response to the drug, infusion reactions, or injection site reactions. The frequency of ADAs was highest with infliximab (25%), intermediate with adalimumab (14%), and lowest with etanercept (1%). The use of concomitant DMARDs (MTX, azathioprine, and others) reduced the likelihood of ADA formation overall by 74%.[76] Much less is known about frequency and effects of ADAs against other kinds of BRMs, which have not been on the market as long as the TNFi.

Paradoxical autoimmune disease Sometimes patients diagnosed with one autoimmune disease later develop new manifestations of a different autoimmune disease. Although this phenomenon was known to occur long before biologic response modifiers were introduced, there appears to be an increase in either incidence or reporting of change of rheumatic disease diagnosis. Recent cases have been reported almost exclusively in adults being treated with TNFi, which may be a function of the longer and more frequent use of TNFi compared with other BRMs, or increased interest in the the phenomenon. As of 2017, the total number of cases of TNFi paradoxical inflammatory reactions in the peer-reviewed literature was 295 among greater than 13,000 patients (about 2%), distributed almost equally among patients treated with infliximab, etanercept, and adalimumab.[77] The most commonly reported association seems to be psoriasis or psoriasiform rash developing in adults being treated with TNFi for IBD, RA, and AS.[78,79] Some patients were able to continue TNFi therapy with addition of topical psoriasis treatment, and most of those who discontinued TNFi therapy had resolution of psoriasis. There is some evidence for a genetic predisposition to this reaction.[80] Conversely, other new-onset inflammatory disorders were described in patients being treated for psoriasis with infliximab, adalimumab, or etanercept in almost equal proportions.[80] New-onset autoimmune renal disease in adult patients taking TNFi for RA, AS, and psoriatic arthritis has also been described.[81]

In the German biologics registry, only 11 of 3071 children with JIA (0.3%) developed IBD while taking etanercept, and combination treatment with etanercept plus MTX seemed to be protective. No patients with systemic JIA or rheumatoid factor positive polyarticular JIA developed IBD.[82] IBD-related arthropathy is considered a spondyloarthropathy (see Pamela F. Weiss and Robert A. Colbert's article, "Juvenile Spondyloarthritis: A Distinct form of Juvenile Arthritis," in this issue), and is the most common extraintestinal manifestation of IBD.[83] It is well known that in patients with IBD, arthritis and other extraintestinal symptoms can occur before onset of GI symptoms.[83] IBD masquerading as JIA (then known as JRA and seronegative enthesitis with arthritis) was a presentation recognized by pediatric rheumatologists long before the advent of BRMs (author, personal experience), and seems very unlikely to represent the development of a paradoxical autoimmune disease.

The development of scleritis[84] has been reported in adults with RA, AS, and psoriatic arthritis taking TNFi. In addition, these investigators reviewed previous reports of 10 patients with JIA who developed uveitis while taking etanercept. Given the known association of autoimmune eye disease with arthritis and particularly of uveitis in children with JIA, most such occurrences seem unlikely to be paradoxical. Adalimumab and infliximab are the preferred TNFi for JIA uveitis unresponsive to topical steroids and MTX, because of an apparent lower success rate with etanercept, according to ophthalmology expert panel recommendations,[85] and some uveitis in JIA is refractory to all TNFi treatment.[64]

There have been scattered reports of a few adult patients with paradoxical autoimmune disease while taking other BRMs including tocilizumab[86] and rituximab.[87] The frequency of true paradoxical events, compared with how often such events would occur in the absence of BRM therapy, has not been sorted out, and the pathogenesis of such reactions has not been elucidated. Such observations highlight the many poorly understood and complex interconnections between genetics, inflammatory mediators, and manifestations of autoimmune disease.

Progressive multifocal leukoencephalopathy This rare, serious, and sometimes fatal brain disorder has been associated with cancer chemotherapy, human immunodeficiency virus infection, RTX treatment, and occasionally certain other BRMs given for rheumatic disease. Progressive multifocal leukoencephalopathy (PML) is caused by JC virus. (It is not Jakob-Creutzfeldt virus; rather, JC stands for the initials of the first patient in which this virus was identified.) Primary JC virus infection is widespread (present in about 75%–80% of adults, with about half of these infections having occurred during childhood), usually causes minimal symptoms, and remains latent in various tissues.[88] Although PML also can occur in people who are not immunosuppressed, strong immunosuppression from disease or treatment can cause the virus to become reactivated and, in rare instances, to also rearrange its genome such that it can cause brain disease. PML has been diagnosed most frequently in patients treated with natalizumab, a monoclonal antibody that inhibits a cell adhesion molecule, which is used for treatment of multiple sclerosis.[88]

Disease screening before starting biologic response modifiers

Except under unusual circumstances, BRMs should not be started in a patient who seems to have an infection of any kind. A careful family and exposure history should be taken to assess risk for certain unusual or opportunistic infections. Risk assessment for the most common of these infections in patients taking BRMs is described next. Based on this information, an infectious disease consultation may be useful to assess the risk of reactivation or initial infection with these organisms.

Mycobacteria Adults taking BRMs are known to be at increased risk for severe infections with *Mycobacteria tuberculosis* (reactivation or initial infection, pulmonary or disseminated) and these infections have also been described in childhood cohorts.[56,89] The American Academy of Pediatrics (AAP) has recommended screening for latent TB in all children who are starting any BRM.[56] Because granulomas serve to sequester latent mycobacteria, the finding in mice that granuloma formation is dependent on TNF may explain the higher apparent risk of TB with TNFi compared with other BRMs. In children, possible exposure to TB through close contacts (including former or current prisoners) or travel should be carefully assessed. The recommended method of direct screening is an interferon-γ release assay (IGRA), although patients younger than age 5 years generally should be screened by a TB skin test because the IGRA performs less well in this age group. Chest radiograph should be done on any patient with a positive TB test, or with a risk factor for latent TB infection. Nontuberculous mycobacteria, such as *Mycobacterium avium*, also cause opportunistic pulmonary and extrapulmonary infections in adults taking BRMs, but there is no accurate screening test. More detailed recommendations for various situations are given in the 2016 report of the AAP Committee on Infectious Diseases.[56]

Hepatitis B Risk factors and immunization status for hepatitis B should be reviewed, and serologies should be considered. In studies of adults taking BRMs, those with positive hepatitis B surface antigen were at greatest risk for reactivation of disease. Those with positive hepatitis B core antibody but negative hepatitis B surface antigen (indicating immunity because of prior infection) were also at higher risk of reactivation. More detailed recommendations about BRMs in children with previous evidence of hepatitis B is given in the AAP Committee on Infections Diseases report.[56] Specific recommendations for children who test positive for past hepatitis C infection have not been published by the committee. Consultation with an infectious disease specialist may be helpful in cases of positive viral hepatitis screening.

Opportunistic infections Certain fungi cause usually mild or asymptomatic pulmonary infection in healthy persons, but can cause severe or fatal infections (reactivated, primary, or disseminated) in immunosuppressed patients. There may be evidence of previous infection on chest radiograph. Some are known to be endemic in certain areas of North America, so locations where the patient has resided or visited are relevant to infection risk. *Histoplasma capsulatum* is a fungus abundant in bird droppings, which is present in the soil of much of the American Midwest and the central provinces of Canada, especially on current or former farmland. Two species of *Coccidioides* live in the soil of California's San Joaquin Valley, other areas of the American Southwest, and northern Mexico. *Blastomyces* is a soil fungus that lives mainly in the soil in the United States and Canada around the Great Lakes, and in the Ohio and Mississippi River valleys. All three organisms cause pneumonitis after inhalation of airborne infectious spores or conidia from disturbed soil and old droppings of birds and bats. Because of the wide exposure to all these organisms in local populations, no specific screening is recommended before starting BRMs, but awareness of the possibility of primary infection or reactivation should be high when caring for patients receiving treatment of rheumatic diseases.[56]

In contrast, the ubiquitous fungus *P jiroveci* is an airborne organism causing asymptomatic or mild infection in most people. As for the previously discussed fungal diseases, routine screening is not recommended.[56] TMP-Sx was shown to be effective in preventing *P jiroveci* pneumonia (PJP) in adults with rheumatic diseases exposed to prolonged high-dose steroids. Although there are little prospective data, guidelines for prophylaxis according to expert opinion take into consideration the high mortality of infection in immunosuppressed patients[90] leading to the suggestion that it be used in patients taking greater than or equal to 20 mg prednisone daily for 4 or more weeks. Adult rheumatic disease patients receiving cyclophosphamide and less than 20 mg daily of prednisone were also at higher risk for PJP infection, leading to the suggestion to also consider PJP prophylaxis in such patients.[91] No specific recommendations have been made for children with rheumatic diseases taking steroid or cyclophosphamide. The AAP Red Book 2015 Report of the Committee on Infectious Diseases recommends the following prophylactic dosing for TMP-Sx in children, unrelated to indication: TMP, 5 mg/kg, with Sx, 25 mg/kg orally, in divided doses twice daily or a single dose once daily, three times per week on consecutive days (eg, Monday-Tuesday-Wednesday). Other options for PJP prophylaxis are also provided.

IMMUNIZATIONS IN CHILDREN WITH RHEUMATIC DISEASES
Why Immunize?

Protecting children with rheumatic diseases from infections is especially important, not only because they may become sicker from infections than healthy children, but also because infections may cause their rheumatic disease to flare. Protection afforded by immunization in these patients may be less than in healthy children, because treatments for disease suppress overall immune responses, not just those associated with autoimmunity.[92] The level and persistence of response to immunization likely varies depending on treatment (eg, MTX seems to have less of an effect than BRMs).[93] Various serologic studies in children with stable rheumatic diseases generally show a rise in specific antibody after immunization, often into a "protective" range, although average antibody levels are not as high as seen in healthy children.[92] There are few studies showing the actual incidence of disease following immunization in healthy children versus those with rheumatic diseases, but the consensus among experts is, to paraphrase, "some immunity is better than no immunity." Children who are very ill from their rheumatic disease do not respond as well as those who are stable, so in sick patients it may be best to postpone immunizations until control of disease is better.

Is Immunization Safe in Children with Rheumatic Diseases?

In general, immunization of children with rheumatic disease does not cause exacerbation of their disease. In the case of killed, inactivated, or subunit vaccines, the risk of adverse outcome from immunization is considered to be significantly less than the risk of adverse outcome from the corresponding infection. However, because of concern for possible vaccine-related infection, experts in the United States[56] and Canada (www.canada.ca/en/public-health/services/immunization/vaccine-preventable-diseases.html) have recommended avoiding immunization with live attenuated vaccines. It is unusual for rheumatic diseases to be diagnosed in the first 6 months of life, so at least most of the closely spaced multiple dose vaccines will have already been given before onset of a disease for which immunosuppressive medication may be needed. Additional recommendations on immunizations in children with altered immunocompetence, including which vaccine for a specified disease is most appropriate for age, is found on the Centers for Disease Control and Prevention Web site at www.cdc.gov/hcp/acip-recs/general-recs/immunocompetence.html.

Immunization guidelines in other countries vary.[94] Given the high risk of varicella zoster in children who are immunosuppressed, one small study in Brazil investigated the utility of administering live attenuated varicella zoster vaccine (VZV) during immunosuppressive treatment. Of 49 children, mostly with JIA, who were all taking MTX (and some taking steroids or BRMs) at the time of immunization, none developed disease flares, or vaccine-associated rash or illness. Their specific antibody levels and their varicella virus–specific T-cell responses were increased by the immunization and responses were similar to healthy control subjects. The study was not powered to study rates of zoster after VZV immunization.[95]

When Should Immunizations Occur?

To achieve the best responses, the AAP recommends whenever possible to bring children up to date on all age-appropriate immunizations (killed and live) before starting immunosuppresant treatment. It is recommended to wait 2 weeks after inactivated or subunit vaccines, and 1 month after live vaccines before starting immunosuppression.[56] This approach should be strongly considered in cases where systemic immunosuppressive treatment can be postponed; for example, patients with JIA whose arthritis can be initially treated with NSAIDs or intra-articular steroid injections, or with uveitis being treated initially with topical steroids. However, many children with rheumatic diseases are so ill at diagnosis, or seem to have such rapidly worsening disease, that risks of delaying treatment seem to outweigh risks of delaying immunization. Once a rheumatic disease is brought under control and, when possible, DMARDs and/or GCS have been tapered to lower doses or discontinued, it is assumed that disease-related and medication-related immunosuppression will have been minimized. At that point, immunizations with non-live vaccines should be given as appropriate (**Table 3**).[56]

How long to wait during or after immunosuppression before giving immunizations?
Little specific information is available about how low the doses of various immunosuppressive medications, alone or in combination, must be to achieve an effective response to various immunizations. Different medications vary in the duration of residual immunosuppression following their complete discontinuation. Recommendations vary, but at least with regard to GCS, it is generally considered that children can develop protective vaccine responses on steroid doses equivalent to prednisone, 10 or 20 mg (or about 2 mg/kg) daily.[56]

Is it worthwhile to reimmunize later?
There is almost no information on whether children who received vaccines at a time when their rheumatic disease was more active, and/or when they were taking more immunosuppressive medications, would benefit from repeating selected immunizations when they are healthier and taking less medication. There are no official recommendations on this topic. Reimmunization should be considered on a case-by-case basis; consultation with a pediatric infectious disease specialist is recommended.

Who Is in Charge of Immunizations?

In addition to vaccines given by PCPs, children may receive vaccines at local health departments, subspecialist offices, pharmacies, emergency departments, and during inpatient hospitalizations. Nonetheless, the PCP is likely to have the most up-to-date information about immunizations that have been given or are due. He or she should take the lead in keeping track and discussing timing of immunizations with the rheumatologist. As in all aspects of health care for children with chronic diseases, excellent communication among providers improves care. Parents, or older patients themselves, should be educated and encouraged to play a part in ensuring that such communication exists.

Immunizing Family Members

Because immediate family members are in close contact with the patient, keeping them up to date on all vaccines limits disease exposure. Live polio and smallpox vaccines are contraindicated for family members, but these vaccinations are not typically given in North America anyway. Family members may receive other live virus vaccines, but in such cases it is best to limit the patient's exposure to the vaccine recipient as much as possible during the time they might transmit disease (see **Table 3**).[56] Rotavirus from the live oral vaccine is transmissible and shed in the stool of infants for up to 2 weeks.[96] Varicella vaccine virus is shed (especially if the recipient has a rash) for up to 4 weeks.[97] Rash from varicella vaccine virus or from zoster ("shingles") vaccine virus, and "shingles" caused by local reactivation, should be covered until it resolves, and contact with immunocompromised patients should be limited. Mumps, measles, and rubella vaccine viruses are not typically transmitted by the recipient, but exposure precautions should still be exercised. There has been some disagreement and change of recommendations on whether live attenuated influenza virus can be

Table 3
Routine Childhood Immunizations in Rheumatic Disease Patients receiving Immunosuppressive Therapy (Steroids, DMARDs, BRMs)

Age Category: Age Due	Non-live Vaccines[a] (Should Be Given)	Live Vaccines[b] (*Should Not* Be Given)
Infancy:		
Birth, 1–2 mo	HepB	
2, 4 or 2, 4, 6 mo	HiB[d]	RV[c,d]
2, 4, 6 mo	DTaP[e], PCV13	
2, 4, 6–18 mo	IPV	
≥6 mo	IIV (2 doses separated by 4 wk, then 1 dose yearly)	
6–18 mo	HepB	
12–15 mo	PCV13, HiB	MMR[c], VAR[c]
12–24 mo	HepA (2 doses separated by 6–18 mo)	
15–18 mo	DTaP[e]	
Childhood:		
Yearly	IIV	LAIV[c]
≥2 y	PPSV23 #1 (≥8 wk after PCV13)	
≥7 y	PPSV23 #2 (5 y after dose #1)	
4–6 y	DTaP[e], IPV, HepB	MMR[c], VAR[c]
Adolescence:		
Yearly	IIV	LIAV[c]
11–12 y	MenACWY, Tdap[e] HPV (2 doses 6–12 mo apart)	
16 y	MenACWY	
16–18 y	MenB (2 doses, 1–6 mo apart)[f]	

For catch-up vaccination schedules and special situations, see: https://www.cdc.gov/vaccines/schedules/hcp/imz/child-adolescent.html.

Abbreviations: DTaP, Diphtheria and Tetanus toxoid, acellular Pertussus; HepA, Hepatitis A; HepB, Hepatitis B virus; HiB, Hemophylus influenzae type B; HPV, human papillomavirus vaccine; IIV, Inactivated Influenza Vaccine (or subunit vaccine); IPV, Inactivated Poliovirus; LAIV, Live Attenuated Influenza Vaccine; MenA,C,W,Y, Meningococcus serotypes A,C,W,Y; MenB, Meningococcus serotypeB; MMR, Measles, Mumps, Rubella; PCV13, Pneumooccal Conjugate 13-valent; PPSV23, Pneumococcal Polysaccharide 23-valent; RV, Rotavirus; Tdap, Tetanus toxoid, diphtheria toxoid reduced dose, acellular pertussis reduced dose; VAR, Varicella

[a] Non-live vaccines should be given ≥2 wk before starting immunosuppression, or when on stable or weaning dose of DMARD or BRM, dose of GCS ≤20 mg/day or 2 mg/kg/day if weight <10 kg, and disease stable or improving. Suppression of vaccine response after stopping these medications varies, and may be >6 mo after cessation of B-lymphocyte-depleting therapies.

[b] Live vaccines may be given ≥4 wk before starting immunosuppression.

[c] Avoid close contact with those who receive live vaccines, including Zoster vaccine in elderly. Cover vaccine-related rashes until resolved.

[d] Number of doses depends on brand of these vaccines.

[e] For patients with autoimmune central nervous system disease, avoid pertussis vaccine; give DT in place of DTap, or Td in place of Tdap.

[f] Interval between doses depends on brand of vaccine.

given to family members, with some experts recommending killed or synthetic vaccines instead. It may be simpler and safer to give the entire family the intramuscular killed influenza vaccine. Good hygiene, such as handwashing and sequestration of body waste and fluids, should be practiced at all times.

SUMMARY

Within the last 20 years, the options for treating children with rheumatic diseases have expanded tremendously. Clinicians have begun to actualize the opportunity for more effective treatment, with less morbidity and mortality, through the appropriate use of BRMs alone or in combination with older antirheumatic drugs. Awareness, recognition, and prevention of possible toxic, metabolic, and infectious side effects is essential for the safe use of these therapies. Rheumatologists, PCPs, hospital providers, other members of the health care team, and well-informed families all play a part in medication safety.

REFERENCES

1. Favier LA, Taylor J, Loiselle Rich K, et al. Barriers to adherence in juvenile idiopathic arthritis: a multicenter collaborative experience and preliminary results. J Rheumatol 2018. [Epub ahead of print].
2. Kok VC, Horng JT, Huang JL, et al. Population-based cohort study on the risk of malignancy in East Asian children with juvenile idiopathic arthritis. BMC Cancer 2014;14:634.
3. Beukelman T, Xie F, Chen L, et al. Risk of malignancy associated with paediatric use of tumour necrosis factor inhibitors. Ann Rheum Dis 2018. [Epub ahead of print].
4. Nordstrom BL, Mlnes D, Gu Y, et al. Risk of malignancy in children with juvenile idiopathic arthritis not treated with biologic agents. Arthritis Care Res (Hoboken) 2012;64(9):1357–64.
5. Wiseman AC. Immunosuppressive medications. Clin J Am Soc Nephrol 2016; 11(2):332–43.
6. McLean-Tooke A, Aldridge C, Waugh S, et al. Methotrexate, rheumatoid arthritis and infection risk: what is the evidence? Rheumatology (Oxford) 2009;48(8):867–71.
7. Doaty S, Agrawal H, Bauer E, et al. Infection and lupus: which causes which? Curr Rheumatol Rep 2016;18(3):13.
8. Beukelman T, Xie F, Chen L, et al. Rates of hospitalized bacterial infection associated with juvenile idiopathic arthritis and its treatment. Arthritis Rheum 2012; 64(8):2773–80.
9. Danza A, Ruiz-Irastorza G. Infection risk in systemic lupus erythematosus patients: susceptibility factors and preventive strategies. Lupus 2013; 22(12):1286–94.
10. Crofford LJ. Use of NSAIDs in treating patients with arthritis. Arthritis Res Ther 2013;15(Suppl 3):S2.
11. Manohar VS, Vinay M, Jayasree T, et al. Prescribing pattern of gastroprotective agents with non-steroidal anti-inflammatory drugs. J Pharmacol Pharmacother 2013;4(1):59–60.
12. Zhang X, Donnan PT, Bell S, et al. Non-steroidal anti-inflammatory drug induced acute kidney injury in the community dwelling general population and people with chronic kidney disease: systematic review and meta-analysis. BMC Nephrol 2017;18(1):256.
13. Liu D, Ahmet A, Ward L, et al. A practical guide to the monitoring and management of the complications of systemic corticosteroid therapy. Allergy Asthma Clin Immunol 2013;9(1):30.
14. Singh JA, Hossain A, Kotb A, et al. Risk of serious infections with immunosuppressive drugs and glucocorticoids for lupus nephritis: a systematic review and network meta-analysis. BMC Med 2016;14(1):137.
15. Aljebab F, Choonara I, Conroy S. Systematic review of the toxicity of long-course oral corticosteroids in children. PLoS One 2017;12(1):e0170259.

16. Hiraki LT, Feldman CH, Marty FM, et al. Serious infection rates among children with systemic lupus erythematosus enrolled in Medicaid. Arthritis Care Res (Hoboken) 2017;69(11):1620–6.

17. Kimura Y, Fieldston E, Devries-Vandervlugt B, et al. High dose, alternate day corticosteroids for systemic onset juvenile rheumatoid arthritis. J Rheumatol 2000; 27(8):2018–24.

18. Young CM, Shiels WE 2nd, Coley BD, et al. Ultrasound-guided corticosteroid injection therapy for juvenile idiopathic arthritis: 12-year care experience. Pediatr Radiol 2012;42(12):1481–9.

19. Caplan A, Fett N, Rosenbach M, et al. Prevention and management of glucocorticoid-induced side effects: a comprehensive review: ocular, cardiovascular, muscular, and psychiatric side effects and issues unique to pediatric patients. J Am Acad Dermatol 2017;76(2):201–7.

20. Shea B, Swinden MV, Tanjong Ghogomu E, et al. Folic acid and folinic acid for reducing side effects in patients receiving methotrexate for rheumatoid arthritis. Cochrane Database Syst Rev 2013;(5):CD000951.

21. Cronstein BN, Sitkovsky M. Adenosine and adenosine receptors in the pathogenesis and treatment of rheumatic diseases. Nat Rev Rheumatol 2017;13(1): 41–51.

22. Vena GA, Cassano N, Iannone F. Update on subcutaneous methotrexate for inflammatory arthritis and psoriasis. Ther Clin Risk Manag 2018;14:105–16.

23. Klein A, Kaul I, Foeldvari I, et al. Efficacy and safety of oral and parenteral methotrexate therapy in children with juvenile idiopathic arthritis: an observational study with patients from the German Methotrexate Registry. Arthritis Care Res (Hoboken) 2012;64(9):1349–56.

24. Salliot C, van der Heijde D. Long-term safety of methotrexate monotherapy in patients with rheumatoid arthritis: a systematic literature research. Ann Rheum Dis 2009;68(7):1100–4.

25. Horneff G, Klein A, Oommen PT, et al. Update on malignancies in children with juvenile idiopathic arthritis in the German BIKER Registry. Clin Exp Rheumatol 2016;34(6):1113–20.

26. Kwon OC, Lee JS, Kim YG, et al. Safety of the concomitant use of methotrexate and a prophylactic dose of trimethoprim-sulfamethoxazole. Clin Rheumatol 2018. [Epub ahead of print].

27. Beukelman T, Patkar NM, Saag KG, et al. 2011 American College of Rheumatology recommendations for the treatment of juvenile idiopathic arthritis: initiation and safety monitoring of therapeutic agents for the treatment of arthritis and systemic features. Arthritis Care Res (Hoboken) 2011;63(4):465–82.

28. Kocharla L, Taylor J, Weiler T, et al. Monitoring methotrexate toxicity in juvenile idiopathic arthritis. J Rheumatol 2009;36(12):2813–8.

29. Yazici Y. Long-term safety of methotrexate in the treatment of rheumatoid arthritis. Clin Exp Rheumatol 2010;28(5 Suppl 61):S65–7.

30. Silverman E, Mouy R, Spiegel L, et al. Leflunomide or methotrexate for juvenile rheumatoid arthritis. N Engl J Med 2005;352(16):1655–66.

31. Plosker GL, Croom KF. Sulfasalazine: a review of its use in the management of rheumatoid arthritis. Drugs 2005;65(13):1825–49.

32. Zawodniak A, Lochmatter P, Beeler A, et al. Cross-reactivity in drug hypersensitivity reactions to sulfasalazine and sulfamethoxazole. Int Arch Allergy Immunol 2010;153(2):152–6.

33. Rainsford KD, Parke AL, Clifford-Rashotte M, et al. Therapy and pharmacological properties of hydroxychloroquine and chloroquine in treatment of systemic lupus

erythematosus, rheumatoid arthritis and related diseases. Inflammopharmacology 2015;23(5):231–69.

34. Vivino FB, Carsons SE, Foulks G, et al. New treatment guidelines for Sjogren's disease. Rheum Dis Clin North Am 2016;42(3):531–51.

35. Marmor MF, Kellner U, Lai TY, et al, American Academy of Ophthalmology. Recommendations on screening for chloroquine and hydroxychloroquine retinopathy (2016 revision). Ophthalmology 2016;123(6):1386–94.

36. Abdulaziz N, Shah AR, McCune WJ. Hydroxychloroquine: balancing the need to maintain therapeutic levels with ocular safety: an update. Curr Opin Rheumatol 2018;30(3):249–55.

37. Dooley MA, Jayne D, Ginzler EM, et al. Mycophenolate versus azathioprine as maintenance therapy for lupus nephritis. N Engl J Med 2011;365(20):1886–95.

38. Tian SY, Feldman BM, Beyene J, et al. Immunosuppressive therapies for the maintenance treatment of proliferative lupus nephritis: a systematic review and network metaanalysis. J Rheumatol 2015;42(8):1392–400.

39. Levy RA, de Jesus GR, de Jesus NR, et al. Critical review of the current recommendations for the treatment of systemic inflammatory rheumatic diseases during pregnancy and lactation. Autoimmun Rev 2016;15(10):955–63.

40. Alami Z, Agier MS, Ahid S, et al. Pregnancy outcome following in utero exposure to azathioprine: a French comparative observational study. Therapie 2017. [Epub ahead of print].

41. Hyams JS, Dubinsky MC, Baldassano RN, et al. Infliximab is not associated with increased risk of malignancy or hemophagocytic lymphohistiocytosis in pediatric patients with inflammatory bowel disease. Gastroenterology 2017;152(8): 1901–1914 e3.

42. Azzi JR, Sayegh MH, Mallat SG. Calcineurin inhibitors: 40 years later, can't live without. J Immunol 2013;191(12):5785–91.

43. Hoskova L, Malek I, Kopkan L, et al. Pathophysiological mechanisms of calcineurin inhibitor-induced nephrotoxicity and arterial hypertension. Physiol Res 2017;66(2):167–80.

44. Ahlmann M, Hempel G. The effect of cyclophosphamide on the immune system: implications for clinical cancer therapy. Cancer Chemother Pharmacol 2016; 78(4):661–71.

45. Bernatsky S, Ramsey-Goldman R, Joseph L, et al. Lymphoma risk in systemic lupus: effects of disease activity versus treatment. Ann Rheum Dis 2014;73(1):138–42.

46. Hsu CY, Lin MS, Su YJ, et al. Cumulative immunosuppressant exposure is associated with diversified cancer risk among 14 832 patients with systemic lupus erythematosus: a nested case-control study. Rheumatology (Oxford) 2017;56(4): 620–8.

47. Somers EC, Marder W, Christman GM, et al. Use of a gonadotropin-releasing hormone analog for protection against premature ovarian failure during cyclophosphamide therapy in women with severe lupus. Arthritis Rheum 2005;52(9): 2761–7.

48. Gajjar R, Miller SD, Meyers KE, et al. Fertility preservation in patients receiving cyclophosphamide therapy for renal disease. Pediatr Nephrol 2015;30(7):1099–106.

49. Nash P, Ohson K, Walsh J, et al. Early and sustained efficacy with apremilast monotherapy in biological-naive patients with psoriatic arthritis: a phase IIIB, randomised controlled trial (ACTIVE). Ann Rheum Dis 2018;77(5):690–8.

50. Ruperto N, Brunner HI, Zuber Z, et al. Pharmacokinetic and safety profile of tofacitinib in children with polyarticular course juvenile idiopathic arthritis: results of a phase 1, open-label, multicenter study. Pediatr Rheumatol Online J 2017;15(1):86.

51. Coutinho AE, Chapman KE. The anti-inflammatory and immunosuppressive effects of glucocorticoids, recent developments and mechanistic insights. Mol Cell Endocrinol 2011;335(1):2–13.

52. Brunner HI, Ruperto N, Tzaribachev N, et al. Subcutaneous golimumab for children with active polyarticular-course juvenile idiopathic arthritis: results of a multicentre, double-blind, randomised-withdrawal trial. Ann Rheum Dis 2018;77(1):21–9.

53. Ramanan AV, Dick AD, Jones AP, et al. Adalimumab plus methotrexate for uveitis in juvenile idiopathic arthritis. N Engl J Med 2017;376(17):1637–46.

54. Davies R, Southwood TR, Kearsley-Fleet L, et al. Medically significant infections are increased in patients with juvenile idiopathic arthritis treated with etanercept: results from the British society for paediatric and adolescent rheumatology etanercept cohort study. Arthritis Rheumatol 2015;67(9):2487–94.

55. Becker I, Horneff G. Risk of serious infection in juvenile idiopathic arthritis patients associated with tumor necrosis factor inhibitors and disease activity in the German biologics in pediatric rheumatology registry. Arthritis Care Res (Hoboken) 2017;69(4):552–60.

56. Davies HD, Committee on Infectious Diseases. Infectious complications with the use of biologic response modifiers in infants and children. Pediatrics 2016;138(2) [pii:e20161209].

57. Pisetsky DS. Tumor necrosis factor: is it time to change the name? Arthritis Res Ther 2014;16(2):108.

58. Diak P, Siegel J, La Grenade L, et al. Tumor necrosis factor alpha blockers and malignancy in children: forty-eight cases reported to the Food and Drug Administration. Arthritis Rheum 2010;62(8):2517–24.

59. Mariette X, Matucci-Cerinic M, Pavelka K, et al. Malignancies associated with tumour necrosis factor inhibitors in registries and prospective observational studies: a systematic review and meta-analysis. Ann Rheum Dis 2011;70(11):1895–904.

60. Ruperto N, Lovell DJ, Quartier P, et al. Abatacept in children with juvenile idiopathic arthritis: a randomised, double-blind, placebo-controlled withdrawal trial. Lancet 2008;372(9636):383–91.

61. Birolo C, Zannin ME, Arsenyeva S, et al. Comparable efficacy of abatacept used as first-line or second-line biological agent for severe juvenile idiopathic arthritis-related uveitis. J Rheumatol 2016;43(11):2068–73.

62. Ruperto N, Brunner HI, Quartier P, et al. Two randomized trials of canakinumab in systemic juvenile idiopathic arthritis. N Engl J Med 2012;367(25):2396–406.

63. Turnier JL, Brunner HI. Tocilizumab for treating juvenile idiopathic arthritis. Expert Opin Biol Ther 2016;16(4):559–66.

64. Calvo-Rio V, Santos-Gomez M, Calvo I, et al. Anti-interleukin-6 receptor tocilizumab for severe juvenile idiopathic arthritis-associated uveitis refractory to anti-tumor necrosis factor therapy: a multicenter study of twenty-five patients. Arthritis Rheumatol 2017;69(3):668–75.

65. Yokota S, Itoh Y, Morio T, et al. Macrophage activation syndrome in patients with systemic juvenile idiopathic arthritis under treatment with tocilizumab. J Rheumatol 2015;42(4):712–22.

66. Grom AA, Ilowite NT, Pascual V, et al. Rate and clinical presentation of macrophage activation syndrome in patients with systemic juvenile idiopathic arthritis treated with canakinumab. Arthritis Rheumatol 2016;68(1):218–28.

67. Schulert GS, Minoia F, Bohnsack J, et al. Effect of biologic therapy on clinical and laboratory features of macrophage activation syndrome associated with systemic juvenile idiopathic arthritis. Arthritis Care Res (Hoboken) 2018;70(3):409–19.

68. Horneff G, Schulz AC, Klotsche J, et al. Experience with etanercept, tocilizumab and interleukin-1 inhibitors in systemic onset juvenile idiopathic arthritis patients from the BIKER registry. Arthritis Res Ther 2017;19(1):256.

69. Loh NK, Lucas M, Fernandez S, et al. Successful treatment of macrophage activation syndrome complicating adult Still disease with anakinra. Intern Med J 2012;42(12):1358–62.

70. Kahn PJ, Cron RQ. Higher-dose Anakinra is effective in a case of medically refractory macrophage activation syndrome. J Rheumatol 2013;40(5):743–4.

71. Schioppo T, Ingegnoli F. Current perspective on rituximab in rheumatic diseases. Drug Des Devel Ther 2017;11:2891–904.

72. Blair HA, Duggan ST. Belimumab: a review in systemic lupus erythematosus. Drugs 2018;78(3):355–66.

73. Furie RA, Wallace DJ, Aranow C, et al. Long-term safety and efficacy of belimumab in patients with systemic lupus erythematosus: a continuation of the phase 3 United States BLISS-76 trial. Arthritis Rheumatol 2018. [Epub ahead of print].

74. Oon S, Huq M, Godfrey T, et al. Systematic review, and meta-analysis of steroid-sparing effect, of biologic agents in randomized, placebo-controlled phase 3 trials for systemic lupus erythematosus. Semin Arthritis Rheum 2018. [Epub ahead of print].

75. Wolbink GJ, Vis M, Lems W, et al. Development of antiinfliximab antibodies and relationship to clinical response in patients with rheumatoid arthritis. Arthritis Rheum 2006;54(3):711–5.

76. Thomas SS, Borazan N, Barroso N, et al. Comparative immunogenicity of TNF inhibitors: impact on clinical efficacy and tolerability in the management of autoimmune diseases. a systematic review and meta-analysis. BioDrugs 2015;29(4):241–58.

77. Havmose M, Thomsen SF. Development of paradoxical inflammatory disorders during treatment of psoriasis with TNF inhibitors: a review of published cases. Int J Dermatol 2017;56(11):1087–102.

78. Peer FC, Miller A, Pavli P, et al. Paradoxical psoriasiform reactions of anti-tumour necrosis factor therapy in inflammatory bowel disease patients. Intern Med J 2017;47(12):1445–8.

79. Fiorino G, Danese S, Pariente B, et al. Paradoxical immune-mediated inflammation in inflammatory bowel disease patients receiving anti-TNF-alpha agents. Autoimmun Rev 2014;13(1):15–9.

80. Cabaleiro T, Prieto-Perez R, Navarro R, et al. Paradoxical psoriasiform reactions to anti-TNFalpha drugs are associated with genetic polymorphisms in patients with psoriasis. Pharmacogenomics J 2016;16(4):336–40.

81. Piga M, Chessa E, Ibba V, et al. Biologics-induced autoimmune renal disorders in chronic inflammatory rheumatic diseases: systematic literature review and analysis of a monocentric cohort. Autoimmun Rev 2014;13(8):873–9.

82. Barthel D, Ganser G, Kuester RM, et al. Inflammatory bowel disease in juvenile idiopathic arthritis patients treated with biologics. J Rheumatol 2015;42(11):2160–5.

83. Vavricka SR, Rogler G, Gantenbein C, et al. Chronological order of appearance of extraintestinal manifestations relative to the time of IBD diagnosis in the swiss inflammatory bowel disease cohort. Inflamm Bowel Dis 2015;21(8):1794–800.

84. Gaujoux-Viala C, Giampietro C, Gaujoux T, et al. Scleritis: a paradoxical effect of etanercept? Etanercept-associated inflammatory eye disease. J Rheumatol 2012;39(2):233–9.

85. Levy-Clarke G, Jabs DA, Read RW, et al. Expert panel recommendations for the use of anti-tumor necrosis factor biologic agents in patients with ocular inflammatory disorders. Ophthalmology 2014;121(3):785–796 e3.

86. Terreaux W, Masson C, Eschard JP, et al. Incidence of paradoxical reactions in patients treated with tocilizumab for rheumatoid arthritis: data from the French registry REGATE. Joint Bone Spine 2018;85(1):53–7.
87. Thomas L, Canoui-Poitrine F, Gottenberg JE, et al. Incidence of new-onset and flare of preexisting psoriasis during rituximab therapy for rheumatoid arthritis: data from the French AIR registry. J Rheumatol 2012;39(5):893–8.
88. Saribas AS, Ozdemir A, Lam C, et al. JC virus-induced progressive multifocal leukoencephalopathy. Future Virol 2010;5(3):313–23.
89. Davis BP, Ballas ZK. Biologic response modifiers: indications, implications, and insights. J Allergy Clin Immunol 2017;139(5):1445–56.
90. Park JW, Curtis JR, Moon J, et al. Prophylactic effect of trimethoprim-sulfamethoxazole for pneumocystis pneumonia in patients with rheumatic diseases exposed to prolonged high-dose glucocorticoids. Ann Rheum Dis 2017;77(5):644–9.
91. Mecoli CA, Saylor D, Gelber AC, et al. *Pneumocystis jiroveci* pneumonia in rheumatic disease: a 20-year single-centre experience. Clin Exp Rheumatol 2017; 35(4):671–3.
92. Silva CA, Aikawa NE, Bonfa E. Vaccinations in juvenile chronic inflammatory diseases: an update. Nat Rev Rheumatol 2013;9(9):532–43.
93. Stoof SP, Heijstek MW, Sijssens KM, et al. Kinetics of the long-term antibody response after meningococcal C vaccination in patients with juvenile idiopathic arthritis: a retrospective cohort study. Ann Rheum Dis 2014;73(4):728–34.
94. Groot N, Heijstek MW, Wulffraat NM. Vaccinations in paediatric rheumatology: an update on current developments. Curr Rheumatol Rep 2015;17(7):46.
95. Groot N, Pileggi G, Sandoval CB, et al. Varicella vaccination elicits a humoral and cellular response in children with rheumatic diseases using immune suppressive treatment. Vaccine 2017;35(21):2818–22.
96. Anderson EJ. Rotavirus vaccines: viral shedding and risk of transmission. Lancet Infect Dis 2008;8(10):642–9.
97. Pierson DL, Mehta SK, Gilden D, et al. Varicella zoster virus DNA at inoculation sites and in saliva after Zostavax immunization. J Infect Dis 2011;203(11):1542–5.

General Nutrition and Fitness for the Child with Rheumatic Disease

Sharon Bout-Tabaku, MD, MSCE

KEYWORDS

- Obesity • Nutrition • Growth • Supplements • Cardiovascular disease
- Physical fitness • Exercise • Bone health

KEY POINTS

- Because of new medications and aggressive treatment, most children with rheumatic diseases are no longer at high risk for growth failure.
- Children with rheumatic diseases have a risk of long-term poor bone and cardiovascular health outcomes due to both chronic disease and corticosteroid treatment.
- The duration and dose of corticosteroid therapy can often be minimized by using steroid-sparing agents, such as disease-modifying antirheumatic drugs and biologic response modifiers.
- Bone health and compliance with daily calcium and vitamin D supplementation should be monitored.
- Fitness levels are often low, although functional skills are good in children with rheumatic disease. Providers should assess fitness and plan for daily physical activity with a graduated program that may include rehabilitation, group exercise and recreation, and strengthening and conditioning.

INTRODUCTION

Children with rheumatic diseases are at higher risk of poor nutritional outcomes and growth failure due to chronic inflammation. An additional consequence of uncontrolled disease is that arthritis or other manifestations limit both activities of daily living and the ability to exercise. In the long term, chronic inflammation is associated with other comorbidities, such as cardiovascular disease (CVD) and poor bone health.[1] In the past, treatment for control of the most serious diseases, such as systemic juvenile idiopathic arthritis (sJIA), systemic lupus, and dermatomyositis, relied heavily on glucocorticosteroids (GCS), which have may metabolic side effects (also discussed in

Disclosure Statement: The author has no relevant disclosures.
Department of Pediatric Medicine, Sidra Medicine, Qatar Foundation, OPC, Level 2, Al Luqta Street, Education City North Campus, PO Box 26999, Doha, Qatar
E-mail address: sbouttabaku@sidra.org

Pediatr Clin N Am 65 (2018) 855–866
https://doi.org/10.1016/j.pcl.2018.04.009
0031-3955/18/© 2018 Elsevier Inc. All rights reserved.

pediatric.theclinics.com

Dr. Gloria C. Higgins' article, "Complications of Treatments for Pediatric Rheumatic Diseases," in this issue.).

The overall outcomes of childhood rheumatic diseases have improved remarkably in the last 20 years because of more rapid recognition, better understanding of these disease processes, the availability of new medications, and a trend towards more aggressive treatment. Nonetheless, good nutrition, bone health, and physical fitness warrant close attention in these children and are best achieved through collaboration among the primary care provider, other pediatric care providers, and the rheumatologist.

WHAT PHYSIOLOGIC PROCESSES INHIBIT GROWTH IN CHILDREN WITH RHEUMATIC DISEASES?

Chronic systemic inflammation itself results in cachexia, which is associated with poor appetite, increased basal metabolic rate, loss of lean muscle, and inefficient use of stored fat for energy.[2] Occasionally, the chronic disease state is associated with growth hormone resistance, which affects muscle mass and bone density. Tumor necrosis factor (TNF), initially named cachexin,[3] and many other cytokines such as interferon-γ and several interleukins (IL-6, IL-12, IL-17, and IL-23) also inhibit growth through pathways that involve insulin-like growth factor 1, a mediator of growth hormone. In addition, malabsorption and medication side effects can contribute to vitamin and macronutrient deficiencies, poor muscle mass, and abnormally low bone density, respectively.[4]

WHAT ARE THE EFFECTS OF RHEUMATIC DISEASE MEDICATIONS ON GROWTH?

It is well known that chronic high-dose GCS treatment decreases growth velocity. Although the best available growth data are for children with juvenile idiopathic arthritis (JIA), children with other severe rheumatic diseases often did, and sometimes still do, receive prolonged courses of high to moderate dose GCS. In the past, as a result of both their disease processes and prolonged treatment with GCS, a high proportion of children with sJIA and rheumatoid factor–positive polyarticular JIA had growth failure.[5] In an early longitudinal study of children with "juvenile chronic arthritis" followed an average of 15 years until 1981, 10% of patients with systemic arthritis experienced severe growth failure.[6] In a later study, 40% of patients with a history of sJIA who had received at least 2 years of treatment with GCS during childhood, had a final height of at least 2 standard deviations below the mean. In addition, 80% of this cohort failed to reach predicted final height.[7]

The timing of GCS therapy before and during the physiologic growth spurt also affects the degree of growth retardation. Early onset of arthritis was shown to be a contributor to growth failure.[8] In a 2011 study of growth and development in childhood lupus, growth failure determinants included age at first visit less than 13.4 years, and cumulative steroid dose greater than 400 mg/kg.[9]

GROWTH IN JUVENILE IDIOPATHIC ARTHRITIS PATIENTS IS OVERALL IMPROVING

Soon after the advent of TNF inhibitors (TNFi), improvement in the growth of JIA patients treated with these medications became evident. A cohort of patients with severe polyarticular course JIA, followed 2 years before and 2 years after treatment with the TNFi etanercept or infliximab, was described in 2006. Along with the significant decrease in disease activity after introduction of a TNFi, linear growth velocity increased in 76% of patients. The improvement in the growth velocity was the best in patients with the greatest growth retardation.[10] Of the 77% of patients who were taking GCS at the time of starting a TNFi, all were able to significantly decrease their steroid dose. There was, however, no statistical correlation between decrease in steroid dose and the increase in height velocity. Another prospective study examined growth velocity and growth restoration over 3 years in patients with polyarticular or systemic JIA enrolled in a clinical trial of etanercept only or etanercept plus methotrexate (MTX), versus MTX only. The participants in the 2 etanercept groups had significant increases in mean height and weight percentiles during 3 years of study compared to those taking only MTX, and there was no difference in the two etanercept groups with or without MTX.[11] Despite such encouraging results, some children continue to have growth failure after starting a biologic response modifier (BRM), especially those who have unsuccessfully tried multiple different BRM treatments without achieving disease control, and those with sJIA.[12]

More recently, analysis of a national JIA database in Canada revealed that most children given modern treatments from the time of diagnosis of JIA are achieving their growth potential. This large prospective study of about 1100 new-onset JIA patients followed during 2005 to 2010 demonstrated that most had growth patterns like healthy children in the population.[13,14] However, there was variation among subgroups, as rheumatoid factor–positive polyarthritis patients had mild growth impairment, and systemic arthritis patients had a decrease in mean height z scores. Similarly, uncontrolled disease activity and prolonged use of GCS put children at risk for growth failure.[14]

WHAT CAUSES OBESITY IN RHEUMATIC DISEASES?

Caloric intake in excess of caloric expenditure is the primary cause of obesity in humans. A sedentary lifestyle contributes to obesity in children with chronic illness and also in healthy children. However, excessive weight gain is also a well-known metabolic effect of systemic corticosteroids; when they are used for a prolonged period or at high doses, an increase in body mass index (BMI) z score (relative weight adjusted for age and sex), and Cushingoid features are prominent. In a recent study of children with a variety of rheumatic diseases (including JIA, systemic lupus, dermatomyositis, and vasculitis) starting moderate- to high-dose corticosteroids, the BMI z score increased to a peak of 1.29 at an average of 4 months and then decreased with tapering steroid doses. However, only half of the patients returned to within +0.25 SD of their baseline BMI z score by 18 months.[13]

A 2012 a single-center cross-sectional study of American children with JIA revealed an obesity prevalence (BMI >95th percentile) of 18%, which was the same as children in the general population.[15] There was no association of obesity with inflammatory markers. However, in the previously cited Canadian database, the 3-year cumulative incidence of obesity was 10.8%, with highest frequency among sJIA patients at 34%.[14] Among children in the German national pediatric rheumatology database, the use of high-dose GCS, functional limitations, and less frequent physical activity were associated with being overweight. However, between 2003 and 2012, the prevalence of overweight decreased from 14% to 8%, with the greatest change in children with systemic JIA.[16] These weight decreases were associated with higher levels of physical activity and less frequent treatment with high-dose GCS. Although both associations could be the result of better disease control with more modern treatment strategies, causality could not be shown in this type of study.

RHEUMATIC DISEASE WITH OTHER COMORBID DISEASE AND NUTRITION CONCERNS

Other comorbidities that occur with rheumatic diseases can impact nutrition, such as celiac disease and inflammatory bowel disease. Children with these diseases are referred to rheumatology clinics for joint pain and swelling due to peripheral and axial arthritis[17] and enthesitis, as well as for arthralgia. The most commonly described auto-immune rheumatic diseases that are associated with celiac disease are lupus and Sjogren syndrome.[18] Recently, the prevalence of celiac disease in pediatric patients presenting for rheumatic disease evaluation was estimated at 2.0%.[19] Usually symptoms improve or completely abate after following a gluten-free diet. Inflammatory bowel disease is also associated with autoimmune rheumatic disease. In children, one study showed that Crohn disease was associated with more prevalent arthritis and lupus, whereas ulcerative colitis was not strongly associated with these diseases.[20]

Thus, general pediatric and rheumatology care providers should have a high degree of suspicion for these comorbid diseases when rheumatic disease patients present with gastrointestinal symptoms, unexplained weight loss, or poor growth.

BONE HEALTH IN CHILDREN WITH RHEUMATIC DISEASES

Peak skeletal mass acquisition is of concern in children with chronic rheumatic diseases. Failure to develop adequate bone mineralization is common and is characterized by a failure of bone formation. If this happens during puberty when bone mass accrual is at its peak, children do not attain normal skeletal mass. Therapeutic interventions at later times during adolescence cannot reverse inadequate bone mineralization.[21]

Recognition of bone health has always been important for pediatric rheumatologists and the general practitioners who co-manage patients with rheumatic diseases. This awareness has usually centered on the adverse side effects of corticosteroid use, and other known risk factors for bone fragility, such as systemic inflammation, decreased physical activity and weight-bearing exercise, muscle dysfunction, delayed puberty, and poor calcium and vitamin D intake.[22]

Even with the current advances in treatment, both assessment of risk for poor bone health and maintenance of bone health remain active areas of care and management. There are multiple consensus statements and recommendations on bone health that can be synthesized into general principles: children with active inflammation and/or on chronic corticosteroid therapy (3 months or longer), and significant increase in BMI z score in the first 6 months of corticosteroid therapy, should have routine screening of bone health and receive supplementation of calcium and vitamin D.[22] Bone density in children with osteopenia is best monitored by dual-energy X-ray absorptiometry (DXA) according to age-related norms, ideally performed in a pediatric facility. Cholecalciferol supplementation is well tolerated and effective in increasing Vitamin D levels. In addition, results of a small study of adolescent and young adult females with well-controlled juvenile onset systemic lupus erythematosus (SLE) and low Vitamin D levels suggested that Vitamin D replenishment may have a small beneficial effect on lupus activity and fatigue.[23]

DIETARY AND NUTRITION SUPPLEMENTATION

The data on nutrition supplementation in children with rheumatic disease are sparse. However, in clinical practice, families and patients have many questions and often try different interventions ranging from supplementation, to restrictive diets, to "anti-inflammatory" diets. Complementary and alternative medicine (CAM) is commonly used, with frequencies between 34% and 92% in different studies. Dietary modifications and natural health products are among those most commonly used.[24,25]

In children with rheumatic diseases, there was a greater use of CAM among patients who did not have regular follow-up care.[26] In a JIA cohort, taking CAM was associated with subsequent lower global health and physical functioning despite higher adherence to prescribed medications as assessed by the rheumatologist ($P<.05$). Use of

CAM was not associated with subsequent improved quality of life, decreased pain, or disease severity.[27]

Data on diet and nutrition supplementation are abundant in adult studies. Large studies and meta-analyses demonstrate that regular consumption of sugar-sweetened soda, but not diet soda, is associated with increased risk of seropositive rheumatoid arthritis (RA) in women, independent of other dietary and lifestyle factors.[28] Plant-based diets, such as the Mediterranean diet, were shown to have positive effects on pain and disease activity in adults with RA in several large prospective and randomized controlled trials.[29] Fasting and elimination diet studies are few; fasting diets may help with pain and swelling but their effect on disease progression and long-term outcomes is not known.[29]

In growing children, diets including the basic food groups containing sufficient calories, vitamins, and minerals are essential for growth and development, so fasting and elimination diets are not advised. Use of the Mediterranean diet in children showed evidence of improvement in cardiorespiratory fitness and obesity-related diseases, but none related to musculoskeletal health.[30]

The evidence for using marine oil, specifically omega-3 fatty acids, to alleviate pain in arthritis patients is of moderate quality in adults with RA.[29,31] One study demonstrated a possible mechanism for the beneficial effect through the reduction in the concentration of thromboxane B2 in blood of subjects with high risk of CVD. Adults with RA had lower leukotriene B4 content in neutrophils after supplementation with marine-derived omega-3 polyunsaturated fatty acids.[32,33]

Herbal medicine and supplements are also popular among patients, and their use should be recognized and discussed by medical care providers. Some herbal medicines have shown promise for reducing pain and inflammation in rheumatic diseases in adults. There is research on compounds such as g-linolenic acid and plants such as *Harpagophytum procumbens* (devil's claw), *Tanacetum parthenium* (feverfew), *Uncaria tomentosa* (cat's claw), *Urtica dioica* (stinging nettles), and *Zingiber officinale* (ginger).[24] There are a few studies showing improvement in pain, and fewer on active joint disease, related to intake of borage seed oil, curcumin (turmeric), and *Tripterygium wilfordii*, sometimes called the thunder god vine.[29] When evaluating such research and counseling patients, it is important to discuss that herbal products are often combined formulations, which differ in active ingredient content. Furthermore, safety varies according to the geographic source of the plant material, the climate in which they were grown, and the time of harvest, as well as the part of the plant used and (for extracts) the choice of extraction method.[24] Finally, the production, marketing, and sale of most herbal products and dietary supplements are not regulated. There is also a possibility of interactions between herbal products and prescribed medications; for example, lower efficacy of corticosteroids and methotrexate associated with the use of products containing Echinacea. The National Institutes of Health Center for Complementary and Integrative Health has warehoused information that is a good resource for herbal medicines, including their use and safety concerns (https://nccih.nih.gov/health/herbsataglance.htm).

CARDIOVASCULAR OUTCOMES

Poor long-term CVD outcomes are a concern for many children with rheumatic diseases because of their chronic longstanding inflammation, abnormal risk factors as shown by markers of risk such as high C-reactive protein, and because of the strong association in adults who have RA and lupus with poor CVD outcomes.[34] Several studies, summarized by Coulson and colleagues,[35] have shown abnormal lipid profiles in children with various categories of JIA, not all related to corticosteroid treatment. Children with JIA have elevated systolic and diastolic blood pressures compared with healthy controls, although values were within normal levels.[35] In the Atherosclerosis Prevention in Pediatric Lupus Erythematous cohort, an intervention study of statins, at baseline patients had a higher carotid intima-media thickness (CIMT) that was associated with higher BMI, longer disease duration, increasing age, and male sex.[36] In adults with RA, a small study showed that reduction in CIMT was associated with clinical response to TNFi, and a large study demonstrated a greater than 2-fold reduction in first CVD events in patients treated with TNFi compared to those treated with other medications.[37,38] Similarly, a small study of prepubertal children with JIA revealed increased CIMT at diagnosis compared with healthy controls, and after a year of treatment, the greatest improvement in CIMT was in those treated with TNFi therapy.[39] Thus, there is ample evidence to show that children with rheumatic diseases have vascular abnormalities. However, what this means in terms of future cardiovascular risk is not known. It seems likely that effective disease treatment and, when possible, the avoidance of steroids can only be helpful from a cardiovascular standpoint.

GENERAL RECOMMENDATIONS FOR ACHIEVING BETTER NUTRITIONAL OUTCOMES

1. Because of a risk of growth failure and poor nutrition, providers should monitor growth parameters and perform general diet screening regularly.
2. Prescribers should recognize and attempt to mitigate corticosteroid side effects leading to obesity and poor bone and cardiovascular health by use of steroid-sparing agents such as disease-modifying antirheumatic drugs and BRMs to allow reduction of steroid dose and duration.
3. Providers should take a diet history, including use of supplements and herbal medications, and counsel families accordingly.
4. Children should eat regular meals with a balanced diet and suitable portion sizes, and receive nutritional support as needed.
5. Obesity should be treated aggressively with referral to programs for weight management, nutrition, and physical fitness.
6. Providers should screen for low 25-OH vitamin D and supplement as needed for bone health, as well as insure adequate calcium intake by supplementation as needed.
7. For children at risk for fracture due to moderate to high GCS use and obesity, providers should consider DXA imaging of the posterior-anterior spine and total body less head, to assess bone mineral content and areal bone mineral density (https://www.iscd.org/official-positions/2013-iscd-official-positions-pediatric/).

Diet Resources: More specific information and details for families can be found below:

Arthritis Foundation (US): http://www.kidsgetarthritistoo.org/living-with-ja/daily-life/healthy-eating/juvenile-arthritis-nutrition-2.php.
National Rheumatoid Arthritis Society (UK): http://www.jia.org.uk/diet-and-jia.

PHYSICAL FITNESS AND ACTIVITY FOR CHILDREN WITH RHEUMATIC DISEASES

Most studies of physical fitness in children with rheumatic disease have involved JIA patients with mainly joint disease. Some of these studies are applicable to children with other rheumatic diseases. However, it is important to remember that systemic rheumatic diseases including sJIA, lupus, dermatomyositis, and systemic vasculitis often have persistent internal organ or muscle involvement that also limits physical activity. In many such patients, a high level of inflammation causes anemia and constitutional symptoms that also diminish exercise tolerance. Clearly, effective medical treatment of these diseases is essential for improving physical fitness.

It is no surprise that children with JIA (previously known as juvenile rheumatoid arthritis) and polyarticular joint involvement have historically been less physically fit than their peers. A small study in 1992 showed that children with polyarticular JIA achieved poorer scores on a standardized physical fitness test compared to age, sex, and size-matched normally active, healthy children who were not involved in competitive athletics[40]. Ten years later, shortly after the initial approval of a TNFi for treatment of JIA, a meta-analysis of 5 studies of peak oxygen consumption during exercise showed moderate to severe impairment in cardiorespiratory fitness of JIA patients compared to healthy children[41]. In their own subsequent study these investigators demonstrated that the level of physical activity in JIA patients, as measured by an electronic activity monitor and by parental activity rating, was significantly related to cardiorespiratory fitness as measured by peak oxygen consumption during exercise, but not to body composition[42].

In the years following the advent of powerful new medications and more aggressive treatments for polyarticular JIA, anecdotally most pediatric rheumatologists saw impressive improvements in the physical function of many of their JIA patients, including better ability to exercise and sometimes to participate in sports. However, recent studies from Switzerland[43] and Australia[44] comparing children with JIA to healthy peers showed that those with JIA still have reduced total daily physical activity and reduced cardiorespiratory fitness. Only 38% of JIA patients met the recommend goal of 60 minutes of daily moderate to vigorous physical activity (MVPA), as compared to 60% of healthy controls[43]. More recently, even lower achievement of recommended MVPA (4% for JIA patients compared to 16% for controls) was documented in a 2016 study of JIA patients in The Netherlands, who had been treated for their joint disease according to modern guidelines and had low disease activity scores according to their rheumatologist[45]. In this study, lower MVPA correlated with lower self-assessment of overall wellbeing according to the standardized Child Health Assessment Questionnaire, and with higher self-assessment of pain. A recent study from Denmark using accelerometry to measure physical fitness also demonstrated lower levels of fitness in JIA patients compared to healthy controls matched for age and sex. Lower physical activity in the JIA group correlated with low fitness level, higher erythrocyte sedimentation rate, higher overall disease activity, and higher number of joints with swelling or limited range of motion, especially hip and ankle joints[46]. However, unlike the previously mentioned study from The Netherlands[45], there was no relationship between physical activity and pain scores[46]. In a second report involving the same study, the only psychosocial factor identified to be associated with higher physical fitness scores was the patient's specific belief of having control of pain[47].

It is likely that multiple factors contribute to the lower levels of fitness and physical activity in recent studies of JIA patients with low disease activity. Fitness and physical activity go hand-in-hand, each influencing the other. In the previously discussed early study[40] of physical fitness in polyarticular JIA patients, fitness levels were not always related to degree of disease activity as estimated by active joint counts or disease severity scores, leading the authors to hypothesize that lower physical fitness may also be associated with family, physician, and school concerns about potential limitations. In the aforementioned recent study from Australia[44], although the JIA patients did not have any impairment in fundamental movement skills, parents of these children reported significantly more physical and psychosocial impairments in both their children and themselves, compared to the healthy controls and their parents. These results suggest that parental concern about their child's abilities and exercise capacity may lead to discouraging or setting limitations on the child's physical activity.

In addition to socially imposed limitations, fatigue can be a significant problem for JIA patients, and can be the result of both physical and psychological factors. Fatigue is associated with disability and poor self-efficacy. Some interventions to increase overall activity level, reduce perceived disability, and increase self-efficacy may reduce fatigue and improve overall functioning[48].

An appropriate amount of exercise reduces disease-related disability, encourages an active lifestyle, improves bone and cardiovascular health, and does not exacerbate arthritis[49]. In view of the many benefits of exercise, educating children with rheumatic disease and their families on the child's appropriate level of physical activity, and encouraging these children to engage in exercise, is important. Although most will be unable to participate in highly competitive sports activities, a recreational sports team or another exercise activity may be a good fit.

EXERCISE INTERVENTIONS

Although physical therapy has always been important for mobilizing joints with flexion contractures and strengthening muscles around joints, recently a number of aerobic exercise interventions have been developed for JIA patients with a goal of increasing overall physical fitness. One of the first randomized, controlled trials of exercise for JIA patients was conduced by Canadian investigators in 2007. This 12-week, single-blinded study comparing 2 exercise programs (high-intensity aerobics vs qigong) 3 times weekly demonstrated no difference in cardiorespiratory fitness as assessed by peak oxygen uptake and other measures. However, participants in both programs had significant improvement in scores on the Child Health Assessment Questionnaire, and compliance with qigong was better.[50] In 2017, a systematic literature review was conducted to create guidelines on the use of structured physical activity in JIA management. Grade A evidence from randomized randomized clinical trials was found for the following recommendations: (1) Pilates for improving pain, quality of life, functional ability, and range of motion (ROM), (2) a home exercise program for improving quality of life and functional ability, and (3) an aquatic aerobic fitness program for decreasing the number of active joints.

A recent observer-blinded, randomized, controlled trial conducted in 3 centers in The Netherlands studied the effects of a new internet-based program called rheumates@work. The study compared outcomes in an intervention group who participated in a cognitive and physical internet-based training program for 14 weeks combined with 4 group sessions versus a control group who received standard care. They found a positive effect in the intervention group on physical activity, exercise capacity, and participation in school and physical education class in the intervention group, with improvements lasting for 12 months.[51]

Compliance with an exercise program that will carry over to become part of the participants' lifestyle has long been a challenge for both healthy persons and those with disabilities. One recently studied exercise intervention consisted of a "gamified" series of walking contests between groups of healthy adolescents in several schools in Northern Ireland, using pedometers and an internet site. The perception of being a part of a team, peer influence, competition against oneself, and positive reinforcement or incentives were among the factors found to be important for continuing participation[52]. Alternative programs that encourage children onto a lifelong pathway to exercise are being used in many pediatric centers across the United States. These programs focus on the idea that exercise is medicine, and for children, the approach to exercise is through play/recreation. Although specific details of these programs vary, general elements are similar. A typical program targeting children with chronic diseases is developed and supervised by sports medicine physicians, athletic trainers, and physical therapists, who collaborate with a variety of subspecialty providers who refer children. It engages the patients and families in the physical activity program, which aims to change: (1) thoughts and attitudes toward physical activity, (2) habits at home regarding physical activity, (3) functional movement skills and fitness measures, including strength, coordination, balance, and endurance, and (4) confidence to engage in a variety of physical activities with friends and peers. After an initial evaluation, based on baseline function, children are put into a 1:1 rehabilitation program, group exercise and play class, or a strength and conditioning class. Such programs hold promise to be particularly effective in promoting enjoyment of exercise and its incorporation into overall lifestyle for children who are accustomed to being sedentary due to disease or attitudes.

Exercise Program Resources: More specific information and details for physicians can be found below:

http://www.exerciseismedicine.org/support_page.php/physical-activity-health-impact/

http://www.nationwidechildrens.org/play-strong.

GENERAL PRINCIPLES AND RECOMMENDATIONS ON ACTIVITY AND EXERCISE

1. If the child's rheumatic disease is active or flaring, it may be best to hold intense activities until disease is better controlled and/or to discuss further with the pediatric rheumatologist.
2. If the child is improving from an active disease episode or in remission, start discussion about benefits of physical activity globally for weight management, improvement in pain and stiffness, and long-term cardiovascular health.
3. Complete a brief assessment of the child's physical activity in terms of intensity, frequency, and duration per week.
4. Determine the perceptions about exercise and activity abilities and limitation from both child and parents.
5. Plan on whether a home exercise program will be implemented or whether a structured program would be better suited.
6. Recommend daily physical activity based on patient abilities with the ultimate goal of dynamic, high-impact, and resistance activities.
7. Reassess adherence to exercise program, daily activity, and fitness in 3 to 4 months. If there are no significant changes from baseline behavior, recommend referral to a structured program or physical therapist.

Home Exercise Resources: Some examples of online exercise games and dances for children, ways to incorporate physical activity into everyday life for families, age-related guidelines for physical activity, and handouts for physicians can be found below:

www.gonoodle.com/

http://www.kidsgetarthritistoo.org/living-with-ja/daily-life/staying-active/ja-exercise.php.

https://www.nhlbi.nih.gov/health/educational/wecan/get-active/getting-active.htm.

https://www.caringforkids.cps.ca/handouts/physical.activity.

REFERENCES

1. Khalid U, Egeberg A, Ahlehoff O, et al. Incident heart failure in patients with rheumatoid arthritis: a nationwide cohort study. J Am Heart Assoc 2018;7(2) [pii:e007227].

2. Sevilla WMA. Nutritional considerations in pediatric chronic disease. Pediatr Rev 2017;38(8):343–52.
3. Matthys P, Billiau A. Cytokines and cachexia. Nutrition 1997;13(9):763–70.
4. Kyle UG, Shekerdemian LS, Coss-Bu JA. Growth failure and nutrition considerations in chronic childhood wasting diseases. Nutr Clin Pract 2015;30(2):227–38.
5. Simon D, Prieur AM, Quartier P, et al. Early recombinant human growth hormone treatment in glucocorticoid-treated children with juvenile idiopathic arthritis: a 3-year randomized study. J Clin Endocrinol Metab 2007;92(7):2567–73.
6. Stoeber E. Prognosis in juvenile chronic arthritis. Follow-up of 433 chronic rheumatic children. Eur J Pediatr 1981;135(3):225–8.
7. Simon D, Fernando C, Czernichow P, et al. Linear growth and final height in patients with systemic juvenile idiopathic arthritis treated with longterm glucocorticoids. J Rheumatol 2002;29(6):1296–300.
8. Simon D. rhGH treatment in corticosteroid-treated patients. Horm Res 2007; 68(1):38–45.
9. Rygg M, Pistorio A, Ravelli A, et al. A longitudinal PRINTO study on growth and puberty in juvenile systemic lupus erythematosus. Ann Rheum Dis 2012;71(4): 511–7.
10. Tynjala P, Lahdenne P, Vahasalo P, et al. Impact of anti-TNF treatment on growth in severe juvenile idiopathic arthritis. Ann Rheum Dis 2006;65(8):1044–9.
11. Giannini EH, Ilowite NT, Lovell DJ, et al. Effects of long-term etanercept treatment on growth in children with selected categories of juvenile idiopathic arthritis. Arthritis Rheum 2010;62(11):3259–64.
12. Uettwiller F, Perlbarg J, Pinto G, et al. Effect of biologic treatments on growth in children with juvenile idiopathic arthritis. J Rheumatol 2014;41(1):128–35.
13. Shiff NJ, Brant R, Guzman J, et al. Glucocorticoid-related changes in body mass index among children and adolescents with rheumatic diseases. Arthritis Care Res (Hoboken) 2013;65(1):113–21.
14. Guzman J, Kerr T, Ward LM, et al. Growth and weight gain in children with juvenile idiopathic arthritis: results from the ReACCh-Out cohort. Pediatr Rheumatol Online J 2017;15(1):68.
15. Pelajo CF, Lopez-Benitez JM, Miller LC. Obesity and disease activity in juvenile idiopathic arthritis. Pediatr Rheumatol Online J 2012;10(1):3.
16. Schenck S, Niewerth M, Sengler C, et al. Prevalence of overweight in children and adolescents with juvenile idiopathic arthritis. Scand J Rheumatol 2015;44(4): 288–95.
17. Voulgari PV. Rheumatological manifestations in inflammatory bowel disease. Ann Gastroenterol 2011;24(3):173–80.
18. Lerner A, Matthias T. Rheumatoid arthritis-celiac disease relationship: joints get that gut feeling. Autoimmun Rev 2015;14(11):1038–47.
19. Sherman Y, Karanicolas R, DiMarco B, et al. Unrecognized celiac disease in children presenting for rheumatology evaluation. Pediatrics 2015;136(1):e68–75.
20. Shor DB, Dahan S, Comaneshter D, et al. Does inflammatory bowel disease coexist with systemic lupus erythematosus? Autoimmun Rev 2016;15(11): 1034–7.
21. Cassidy JT, Hillman LS. Abnormalities in skeletal growth in children with juvenile rheumatoid arthritis. Rheum Dis Clin North Am 1997;23(3):499–522.
22. Zhang Y, Milojevic D. Protecting bone health in pediatric rheumatic diseases: pharmacological considerations. Paediatr Drugs 2017;19(3):193–211.
23. Lima GL, Paupitz J, Aikawa NE, et al. Vitamin D supplementation in adolescents and young adults with juvenile systemic lupus erythematosus for improvement in

disease activity and fatigue scores: a randomized, double-blind, placebo-controlled trial. Arthritis Care Res (Hoboken) 2016;68(1):91–8.

24. April KT, Walji R. The state of research on complementary and alternative medicine in pediatric rheumatology. Rheum Dis Clin North Am 2011;37(1):85–94.

25. Nousiainen P, Merras-Salmio L, Aalto K, et al. Complementary and alternative medicine use in adolescents with inflammatory bowel disease and juvenile idiopathic arthritis. BMC Complement Altern Med 2014;14:124.

26. Fadanelli G, Vittadello F, Martini G, et al. Complementary and alternative medicine (CAM) in paediatric rheumatology: a European perspective. Clin Exp Rheumatol 2012;30(1):132–6.

27. April KT, Feldman DE, Zunzunegui MV, et al. Longitudinal analysis of complementary and alternative health care use in children with juvenile idiopathic arthritis. Complement Ther Med 2009;17(4):208–15.

28. Hu Y, Costenbader KH, Gao X, et al. Sugar-sweetened soda consumption and risk of developing rheumatoid arthritis in women. Am J Clin Nutr 2014;100(3):959–67.

29. Chen L, Michalsen A. Management of chronic pain using complementary and integrative medicine. BMJ 2017;357:j1284.

30. Goni L, Cuervo M, Milagro FI, et al. Influence of fat intake and BMI on the association of rs1799983 NOS3 polymorphism with blood pressure levels in an Iberian population. Eur J Nutr 2017;56(4):1589–96.

31. Goldberg RJ, Katz J. A meta-analysis of the analgesic effects of omega-3 polyunsaturated fatty acid supplementation for inflammatory joint pain. Pain 2007; 129(1–2):210–23.

32. Senftleber NK, Nielsen SM, Andersen JR, et al. Marine oil supplements for arthritis pain: a systematic review and meta-analysis of randomized trials. Nutrients 2017;9(1) [pii:E42].

33. Jiang J, Li K, Wang F, et al. Effect of marine-derived n-3 polyunsaturated fatty acids on major eicosanoids: a systematic review and meta-analysis from 18 randomized controlled trials. PLoS One 2016;11(1):e0147351.

34. Goodson NJ, Symmons DP, Scott DG, et al. Baseline levels of C-reactive protein and prediction of death from cardiovascular disease in patients with inflammatory polyarthritis: a ten-year followup study of a primary care-based inception cohort. Arthritis Rheum 2005;52(8):2293–9.

35. Coulson EJ, Ng WF, Goff I, et al. Cardiovascular risk in juvenile idiopathic arthritis. Rheumatology (Oxford) 2013;52(7):1163–71.

36. Schanberg LE, Sandborg C, Barnhart HX, et al. Premature atherosclerosis in pediatric systemic lupus erythematosus: risk factors for increased carotid intima-media thickness in the atherosclerosis prevention in pediatric lupus erythematosus cohort. Arthritis Rheum 2009;60(5):1496–507.

37. Del Porto F, Lagana B, Lai S, et al. Response to anti-tumour necrosis factor alpha blockade is associated with reduction of carotid intima-media thickness in patients with active rheumatoid arthritis. Rheumatology (Oxford) 2007;46(7):1111–5.

38. Jacobsson LT, Turesson C, Gulfe A, et al. Treatment with tumor necrosis factor blockers is associated with a lower incidence of first cardiovascular events in patients with rheumatoid arthritis. J Rheumatol 2005;32(7):1213–8.

39. Breda L, Di Marzio D, Giannini C, et al. Relationship between inflammatory markers, oxidant-antioxidant status and intima-media thickness in prepubertal children with juvenile idiopathic arthritis. Clin Res Cardiol 2013;102(1):63–71.

40. Klepper SE, Darbee J, Effgen SK, et al. Physical fitness levels in children with polyarticular juvenile rheumatoid arthritis. Arthritis Care Res 1992;5(2):93–100.

41. Takken T, van der Net J, Helders PJ. Aerobic fitness in children with juvenile idiopathic arthritis: a systematic review. J Rheumatol 2002;29(12):2643–7.
42. Takken T, van der Net J, Kuis W, et al. Physical activity and health related physical fitness in children with juvenile idiopathic arthritis. Ann Rheum Dis 2003;62(9): 885–9.
43. Maggio AB, Hofer MF, Martin XE, et al. Reduced physical activity level and cardiorespiratory fitness in children with chronic diseases. Eur J Pediatr 2010; 169(10):1187–93.
44. Hulsegge G, Henschke N, McKay D, et al. Fundamental movement skills, physical fitness and physical activity among Australian children with juvenile idiopathic arthritis. J Paediatr Child Health 2015;51(4):425–32.
45. Bos GJ, Lelieveld OT, Wineke A, et al. Physical activity in children with juvenile idiopathic arthritis compared to controls. Pediatr Rheumatol Online J 2016; 14(1):42.
46. Norgaard M, Twilt M, Andersen LB, et al. Accelerometry-based monitoring of daily physical activity in children with juvenile idiopathic arthritis. Scand J Rheumatol 2016;45(3):179–87.
47. Norgaard M, Lomholt JJ, Thastum M, et al. Accelerometer-assessed daily physical activity in relation to pain cognition in juvenile idiopathic arthritis. Scand J Rheumatol 2017;46(1):22–6.
48. Armbrust W, Lelieveld OH, Tuinstra J, et al. Fatigue in patients with juvenile idiopathic arthritis: relationship to perceived health, physical health, self-efficacy, and participation. Pediatr Rheumatol Online J 2016;14(1):65.
49. Long AR, Rouster-Stevens KA. The role of exercise therapy in the management of juvenile idiopathic arthritis. Curr Opin Rheumatol 2010;22(2):213–7.
50. Cavallo S, Brosseau L, Toupin-April K, et al. Ottawa panel evidence-based clinical practice guidelines for structured physical activity in the management of juvenile idiopathic arthritis. Arch Phys Med Rehabil 2017;98(5):1018–41.
51. Singh-Grewal D, Schneiderman-Walker J, Wright V, et al. The effects of vigorous exercise training on physical function in children with arthritis: a randomized, controlled, single-blinded trial. Arthritis Rheum 2007;57(7):1202–10.
52. Corepal R, Best P, O'Neill R, et al. Exploring the use of a gamified intervention for encouraging physical activity in adolescents: a qualitative longitudinal study in Northern Ireland. BMJ Open 2018;0:e019663.

Transitions in Rheumatic Disease: Pediatric to Adult Care

Stacy P. Ardoin, MD, MS

KEYWORDS

- Transition • Rheumatology • Adolescent • Young adult self-management
- Chronic disease • Health care outcomes

KEY POINTS

- Young adults with a broad spectrum of rheumatic disease are vulnerable to poor health and outcomes, highlighting the importance of optimizing the transition to adult care.
- Too often, young adults are ill-prepared for adult care and face substantial challenges, including insufficient education and guidance, interruptions in care, and poor health and vocational outcomes.
- The ideal transition to adult rheumatologic care begins in early adolescence when patients, families, and pediatric providers start to prepare young adults to integrate easily into care with a prepared and proactive adult health care team.
- Primary care and rheumatology providers need to develop, study, and implement interventions to improve transition and transfer processes and health care outcomes for young adults.
- Quality improvement approaches such as the Six Core Elements of Health Care Transition offer opportunities to improve transition care for teens and young adults.

INTRODUCTION: WHY IS TRANSITION FROM PEDIATRIC TO ADULT CARE IMPORTANT?

The successful transition of the young adult patient with chronic disease to adult care is an important milestone in pediatric medicine. The ability to transition care, which for many with serious chronic illnesses may not have been possible in previous eras, reflects improved survival because of advances in preventive care and management of acute and chronic illness. In fact, 90% of children with chronic health conditions survive into adulthood, and around 500,000 young adults with special health care needs become adults each year.[1] Among the estimated 18 million adolescents and young adults in the United States 18 to 21 years of age, about one-quarter have chronic health problems, including rheumatic diseases.[2] Unfortunately, the transition from pediatric-centered to adult-centered health care can be a vulnerable period for young

Disclosure Statement: The author has no relevant disclosures.
Pediatric Rheumatology, Nationwide Children's Hospital, 700 Children's Drive, Columbus, OH 43205, USA
E-mail address: stacy.ardoin@nationwidechildrens.org

Pediatr Clin N Am 65 (2018) 867–883
https://doi.org/10.1016/j.pcl.2018.04.007
0031-3955/18/© 2018 Elsevier Inc. All rights reserved.

adults with rheumatic and other chronic diseases. Hazards include gaps in continuity of care, poor treatment adherence, delays in establishing adult care, differences between adult and pediatric health care systems, inconsistent availability of appropriately trained adult providers, self-management challenges, and unstable medical conditions. The 2014 Institute of Medicine report, "Investing in Health and Well Being of Young Adults," highlights the transition from pediatric to adult health care as an important component of improving the health of young adults, particularly those who have chronic disease.[2]

Without needed support and input from adult and pediatric providers through the transition process, young adults often experience decreased quality of care, increased health care costs, and poor health.[3] Young adults are more likely to use the emergency department and to have lower health status and higher mortality compared with older and younger cohorts.[3–9] The situation is even worse for minority and impoverished adolescents and young adults, who report being less likely to receive transition counseling, which likely contributes to health disparities for these populations.[7]

Childhood-Onset Rheumatic Diseases Become Adult Problems

Most childhood-onset rheumatic diseases persist into adulthood. For example, more than half of the patients with juvenile idiopathic arthritis (JIA) experience active disease in adulthood, requiring ongoing management of immunosuppressive medications.[10–12] Young adults with JIA are at increased risk to drop out of medical care, and some adult rheumatologists express discomfort in the medical management of JIA.[13–16] Childhood-onset lupus is always a lifelong disorder. It is associated with high acuity and frequent hospitalization, risks of disability even in childhood, and higher morbidity and mortality compared with adult-onset lupus.[17–20] Transitioning young adults with lupus are at risk for significant gaps in care.[20] North American parents of youth with inflammatory myopathies report low awareness of transition policy and lack of a transition plan or medical summary.[21] In a retrospective, single-center study of 31 patients with a variety of chronic rheumatic diseases, 58% had active disease when transferring to adult providers, 30% were hospitalized for disease flare in the year before transfer, and 30% experienced an increase in disease activity in the posttransfer year.[22]

Many young adults with chronic disease are also less likely to achieve college education and maintain employment and will have lower income compared with those without chronic disease.[23] Young adults with JIA tend to have higher rates of unemployment, with some studies showing lower and others showing comparable education attainment compared with the general population.[24–27] Those with childhood-onset lupus similarly have less employment than their peers despite similar education.[28] Young adults with rheumatic disorders report problems with absenteeism, job disruptions due to illness, and productivity loss.[29] They also express concerns about employers' attitudes toward young adults with chronic diseases.[30]

WHAT ARE THE BARRIERS TO SUCCESSFUL TRANSITION?

Several national surveys demonstrate that most adolescents, young adults, and their parents are inadequately prepared for the transition to adult care.[1–5] Although some of the barriers to successful transition to adult care are disease specific, most young adults experience similar challenges across the spectrum of chronic diseases. A recent systemic review examining 57 disease-specific chronic illness transition studies identified the following common thematic barriers to transition: health care access/insurance; patient, parent, and provider beliefs/expectations; relationships; and young adult and provider knowledge, skills, and efficacy.[31] In addition, the neurologic and psychosocial development of adolescents and young adults, and problems with treatment adherence, are challenges to the transition process.

Insurance and Access to Care

Before the 2010 Patient Protection and Affordable Health Care Act (ACA) in the United States, approximately 50% of young adults reported gaps (on average lasting 15 months) in insurance coverage.[32] The ACA expanded parental coverage for young adults up to age 26 years, so that the issue of inadequate coverage is shifted to 26- to 34-year-olds who are now the least likely to have reliable health care insurance.[33] Compared with older counterparts, young adults are more likely to "churn" or change insurance frequently, introducing potential for delays in care because of required changes in providers or health care systems.[32] Other challenges young adults face include finding conveniently located, qualified adult providers who accept their insurance, affording out of pocket medical costs and high deductibles, lack of confidence navigating insurance systems, and increased utilization of emergency departments for routine health concerns.

Beliefs and Expectations

Young adults and their families often have negative beliefs and expectations about adult care, and unfortunately pediatric providers sometimes promote these beliefs. The differences between adult and pediatric care models can produce a significant "culture shock" if young adults are not appropriately prepared for transition. As outlined in **Fig. 1**, the approaches in pediatric and adult health care differ. For example, a young adult who is used to a pediatric provider offering a longer appointment time may not appreciate the necessarily shorter visit with an adult provider and may perceive that quality of care is lower, regardless of outcomes. The adult provider may emphasize autonomy, efficiency, and respect for the patient's time. Adult providers may describe young adult patients as ill prepared, dependent on parents, and "needy," whereas both young adults and pediatric providers may view adult providers as disinterested or distant. The discordant expectations surrounding adult and pediatric care, if not negotiated properly, can contribute to challenges in young adults' integration into adult care.

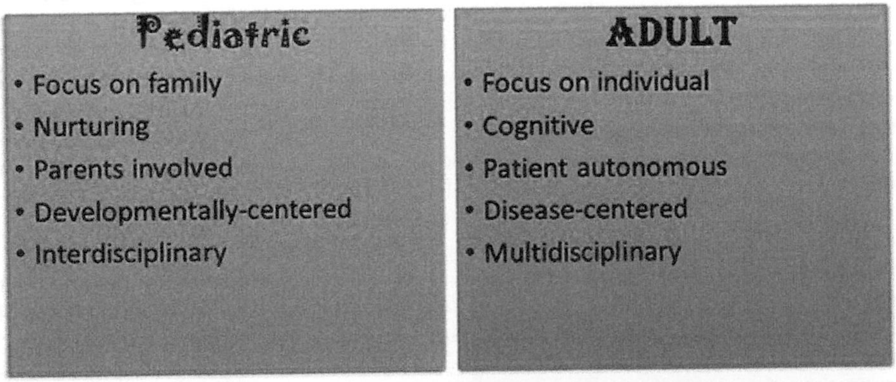

Pediatric	ADULT
• Focus on family	• Focus on individual
• Nurturing	• Cognitive
• Parents involved	• Patient autonomous
• Developmentally-centered	• Disease-centered
• Interdisciplinary	• Multidisciplinary

Fig. 1. The approaches to care in pediatric and adult health care differ, and if appropriate education and expectation setting do not occur during the transition process, the resultant "culture shock" can introduce the young adult transitioning to adult care.

Relationships

Adolescents and young adults with chronic rheumatic disease have often developed strong attachments to pediatric providers and can understandably be reluctant to leave a familiar and comforting environment.[34] Pediatric providers can also be reluctant to "let go," which can frustrate the transition process. Thus, the transition to adult care can be viewed by patients, families, and providers as a negative event than as an accomplishment. When a young adult sees an adult provider for the first time, it can be challenging for the adult provider to quickly establish the rapport and trust that existed in the long-term relationship with the pediatric provider. When adult providers fail to take some time to get to know young adult patients, they miss opportunities to gain young adults' trust and confidence.

Knowledge, Skills, and Efficacy

Adult providers report that young adults entering adult care often lack knowledge about their disease history, medications, and the transition process.[34,35] These knowledge deficits are compounded when appropriate medical records are not shared between providers. Unfortunately, poor adherence to treatment regimens and visit schedules is common among young adults, especially those who lack self-management skills and health literacy.[35] Adult rheumatology practices may have less access to ancillary support, such as social workers, who can support struggling young adults or devote time to tracking down patients who do not show for appointments. In addition, adult providers may lack training and confidence concerning caring for young adults and miss opportunities to assess and encourage young adults' self-care abilities. Many adult providers in private practice have limited appointment time, and those in academic institutions may lack institutional support for longer appointments to help accomplish successful transition. Further, most do not have established protocols for integrating young adults into their practice. Adult providers who assume care of youth with chronic disease often do not receive a summary of the medical records or educational information about the special needs of young adults with pediatric-onset diseases. Sharing of electronic medical records and summaries may help with this barrier.

Neurodevelopment

It comes as no surprise to parents and pediatric care providers that the adolescent/young adult brain functions differently from that of a young child or an older adult. Adolescents and young adults are well known for their creativity, emotionality, impulsiveness, risk-taking behavior, and heightened sensitivity to acceptance and rejection.[36] Longitudinal structural and functional brain magnetic resonance imaging studies provide neurodevelopmental insight for these behaviors. The brain undergoes tremendous change between the ages of 11 and 25 years, including the expansion and later pruning of gray matter, marked synaptic proliferation and remodeling in the prefrontal cortex, and enhanced sensitivity to dopamine.[36–39] As a consequence, adult-oriented executive function, emotional regulation, and decision-making care are not at their full capacity until the age of late 20s. In addition, adolescents and young adults with chronic health conditions, and especially those with disability, are at enhanced risk for mental health disorders including anxiety and depression, which may further affect neurodevelopment and behaviors.[40] These findings have particularly important implications for medical management of young adults in the areas of adherence to treatment plans and negotiation of risk-taking behaviors in the setting of potentially toxic and teratogenic medications.

Adherence to Treatment

Available evidence and clinical experience suggest that adolescents and young adults are at particular risk for nonadherence to treatment, particularly medications.[41,42] Medication adherence is challenging to measure, and available strategies include patient self-report, provider assessment, pill counts, and refill tracking.[43] Of note, health care providers are poor in estimating patients' adherence.[44] In certain instances, laboratory values can serve as surrogate markers of adherence, including hemoglobin A1C levels in diabetics, viral loads in those with human immunodeficiency virus, and medication levels in transplant recipients. Measurements of hydroxychloroquine, mycophenolate, and 6-mercaptopurine levels have been used to estimate adherence in lupus patients.[45–47] Commonly cited reasons for nonadherence include forgetting to take or refill medication, difficulty in obtaining refills, medical regimen complexity, and out-of-pocket medication costs.[48] Rigorously studied interventions to improve medication adherence in adolescents and young adults are lacking, and creative interventions such as text reminders and financial incentives have shown mixed and often disappointing results.[49–51] Available evidence suggests that routine electronic feedback to providers about medication nonadherence (eg, reporting delinquent medication refills) may lead to improvements in adherence but has not been shown to improve clinical outcomes.[52] Other forms of nonadherence including failure to comply with treatment visits, laboratory monitoring, exercise regimens, and behavioral recommendations are also important but less well studied. Overall, although adherence to treatment regimens is very important in adolescents and young adults, clearly effective interventions to improve adherence remain an unmet need.

ASSESSING YOUNG ADULTS' TRANSITION READINESS AND NEEDS
Assessing Readiness to Transition in Adolescents and Young Adults

In current practice, young adults are often ill-prepared or transfer abruptly and are not capable of functioning independently in the adult health care system. Several generic- and condition-specific tools have been developed and validated to assess adolescents' and young adults' preparedness to function in an adult model of care.[53,54] Examples of disease neutral tools include the Transition Readiness Assessment Questionnaire (TRAQ),[55] the TRxANSITION Scale, and the Am I ON TRAC for Adult Care questionnaire.[56] A Got Transition tool is also available (www.gottransition.org); this program will be discussed in more detail in later section. Common to all transition readiness measures are questions aimed at assessing young adults' experience and comfort in interacting independently with providers, obtaining and taking medications consistently, and negotiating insurance and health care systems. The Patient Activation Measure (PAM) correlates with transition readiness.[57] The Readiness for Adult Care in Rheumatology (RACER) questionnaire is specific to this subspecialty.[53,58] Administration and tabulation of scorable transition readiness assessments can be billed by providers as health care assessments. Although higher scores on transition readiness instruments have not clearly been linked to successful transition or other transition outcomes,[57] their utility for the primary care or rheumatology provider is in using them regularly to facilitate ongoing transition dialogue, needs assessment, and planning with patients and their families.

What Do Young Adults with Rheumatic Disease Want?

When surveyed, adolescents and young adults with rheumatic disease indicate that they prioritize having adult health care providers who view them as a person and not a diagnosis want confidentiality and independence in their care and medical information.[59–65] They are interested in knowing about the adult provider's training and how to access adult health care. Young adults often prefer to adopt newer health care technology and communication platforms, such as electronic portals or texting, and may be unresponsive to information shared by telephone or mail.[59–65]

MODELS FOR TRANSITION TO ADULT CARE

Generally, structured transition programs emphasize adolescent and young adult education, self-efficacy, decision-making, and self-advocacy. As shown in **Fig. 2**, the transition to adult care is a gradual process and as the adolescent matures, communication and decision-making are increasingly directed toward the patient than focused primarily on the parent. Optimally, the transfer of care occurs at a time when disease is well controlled, and for patients who have multiple health care providers, it is best if transitions to adult providers occur in a staggered fashion. Overall, the strategy is to support adolescent and young adults' competence, confidence, and independence in self-management and coping. The transfer of care to an adult provider is the endpoint of the transition and, ideally, the young adult is seamlessly integrated into an adult practice.

There is a broad menu of approaches to managing transition, which includes disease-specific clinics, young adult clinics, collaboration with dual adult and pediatric trained providers, and use of transition coordinators to bridge adult and pediatric clinics. Most of the programs described in the literature are small, resource-intensive, highly dependent on specific local resources or grant funding, and likely not scalable to larger populations. Recent systematic reviews show that structured transition interventions in rheumatic and other diseases have achieved statistically significant positive results, but the overall quality of studies is low because of small size, opportunities for bias, nonrandomization, inadequate descriptions of interventions, variability in definitions of successful transition, and inconsistent outcome measurement.[60,61,63–66] Very few transition studies have a "triple aim" approach, which requires evaluation of patient experience, population health, and health care cost.[3] In a technical brief, the US Agency for Healthcare Research and Quality has recognized that the limited evidence base hinders determination of optimal transition interventions.[67]

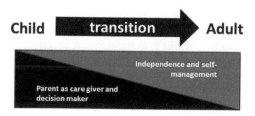

Fig. 2. The transition from pediatric to adult care is a gradual process, ideally beginning at age 12 to 14 years, during which the adolescent learns self-management skills and becomes more independent. As a result, self-care responsibilities and decision-making shift from parent to young adult. Transfer of care to an adult provider occurs at the end of the transition process.

HOW ARE WE DOING IN RHEUMATOLOGY?
State of Current Transition Processes for Adolescents and Young Adults with Rheumatic Disease

Pediatric and adult rheumatology providers have expressed dissatisfaction with the current state of transition processes for childhood-onset rheumatic disease. A survey of members of Childhood Arthritis and Rheumatology Research Alliance (CARRA), an organization that represents more than 90% of North American pediatric rheumatology providers, showed that 56% of respondents found current transition practices unsatisfactory; 90% lacked familiarity with the American Academy of Pediatrics (AAP), American College of Physicians (ACP), and American Academy of Family Physicians (AAFP) transition recommendations (discussed in later section); and only 8% reported using a formal transition policy in their practice.[68] The most commonly reported barriers to implementing transition processes included poor provider training, limited time, low reimbursement, and inadequate access to resources and personnel. Most respondents (>80%) agreed with a need for rheumatology-specific guidelines for transition.[68] Recent surveys of European pediatric rheumatology providers identified similar results.[69,70] A 2014 survey of adult rheumatology providers who were American College of Rheumatology members identified poor familiarity with transition guidelines and lack of formal processes to integrate young adults into adult practices. Many (48%) stated that the medical history information they received from pediatric providers was inadequate, and more than 80% expressed a need for tools and guidelines to help with transition of young adults.[71]

Do Transition Interventions Work in Rheumatology?

Although limited data are available concerning evidence-based transition improvement processes for adolescents and young adults with rheumatic disease, successful transition interventions in rheumatology have been described. For example, in the United Kingdom, a multisite, controlled trial evaluating a structured transition support program for adolescent and young adult JIA showed improvements in knowledge about JIA, use of transition plans, attendance rates at rheumatology appointments, and willingness to undergo joint injections without sedation.[72] In the United States, small, single-center structured transition program interventions have improved rates of successful transfer of care to adult providers in patients with rheumatic disease.[73,74]

Most available studies, however, indicate that youth with rheumatic disease usually transition successfully to adult providers at best about half of the time. For example, in a three-year follow up of 16- to 23-year-olds with rheumatic and other chronic diseases receiving nonstructured transitional care, only 48% successfully transferred to adult care.[57] Even in the setting of a coordinated Canadian rheumatology transition program, 52% of young adults with JIA failed to see an adult rheumatologist or experienced more than 1-year gap in care.[75] Similarly, in a UK structured transition program, 57% of young adults with rheumatic disease did not satisfy predefined criteria for successful transfer of care to adult providers.[76] Thus, even with interventions and deliberate planning, transition outcomes are often disappointing, suggesting that current approaches and practices do not adequately address the vulnerabilities associated with adolescent and young adult neurodevelopmental and psychosocial development and health care navigation.

Transition intervention studies in rheumatology and other chronic diseases tend to focus on satisfaction, quality of life outcomes, or rates of transfer to adult care. A critically important gap in current knowledge is whether transition process interventions can improve actual disease outcomes such as joint health in JIA, renal survival in systemic lupus erythematosus, or overall mortality. Outcome improvements after transition interventions have been demonstrated in small studies of renal graft survival in the setting of renal transplantation and in hemoglobin A1C levels in diabetes.[77–79]

ROLE OF PRIMARY CARE PROVIDERS IN TRANSITION TO ADULT CARE

Adult and pediatric primary care providers play vital roles in ensuring the successful transition to adult care.[73] Limited available data suggest that, as in rheumatology practices, structured transition processes are often absent in primary care practices.[80] Transfer from US pediatric to adult primary care tends to occur later than recommended and is susceptible to the same gaps in care characteristic of subspecialty transition care.[81] Pediatric rheumatologists often see their patients more frequently than primary care providers do and may assume preventive care responsibilities, such as overseeing immunizations, performing sports physicals, and counseling on contraception. Although providing these preventive services in the subspecialty clinic can be convenient to families, it can also discourage the connection to the primary care provider and set up unrealistic expectations that adult subspecialists will function as primary care providers. In some studies, adult primary care providers express lack of interest or confidence in accepting young adults with chronic health conditions.[81–83] Primary care transition models for complicated patients can include complex care clinics, young adult transition clinics, and dual internal medicine and pediatrics trained primary care providers. The need to develop appropriate self-management skills remains even when a young adult stays with the same provider during transition.

Transitioning adolescents and young adults with rheumatic diseases also need guidance concerning realistic and educational and vocational expectations, given their higher likelihood of unemployment and job maintenance and performance issues. In US public high schools, resources such as 504 plans and individualized educational plans are often needed. Providers can encourage linkage with disability services in the university setting. Referral to vocational rehabilitation can help young adults find appropriate employment, and adult providers can provide letters supporting needed accommodations to employers.

GUIDELINES AND SYSTEMS-BASED APPROACHES TO TRANSITION IMPROVEMENT

A 2012 joint clinical report from the AAP, ACP, and AAFP provides guidance to primary and specialty care providers concerning how best to support adolescents and young adults through the transition process, with specific age-specific recommendations (**Fig. 3**).[84] These guidelines suggest that the process of transition planning begins at age 12 to 14 years, with a gradual preparation for adult care over the ensuing years, and that the actual transfer to adult care providers occurs between the ages of 18 and 22 years. More recently, the European League against Rheumatism (EULAR) and Pediatric Rheumatology European Society (PRES) provided rheumatology-specific guidelines for the transfer from pediatric to adult care, which are summarized in **Box 1**.[85]

Building upon the 2012 AAP, AAFP, and ACP clinical report, and to address the unmet needs of adolescents and young adults, Got Transition: The Center for Health Care Transition Improvement was founded. It is a US national center for health care transition funded by the Maternal and Child Health Bureau and The National Alliance to Advance Alliance Health, which has developed a systematic, quality improvement–

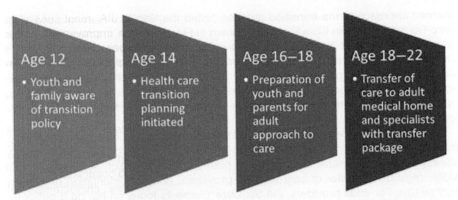

Fig. 3. The 2011 joint recommendations from the American Academy of Pediatrics, American College of Physicians, and American Association of Family Practitioners provide age-based guidelines for the transition process. These recommendations apply to primary care providers and to specialists. (*Data from* American Academy of Pediatrics, American Academy of Family Physicians, American College of Physicians, Transitions Clinical Report Authoring Group, Cooley WC, Sagerman PJ. Supporting the health care transition from adolescence to adulthood in the medical home. Pediatrics 2011;128(1):182–200.)

Box 1
Summary of European League against Rheumatism/Pediatric Rheumatology European Society recommendations and standards for transitioning young adults with rheumatic disease

- Young adults need access to high-quality, transitional care

- Transition preparation must start as early as possible in adolescence

- Direct communication is needed between stakeholders (adolescent, young adult, parent, adult, and pediatric rheumatology providers) during the transition process

- Transition processes and progress should be planned with family and documented in medical record

- Adult and pediatric care services need to have a written transition policy

- There should be a written description of the transition multidisciplinary care team, and this team should include a transition coordinator

- Transition processes must be adolescent/young adult focused and developmentally appropriate

- A transfer document must be prepared

- Health care teams involved in transition must have appropriate training in adolescent care and childhood-onset rheumatic diseases

- There must be secure funding for resources to provide transition services to young adults with rheumatic disease

- There must be a freely accessible electronic-based platform to host recommendations and standards for transitional care

- Increased evidence-based knowledge is needed to improve outcomes for young adults with rheumatic disease

(*Data from* Foster HE, Minden K, Clemente D, et al. EULAR/PReS standards and recommendations for the transitional care of young people with juvenile-onset rheumatic diseases. Ann Rheum Dis 2017;76(4):639–46.)

oriented approach to the transition process called the Six Core Elements of Health Care Transition. The Six Core Elements (shown in **Fig. 4**) provide practical and flexible recommendations for adult and pediatric primary and specialty care providers to implement in clinical practice. Adult and pediatric primary care and rheumatology providers can elect to implement all or select core elements, depending on available resources and population needs. Flexibility and creativity are encouraged in determining optimal ways to operationalize the six core elements in different institutions and clinical settings.

For pediatric providers, the Six Core Elements involve providing a transition policy, tracking and monitoring individuals going through the transition process, regularly assessing transition readiness, transition planning to encourage self-management skills, organized transfer of care to adult providers, and documentation of transfer completion. For adult providers, the Six Core Elements focus on having a policy for integrating young adults into practice, tracking and monitoring young adults' self-management progress, and providing ongoing care. Got Transition's comprehensive website (www.gottransition.org) offers several downloadable sample tools that can be customized for use in a variety of clinical settings. In addition, information concerning appropriate billing for transition-related clinical care is provided on the website. In concert with a multidisciplinary ACP effort, the American College of Rheumatology (ACR) developed transition resources to assist adult and pediatric providers in implementing the Six Core Elements (https://www.rheumatology.org/Practice-Quality/Pediatric-to-Adult-Rheumatology-Care-Transition). These ACR resources include a customizable draft transition policy and adult practice welcome letter, JIA and lupus medical summary templates, and condition fact sheets for adult providers. Additional websites that provide educational support to patients and families about transition include the following: The Arthritis Foundation (http://www.kidsgetarthritistoo.org/resources/transition-toolkit.php), the Lupus Foundation of America (http://www.lupus.org/resources/15-questions-transitioning-from-pediatric-to-adult-care), and the University of Florida transition program (https://hscj.ufl.edu/jaxhats/toolkit/).

A pilot project incorporating the Six Core Elements of health transition into a US Medicaid managed health care plan demonstrated feasibility.[86] A health care transition learning collaborative of primary and subspecialty care practices in Washington, DC, Boston, Denver, Wisconsin, and New Hampshire implemented the six core elements using quality improvement methodology. The tools were

Six Core Elements Approach to Health Care Transition

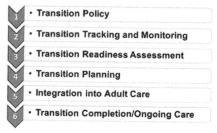

1. • Transition Policy
2. • Transition Tracking and Monitoring
3. • Transition Readiness Assessment
4. • Transition Planning
5. • Integration into Adult Care
6. • Transition Completion/Ongoing Care

Fig. 4. The Six Core Elements Approach to Health Care Transition includes development of transition policy, tracking and monitoring of transition progress, assessment of transition readiness, transition planning, integration of the young adult into an adult care model, and monitoring transition completion and ongoing adult care.

feasible to implement, and measurable improvements in transition and transfer processes were observed.[87,88] The Six Core Elements have been adopted at a large pediatric medical center in collaboration with adult care colleagues, resulting in the availability of tools in the electronic medical record to assess and track transition readiness and progress and creation and sharing of medical summaries.[88]

PUTTING IT ALL TOGETHER

In order to provide a practical example of how the Six Core Elements can be implemented into an academic subspecialty clinic or general pediatric practice, the following scenario is offered: the practice or division has several providers that may include physicians and nurse practitioners. A social worker serves as the transition coordinator. The practice develops a transition quality improvement team including administrative staff, a nurse, some of the pediatric care providers, an adult care provider from each of the few practices to which patients are most often referred, and the social worker who oversees transition projects. In an academic division, this team would also include a fellow. With parent and family input, a transition policy is developed (using ACR and Got Transition templates; see sample **Fig. S1**), which requires notification of patients and families that starting at age 14 years, providers will focus on fostering teen self-management skills. Families are also prepared that sometime between ages 18 and 22 years, the transfer to adult care will occur.

An information transition packet and annual self-management and transition readiness assessment visits with a nurse practitioner or other team member are offered to adolescents and young adults 14 years of age and older. At these self-management visits, transition readiness is assessed with a tool such as the Transition Readiness Assessment Questionnaire in order to identify strengths and opportunities for improvement and to develop specific plans to improve transition readiness. For example, the adolescent or young adult may set a goal to start requesting prescription refills or schedule future clinic appointments independently. At clinic visits, adolescents and young adults see care providers without a parent for at least a portion of the visit. At age 18 years, young adults are asked if they wish to provide consent for medical information to be shared with parent or guardian. Guardianship needs are addressed for young adults who have cognitive impairments.

If there is an electronic medical record, the practice or division develops tools to allow easy tracking of transition activities in the electronic medical record. Young adults who are expected to transfer to adult care within 12 months enter a transition registry, which initiates a structured process of identifying and scheduling an appointment with an adult provider, creating a medical summary and transfer letter (using the ACR and Got Transition templates; see sample **Fig. S2**), providing a transfer packet to the patient and adult provider and tracking to assure attendance at the initial appointment with the adult care provider is kept.

Adult providers are surveyed annually concerning the quality of medical records received and knowledge deficits observed in transitioning young adults. For subspecialty patients who take infusions, a transfer infusion roadmap is developed in collaboration with adult subspecialty colleagues and is provided to the adult care provider and the patient. The team also develops processes for young adults with cognitive impairment who may require guardianship, specifically trained adult providers, and other support, using resources available at the Got Transition website. Smaller primary care practices and subspecialty centers could adopt similar approaches to implementing the six core elements, scaling the interventions according to available resources.

Programs such as the one described earlier have the best chance of success if the following conditions are in place:

1. Everybody in the practice supports the transition effort, including those who are not members of the transition team.
2. A member of the team has direct responsibility for insuring that the transition project operates as desired (in the example, it is the social worker).
3. Meetings to assess progress with the transition project are held regularly.
4. Quality improvement is practiced by making small changes in policy or procedure and assessing their success.
5. Parents and patients are given the opportunity for feedback on the transition program.

SUMMARY

It is not easy becoming an adult, especially for young adults with chronic rheumatic diseases who are at risk for continued active disease, morbidity, mortality, interruptions in care, mental health challenges, and suboptimal vocational outcomes. Starting early in adolescence, encouragement, education, and multidisciplinary support are needed from providers so that young adults can become confident in successfully navigating increasingly complex health care systems. Effective, feasible, evidence-based transition interventions that consider cost, satisfaction, disease outcomes, treatment adherence, and complex young adult neurodevelopment are needed to establish best practice transition processes. Fortunately, a growing interest in transition research, quality improvement, and advocacy promises a brighter future. Adoption of concepts such as the Six Core Elements of Health Care Transition may provide opportunities to promote creative, flexible, effective interventions that promote health resilience and improve outcomes for young adults grappling with rheumatologic disease.

SUPPLEMENTARY DATA

Supplementary data related to this article can be found online at https://doi.org/10.1016/j.pcl.2018.04.007.

REFERENCES

1. Lotstein DS, McPherson M, Strickland B, et al. Transition planning for youth with special health care needs: results from the national survey of children with special health care needs. Pediatrics 2005;115(6):1562–8.
2. Bonnie R, Stroud C, Breiner H, editors. Investing in health and well being of young adults. 1st edition. Washington, DC: National Academies Press; 2014.
3. McManus MA, Pollack LR, Cooley WC, et al. Current status of transition preparation among youth with special needs in the united states. Pediatrics 2013;131(6): 1090–7.
4. Sawicki GS, Whitworth R, Gunn L, et al. Receipt of health care transition counseling in the national survey of adult transition and health. Pediatrics 2011; 128(3):e521–9.
5. Sawicki GS, Garvey KC, Toomey SL, et al. Preparation for transition to adult care among medicaid-insured adolescents. Pediatrics 2017;140(1) [pii:e20162768].

6. Neinstein LS, Irwin CE Jr. Young adults remain worse off than adolescents. J Adolesc Health 2013;53(5):559–61.

7. Lotstein DS, Kuo AA, Strickland B, et al. The transition to adult health care for youth with special health care needs: do racial and ethnic disparities exist? Pediatrics 2010;126(Suppl 3):S129–36.

8. Cohen E, Gandhi S, Toulany A, et al. Health care use during transfer to adult care among youth with chronic conditions. Pediatrics 2016;137(3):e20152734.

9. Rachas A, Tuppin P, Meyer L, et al. Excess mortality and hospitalizations in transitional-age youths with a long-term disease: a national population-based cohort study. PLoS One 2018;13(3):e0193729.

10. Hersh A, von Scheven E, Yelin E. Adult outcomes of childhood-onset rheumatic diseases. Nat Rev Rheumatol 2011;7(5):290–5.

11. Relas H, Luosujarvi R, Kosola S. Outcome of transition phase patients with juvenile idiopathic arthritis. Mod Rheumatol 2018;1–6 [Epub ahead of print].

12. Prior M, McManus M, White P, et al. Measuring the "triple aim" in transition care: a systematic review. Pediatrics 2014;134(6):e1648–61.

13. van Pelt PA, Dolhain RJEM, Kruize AA, et al. Disease activity and dropout in young persons with juvenile idiopathic arthritis in transition of care: a longitudinal observational study. Clin Exp Rheumatol 2018;36(1):163–8.

14. van Mater H, Balevic SJ, Freed GL, et al. Prescribing for children with rheumatic disease: perceived treatment approaches between pediatric and adult rheumatologists. Arthritis Care Res (Hoboken) 2018;70(2):268–74.

15. Minden K. Adult outcomes of patients with juvenile idiopathic arthritis. Horm Res 2009;72(Suppl 1):20–5.

16. Vidqvist KL, Malin M, Varjolahti-Lehtinen T, et al. Disease activity of idiopathic juvenile arthritis continues through adolescence despite the use of biologic therapies. Rheumatology (Oxford) 2013;52(11):1999–2003.

17. Son MB, Johnson VM, Hersh AO, et al. Outcomes in hospitalized pediatric patients with systemic lupus erythematosus. Pediatrics 2014;133(1):e106–13.

18. Hersh AO, Case SM, Son MB. CARRA Registry Investigators. Predictors of disability in a childhood-onset systemic lupus erythematosus cohort: results from the CARRA legacy registry. Lupus 2018;27(3):494–500.

19. Tucker LB, Uribe AG, Fernandez M, et al. Adolescent onset of lupus results in more aggressive disease and worse outcomes: results of a nested matched case-control study within LUMINA, a multiethnic US cohort (LUMINA LVII). Lupus 2008;17(4):314–22.

20. Son MB, Sergeyenko Y, Guan H, et al. Disease activity and transition outcomes in a childhood-onset systemic lupus erythematosus cohort. Lupus 2016;25(13):1431–9.

21. Katz JD, Mamyrova G, Agarwal S, et al. Parents' perception of self-advocacy of children with myositis: an anonymous online survey. Pediatr Rheumatol Online J 2011;9(1):10.

22. Hersh AO, Pang S, Curran ML, et al. The challenges of transferring chronic illness patients to adult care: reflections from pediatric and adult rheumatology at a US academic center. Pediatr Rheumatol Online J 2009;7:13.

23. Maslow GR, Haydon A, McRee AL, et al. Growing up with a chronic illness: social success, educational/vocational distress. J Adolesc Health 2011;49(2):206–12.

24. Schlichtiger J, Haas JP, Barth S, et al. Education and employment in patients with juvenile idiopathic arthritis - a standardized comparison to the German general population. Pediatr Rheumatol Online J 2017;15(1):45.

25. Flato B, Lien G, Smerdel A, et al. Prognostic factors in juvenile rheumatoid arthritis: a case-control study revealing early predictors and outcome after 14.9 years. J Rheumatol 2003;30(2):386–93.

26. Oen K, Malleson PN, Cabral DA, et al. Disease course and outcome of juvenile rheumatoid arthritis in a multicenter cohort. J Rheumatol 2002;29(9):1989–99.

27. Peterson LS, Mason T, Nelson AM, et al. Psychosocial outcomes and health status of adults who have had juvenile rheumatoid arthritis: a controlled, population-based study. Arthritis Rheum 1997;40(12):2235–40.

28. Lawson EF, Hersh AO, Trupin L, et al. Educational and vocational outcomes of adults with childhood- and adult-onset systemic lupus erythematosus: nine years of followup. Arthritis Care Res (Hoboken) 2014;66(5):717–24.

29. Jetha A, Badley E, Beaton D, et al. Unpacking early work experiences of young adults with rheumatic disease: an examination of absenteeism, job disruptions, and productivity loss. Arthritis Care Res (Hoboken) 2015;67(9):1246–54.

30. Hanson H, Hart RI, Thompson B, et al. Experiences of employment among young people with juvenile idiopathic arthritis: a qualitative study. Disabil Rehabil 2017; 40(16):1–8.

31. Gray WN, Schaefer MR, Resmini-Rawlinson A, et al. Barriers to transition from pediatric to adult care: a systematic review. J Pediatr Psychol 2017.

32. Philip R Lee Institute for Health Care Policy. Health insurance churning among young adults. Available at: https://healthpolicy.ucsf.edu/health-insurance-churning-among-young-adults. Accessed January 19, 2018.

33. Kotagal M, Carle AC, Kessler LG, et al. Limited impact on health and access to care for 19- to 25-year-olds following the patient protection and affordable care act. JAMA Pediatr 2014;168(11):1023–9.

34. Peter NG, Forke CM, Ginsburg KR, et al. Transition from pediatric to adult care: internists' perspectives. Pediatrics 2009;123(2):417–23.

35. Crowley R, Wolfe I, Lock K, et al. Improving the transition between paediatric and adult healthcare: a systematic review. Arch Dis Child 2011;96(6):548–53.

36. Colver A, Longwell S. New understanding of adolescent brain development: relevance to transitional healthcare for young people with long term conditions. Arch Dis Child 2013;98(11):902–7.

37. Chung WW, Hudziak JJ. The transitional age brain: "the best of times and the worst of times". Child Adolesc Psychiatr Clin N Am 2017;26(2):157–75.

38. Snook L, Paulson LA, Roy D, et al. Diffusion tensor imaging of neurodevelopment in children and young adults. Neuroimage 2005;26(4):1164–73.

39. Lebel C, Beaulieu C. Longitudinal development of human brain wiring continues from childhood into adulthood. J Neurosci 2011;31(30):10937–47.

40. Ferro MA, Gorter JW, Boyle MH. Trajectories of depressive symptoms during the transition to young adulthood: the role of chronic illness. J Affect Disord 2015;174: 594–601.

41. Witkop ML, McLaughlin JM, Anderson TL, et al. Predictors of non-adherence to prescribed prophylactic clotting-factor treatment regimens among adolescent and young adults with a bleeding disorder. Haemophilia 2016;22(4):e245–50.

42. Borus JS, Laffel L. Adherence challenges in the management of type 1 diabetes in adolescents: prevention and intervention. Curr Opin Pediatr 2010;22(4): 405–11.

43. Osterberg L, Blaschke T. Adherence to medication. N Engl J Med 2005;353(5): 487–97.

44. Clyne W, McLachlan S, Mshelia C, et al. "My patients are better than yours": optimistic bias about patients' medication adherence by european health care professionals. Patient Prefer Adherence 2016;10:1937–44.

45. Koneru S, Kocharla L, Higgins GC, et al. Adherence to medications in systemic lupus erythematosus. J Clin Rheumatol 2008;14(4):195–201.

46. Mok CC. Therapeutic monitoring of the immuno-modulating drugs in systemic lupus erythematosus. Expert Rev Clin Immunol 2017;13(1):35–41.

47. Costedoat-Chalumeau N, Pouchot J, Guettrot-Imbert G, et al. Adherence to treatment in systemic lupus erythematosus patients. Best Pract Res Clin Rheumatol 2013;27(3):329–40.

48. Nevins TE, Nickerson PW, Dew MA. Understanding medication nonadherence after kidney transplant. J Am Soc Nephrol 2017;28(8):2290–301.

49. Linnemayr S, Huang H, Luoto J, et al. Text messaging for improving antiretroviral therapy adherence: no effects after 1 year in a randomized controlled trial among adolescents and young adults. Am J Public Health 2017;107(12):1944–50.

50. Choudhry NK, Krumme AA, Ercole PM, et al. Effect of reminder devices on medication adherence: the REMIND randomized clinical trial. JAMA Intern Med 2017;177(5):624–31.

51. Wong CA, Miller VA, Murphy K, et al. Effect of financial incentives on glucose monitoring adherence and glycemic control among adolescents and young adults with type 1 diabetes: a randomized clinical trial. JAMA Pediatr 2017;171(12):1176–83.

52. van Heuckelum M, van den Ende CHM, Houterman AEJ, et al. The effect of electronic monitoring feedback on medication adherence and clinical outcomes: a systematic review. PLoS One 2017;12(10):e0185453.

53. Stinson J, Kohut SA, Spiegel L, et al. A systematic review of transition readiness and transfer satisfaction measures for adolescents with chronic illness. Int J Adolesc Med Health 2014;26(2):159–74.

54. White PH, Ardoin S. Transitioning wisely: improving the connection from pediatric to adult health care. Arthritis Rheumatol 2016;68(4):789–94.

55. Sawicki GS, Lukens-Bull K, Yin X, et al. Measuring the transition readiness of youth with special healthcare needs: validation of the TRAQ–transition readiness assessment questionnaire. J Pediatr Psychol 2011;36(2):160–71.

56. Moynihan M, Saewyc E, Whitehouse S, et al. Assessing readiness for transition from paediatric to adult health care: revision and psychometric evaluation of the am I ON TRAC for adult care questionnaire. J Adv Nurs 2015;71(6):1324–35.

57. Jensen PT, Paul GV, LaCount S, et al. Assessment of transition readiness in adolescents and young adults with chronic health conditions. Pediatr Rheumatol Online J 2017;15(1):70.

58. Spiegel L. Pediatric to adult care transition challenging for patients with JIA. Rheumatologist 2015;9(5). Available at: http://www.the-rheumatologist.org/article/pediatric-to-adult-care-transition-challenging-for-patients-with-jia/. Accessed December 11, 2018.

59. Fegran L, Hall EO, Uhrenfeldt L, et al. Adolescents' and young adults' transition experiences when transferring from paediatric to adult care: a qualitative meta-synthesis. Int J Nurs Stud 2014;51(1):123–35.

60. Shaw KL, Southwood TR, McDonagh JE, British Society of Paediatric and Adolescent Rheumatology. Young people's satisfaction of transitional care in adolescent rheumatology in the UK. Child Care Health Dev 2007;33(4):368–79.

61. Wells CK, McMorris BJ, Horvath KJ, et al. Youth report of healthcare transition counseling and autonomy support from their rheumatologist. Pediatr Rheumatol Online J 2012;10(1):36.

62. Applebaum MA, Lawson EF, von Scheven E. Perception of transition readiness and preferences for use of technology in transition programs: teens' ideas for the future. Int J Adolesc Med Health 2013;25(2):119–25.

63. Coyne B, Hallowell SC, Thompson M. Measurable outcomes after transfer from pediatric to adult providers in youth with chronic illness. J Adolesc Health 2017;60(1):3–16.

64. Campbell F, Biggs K, Aldiss SK, et al. Transition of care for adolescents from paediatric services to adult health services. Cochrane Database Syst Rev 2016;(4):CD009794.

65. Clemente D, Leon L, Foster H, et al. Systematic review and critical appraisal of transitional care programmes in rheumatology. Semin Arthritis Rheum 2016; 46(3):372–9.

66. Gabriel P, McManus M, Rogers K, et al. Outcome evidence for structured pediatric to adult health care transition interventions: a systematic review. J Pediatr 2017;188:263–9.e15.

67. McPheeters M, Davis AM, Taylor JL, et al. Transition care for children with special health care needs. Technical Brief, Number 15. Agency for Health Care Research and Quality; 2014. Available at: https://effectivehealthcare.ahrq.gov/sites/default/files/pdf/children-special-needs-transition_technical-brief.pdf.

68. Ronis T, Ardoin SP, White PH, et al. Transitioning youth with rheumatic conditions: perspectives of pediatric rheumatology providers in the United States and Canada. J Rheumatol 2014;41(4):768–79.

69. Clemente D, Leon L, Foster H, et al. Transitional care for rheumatic conditions in Europe: current clinical practice and available resources. Pediatr Rheumatol Online J 2017;15(1):49.

70. Hilderson D, Moons P, Westhovens R, et al. Attitudes of rheumatology practitioners toward transition and transfer from pediatric to adult healthcare. Rheumatol Int 2012;32(12):3887–96.

71. Zisman D, White P, Chira P, et al. US adult rheumatologists perspective on the transition process for young adults with rheumatic conditions. Arthritis Rheum 2015;67(suppl 10). Available at: http://acrabstracts.org/abstract/us-adult-rheumatologists-perspective-on-the-transition-process-for-young-adults-with-rheumatic-conditions/.

72. Robertson LP, McDonagh JE, Southwood TR, et al, British Society of Paediatric and Adolescent Rheumatology. Growing up and moving on. A multicentre UK audit of the transfer of adolescents with juvenile idiopathic arthritis from paediatric to adult centred care. Ann Rheum Dis 2006;65(1):74–80.

73. Jensen PT, Karnes J, Jones K, et al. Quantitative evaluation of a pediatric rheumatology transition program. Pediatr Rheumatol Online J 2015;13:17.

74. Rettig P, Athreya BH. Adolescents with chronic disease. transition to adult health care. Arthritis Care Res 1991;4(4):174–80.

75. Hazel E, Zhang X, Duffy CM, et al. High rates of unsuccessful transfer to adult care among young adults with juvenile idiopathic arthritis. Pediatr Rheumatol Online J 2010;8:2.

76. Chanchlani N, McGee M, McDonaugh JE. Informational continuity is integral for successful transition of adolescents to adult care. J Rheumatol 2015;43:901–2.

77. Prestidge C, Romann A, Djurdjev O, et al. Utility and cost of a renal transplant transition clinic. Pediatr Nephrol 2012;27(2):295–302.

78. Harden PN, Walsh G, Bandler N, et al. Bridging the gap: an integrated paediatric to adult clinical service for young adults with kidney failure. BMJ 2012;344:e3718.

79. Cadario F, Prodam F, Bellone S, et al. Transition process of patients with type 1 diabetes (T1DM) from paediatric to the adult health care service: a hospital-based approach. Clin Endocrinol (Oxf) 2009;71(3):346–50.

80. Maddux MH, Ricks S, Bass J. Preparing patients for transfer of care: practices of primary care pediatricians. J Community Health 2015;40(4):750–5.

81. Wisk LE, Finkelstein JA, Sawicki GS, et al. Predictors of timing of transfer from pediatric- to adult-focused primary care. JAMA Pediatr 2015;169(6):e150951.

82. McLaughlin SE, Machan J, Fournier P, et al. Transition of adolescents with chronic health conditions to adult primary care: factors associated with physician acceptance. J Pediatr Rehabil Med 2014;7(1):63–70.

83. Okumura MJ, Heisler M, Davis MM, et al. Comfort of general internists and general pediatricians in providing care for young adults with chronic illnesses of childhood. J Gen Intern Med 2008;23(10):1621–7.

84. American Academy of Pediatrics, American Academy of Family Physicians, American College of Physicians, Transitions Clinical Report Authoring Group, Cooley WC, Sagerman PJ. Supporting the health care transition from adolescence to adulthood in the medical home. Pediatrics 2011;128(1):182–200.

85. Foster HE, Minden K, Clemente D, et al. EULAR/PReS standards and recommendations for the transitional care of young people with juvenile-onset rheumatic diseases. Ann Rheum Dis 2017;76(4):639–46.

86. McManus M, White P, Pirtle R, et al. Incorporating the six core elements of health care transition into a medicaid managed care plan: lessons learned from a pilot project. J Pediatr Nurs 2015;30(5):700–13.

87. McManus M, White P, Barbour A, et al. Pediatric to adult transition: a quality improvement model for primary care. J Adolesc Health 2015;56(1):73–8.

88. Hickam T, White PH, Modrcin A, et al. Implementing a nationally recognized pediatric-to-adult transitional care approach in a major children's hospital. Health Soc Work 2018;43(1):3–6.

Moving?

Make sure your subscription moves with you!

To notify us of your new address, find your **Clinics Account Number** (located on your mailing label above your name), and contact customer service at:

Email: **journalscustomerservice-usa@elsevier.com**

800-654-2452 (subscribers in the U.S. & Canada)
314-447-8871 (subscribers outside of the U.S. & Canada)

Fax number: **314-447-8029**

Elsevier Health Sciences Division
Subscription Customer Service
3251 Riverport Lane
Maryland Heights, MO 63043

*To ensure uninterrupted delivery of your subscription, please notify us at least 4 weeks in advance of move.

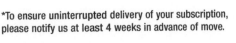